Fantasies of Femininity:
Reframing the Boundaries of Sex

JANE M. USSHER

PENGUIN BOOKS

For Jan

PENGUIN BOOKS

Published by the Penguin Group
Penguin Books Ltd, 27 Wrights Lane, London w8 5tz, England
Penguin Books USA Inc., 375 Hudson Street, New York, New York 10014, USA
Penguin Books Australia Ltd, Ringwood, Victoria, Australia
Penguin Books Canada Ltd, 10 Alcorn Avenue, Toronto, Ontario, Canada m4v 3b2
Penguin Books (NZ) Ltd, 182–190 Wairau Road, Auckland 10, New Zealand

Penguin Books Ltd, Registered Offices: Harmondsworth, Middlesex, England

Published in Penguin Books 1997
10 9 8 7 6 5 4 3 2 1

Set in 10/12pt Monotype Bembo
Typeset by Rowland Phototypesetting Ltd, Bury St Edmunds, Suffolk
Printed in England by Clays Ltd, St Ives plc

PENGUIN BOOKS

Fantasies of Femininity

Jane Ussher was born in Derby in 1961. After a first degree in psychology, she completed a Ph.D. on women's experiences of premenstrual syndrome (PMS), and then trained as a clinical psychologist. She taught for some years in the School of Cultural and Community Studies at Sussex University and is now a senior lecturer in psychology, as well as research director of the Women's Health Research Unit, at University College London. She also works part time in the National Health Service in Women's Health. She has contributed articles to a number of newspapers and magazines, and her other books include *The Psychology of the Female Body*; *Women's Madness: Misogyny or Mental Illness, Psychological Perspectives on Sexual Problems*; *The Psychology of Women's Health Care* and *Gender Issues in Clinical Psychology* (both with Paula Nicolson); and *Body Talk: The Material Discursive Regulation of Sexuality, Madness and Reproduction*.

Jane Ussher lives in London and Sussex.

CONTENTS

ACKNOWLEDGEMENTS

Fantasies of Femininity has had an indecently lengthy gestation, during which time the support and encouragement of a number of friends and colleagues has been invaluable. The idea for the book was conceived when I was working in the school of Cultural and Community Studies at the University of Sussex, where an initial series of interviews were conducted by myself and Damaris Stuart-Williams. The questions we addressed to the women we talked to were those I had myself been struggling with since adolescence: What does it mean to be 'woman'? How do women reconcile the contradictions inherent in sexual relationships with men? How can we account for the violent side of sex? When I discovered, after a number of years of writing and researching, that the answers to these questions were not quite what I had first thought, a radical rethink – and rewrite – was required. Throughout this time, Margaret Bluman acted as a sympathetic and tolerant editor, enduring endless evenings discussing the vagaries of post-modern femininity and sex, without ever appearing disinterested. For this I thank her.

For many and varied forms of inspiration, and practical assistance over recent years, my thanks go to: Mairead Ussher, Paula Nicolson, Stephen Frosh, Janet Sayers, Isabel Tamblyn, Lucy Yardley, Myra Hunter, Hélène Joffe, Yael Goetz, Nicola Horton, Ruth Leigh, Jo Bower, Chris Dewberry, Sue Thorpe, Alison Madgwick and Lynn Clemence. Other members of the Women's Health Research Unit at UCL – Alison Dixon, Jane Weaver, Christine Rutter, Margaret Carris, Mette Knudson and Susannah Browne – have provided a forum for productive thought and discussion. I have drawn on interviews conducted by Damaris Stuart-Williams, Fahimeh Shanghai, Gary Wilson-

Taylor, Katherine Johnson, Helen Malson, Catherine Swann, Ben Gurney-Smith, Deborah Picker, Kerry Clarke and Julie Mooney-Somers. I am grateful to each for this.

I have been inspired by the ideas and arguments of many academic theorists and critics in a range of disciplines whilst conducting the research for this book. In plundering, distilling and reworking their writings in order to address my own questions, I hope I have not misrepresented or detracted from the elegance and eloquence of their original work. The writings of several people have been indispensable: Karen Horney, Michel Foucault, Angela McRobbie, Sue Lees, Lynda Nead, Griselda Pollock, Valerie Walkerdine, Lynne Segal, Ann Kaplan, Judith Butler, Stephen Frosh, Susan Estrich, Susan Douglas, Zsusanna Adler, Jeffrey Weeks, Lillian Faderman and Marjorie Garber.

Finally, and above all, my thanks go to Jan Burns, with whom I have been debating the 'woman question' for the last thirteen years, and who has recently lived with this book as closely as I, providing intellectual inspiration, encouragement through moments of despondency, an enduring sense of humour and, when all else failed, food. But it is not cooking that inspired my dedication of this book to Jan. It is the fact that she helped me to unravel the meaning of fantasies of femininity in a way that no one else could. Without this, I would have produced a very different book.

'Throughout history people have knocked their heads against the riddle of femininity . . . Nor will you have escaped worrying over this problem – those of you who are men; to those of you who are women this will not apply – you are yourselves the problem.

SIGMUND FREUD, 1856–1939

'Eve, she, petticoat, skirt; girl, virgin, maiden; ma'am, spinster; lady, bride, matron; spouse, mother, parent; wench, lass, nymph; dame; teacher; blonde, brunette; sweetheart, bird; loved one; moll, doll, broad, mistress; loose woman; quean, shrew, virago, Amazon.'

Roget's Thesaurus on 'woman'

'Gender is an act . . . which is open to splitting, self parody, self-criticism, and those hyperbolic exhibitions of "the natural" that, in their very exaggeration, reveal its fundamentally phantasmatic status.'

JUDITH BUTLER, 1990

'Womanliness . . . could be assumed and worn as a mask, both to hide the possession of masculinity and to avert the reprisals expected if she was found to possess it.'[1]   JOAN RIVERE, 1929[2]

Imagining 'woman' – imagining sex

Close your eyes and imagine 'woman'. It is hard not to imagine sex.

Turn to the myriad representations of 'woman' that pervade our daily lives – to art, film, mass media imagery, literature or pornography. What you will see is sex.

Then look at the rules of femininity that define how girls become 'woman', taught to them by parents, teachers or through teenage magazines. The only mention of sex is 'don't' – until very recently, at least.

A conundrum.

It is this conundrum, simultaneously fascinating and frustrating – particularly for those who live it – that is the focus of this book. It takes us on a journey through the many images of 'woman' and 'sex', which circulate in the symbolic sphere and are so ubiquitous and familiar that we take them for granted as real or true. They are not.

The book also explores the material consequences of these sexualized images – in terms of the demarcation of the boundaries of femininity and masculinity; the negotiation of sexual power and pleasure; and the creation of legislation which regulates how we 'do' sex (and what we deem a sexual crime or perversion). Representations have real effects.

At the heart of this journey lies a series of questions: Why have images of 'woman' come to be so strongly associated with sex, either as its embodiment or its negation? In whose interests are they created? Whose concerns do these sexualized images reflect? What is their influence on the lived experience of women, and of men? Are they a reflection of what women really are, or a fantasy about what 'woman' is (or should be)? Why are the boundaries of 'sex' so defined?

This is both a personal journey on the part of a woman who is continuously faced with the contradictions of sex, and a scholarly quest, a foray into the many critiques of sexualized images which have gone before. These two levels of analysis are irrevocably intertwined. No one who writes on or researches into the subject of sexuality or femininity can claim neutrality or disinterest, however learned or abstract their rhetorical style. Both sexuality and gender are central to all our lives. Indeed, they appear to be subjects which completely consume our minds – at least if we take the continuing proliferation of images of sex and sexuality in the mass media as indicators of popular concern.

Arguably, what most of us are consumed with is a desire to *really* know both the essence of sex and what it is to be 'woman'. As Sigmund Freud famously commented, 'throughout history people have knocked their heads against the riddle of femininity.' His life's work was devoted to the subject. He was not alone. Many other writers, artists, poets and philosophers seem to have been preoccupied with the mysteries of feminine sexuality. Perhaps the answers they sought will never be found. For, like desire itself, fascination with this subject is maintained by the very fact that satisfaction is rarely achieved; enlightenment or knowledge always seems to be just out of reach.

Yet what we *can* unravel is the conundrum of the contradictory visions of feminine sexuality: the fact that representations of 'woman' seethe with sexuality yet for centuries women have been condemned for exploring their own sexual desires. Or the fact that the scripts of femininity that girls are taught to follow in the process of becoming 'woman' focus on heterosexual love, whereas the 'woman' we see frozen in the masculine gaze is a creature consumed (and controlled) by sex.

To unravel this conundrum and answer the questions I have posed above, I examine in this book the fantasies of femininity that underlie dominant representations of 'woman' and attempt to uncover the reasons for their particular configuration. I focus on mass media imagery aimed at women, and on art, film and pornography. I have chosen these particular genres because they are perhaps the most pervasive, the most powerful, and because they have been subjected to extensive analysis and critique. Others have looked to different arenas, such as literature, advertising or music. I will allude to this work in passing.[3]

In order to demonstrate that these representations are not merely ethereal concepts, that they have direct material effects on the daily lives of women and girls, I also examine the way in which the meaning of 'woman' and 'sex' is regulated by the law, by sexual science, and by legal and social commentary on sexual violence. Arguably, sex laws contain and constrain us, elevating a narrow and sexualized view of 'woman' to the status of truth. Medicine and psychology act to pathologize us, and treat us, in many ways reifying the status of 'woman' promulgated in the mass media, as the second, receptive, sex. Sexual violence is the most concrete and chilling example of the material regulation of sexuality and the bodies of individual women. Dominant representations of sexual violence often position it as 'sex' or see it as the woman's fault. What this reveals about 'sex' and the power relations between women and men speaks volumes. When we ask the question *why* sexual violence is so ubiquitous and often goes unpunished, we are left with uncomfortable reflections on the very nature of heterosexual sex and romance, on the very notion of what it is to be 'woman' and 'man'.

In the course of examining how women manage to reconcile the inherent contradictions in becoming 'woman' I have interviewed many women over the last five years,[4] asking them how they feel about being 'woman' and how they negotiate the boundaries of 'sex'. I have also interviewed men. It is a point of some controversy, but I would argue that to understand what it is to be 'woman' we also have to look at what it is to be 'man', at men's fantasies, fears and desires in relation to women, and at their own (mythical) phallic sexuality. This is not purely to include men or to argue that any theoretical or empirical analysis is incomplete if it focuses solely on women.[5] It is to argue that femininity is irrevocably situated in relation to the psychic and mythical forces that determine what it is to be 'man', sited in relation to the fictions and fantasies that underlie so much of what is dominant and positioned as truth in the phallocentric sphere.

The journey begins with fairy stories but ends with sexual murder. This is no anodyne tale. Nor is it a depressing analysis of woman as victim: Even as we examine representations of 'woman' in teenage magazines, romantic fiction, television soap opera, art, film noir, hard-core porn, theories of sexual problems, laws on homosexuality and scientific explanations of 'normal sex', we must not forget that femininity is not inevitable or fixed – it is multifaceted and always open to interpretation or change. A woman may play the part to perfection. But that doesn't make it real or authentic. Even the perfect performance of femininity may mask resistance or transgression.

Images of sexuality and femininity are complicated and contradictory. We should take nothing for granted. Much of what we think we *know* about 'woman' and 'sex' may be exposed as myth, not truth. What we see is not always what we are, or what we get. This realization may be an unsettling experience. But that is the purpose of this book.

NOTES

1. Butler, Judith, *Gender Trouble: Feminism and the Subversion of Identity*, London: Routledge, 1990, p. 147.

2. Rivere, Joan, 'Womanliness as Masquerade,' *International Journal of Psychoanalysis*, vol. 10; reprinted in Burgin, V., Donald, J. & Kaplan, C., *Formations of Fantasy*, London: Methuen, 1986, pp. 35–44.

3. I will focus on those representations of 'woman', which are associated with sexuality, as I want to examine how and why constructions of 'woman' and of 'sex' are irrevocably intertwined. I cannot cover every possible permutation or connotation; I have focused on certain themes and myths which are persistent and ubiquitous. My selection comes from the repetition of images and stories about 'woman' and about 'sex' over different contexts, and across different points in time. Ann Kaplan has adopted a similar approach in her selection of representations of motherhood, an area I have not covered in detail, as it has been covered so thoroughly elsewhere. See Kaplan, Ann, *Motherhood and Representation. The Mother in Popular Culture and Melodrama*, London: Routledge, 1992.

4. The majority of the interviews were conducted by myself; some were conducted by research assistants or graduate students working with me (see acknowledgements). Unless otherwise noted, the interviews quoted in the text were conducted by myself. Over a five-year period, 148 women and 120 men were interviewed. The age range was 18 to 53, and there was a normal distribution across social class. Two-thirds of the men and one-half of the women were self-identified as heterosexual; the remainder identified as gay, lesbian or bisexual. I have used the interviews to inform my thinking

and thus the arguments made in the book, drawing on them directly to illustrate particular points. However, this book is not presented as, nor intended to be, a piece of empirical research, or a systematic analysis of qualitative data (this will take place elsewhere). The interviews focused on women and men's interpretation of representations of sexuality; their sexual behaviour; and their negotiation of their own sexual subjectivity.

5. There have been many debates in disciplines such as psychology about the practice of basing general theories about *people* on samples that consist solely of men (see Squire, Corrine, *Significant Differences: Feminism in Psychology*, London: Routledge, 1989, for a review). The irony is that whilst many psychological theories are based solely on male samples, such as the work of Kohlberg, where boys were the sole object of study for theories of moral development (see Gilligan, Carol, *In a Different Voice: Psychological Theory and Women's Development*, Cambridge, MA: Harvard University Press, 1982), this is rarely seen as a problem by the establishment. In contrast, feminists who attempt to study women are often asked 'What about men?' Feminist scholars and researchers have argued that it is important and valid for us to be able to focus our gaze solely on the experience of women.

CHAPTER ONE

The Script of Femininity: Sex, Romance and Beauty

Oh God, let me forget the things he said.
Let me not lie another night awake
Repeating the promises he made,
Freezing and burning for his faithless sake;
Seeing his face, feeling his hand once more
Loosen my braided hair until it fell
Shining and free; remembering how he swore
A single strand might lift a man from Hell . . .

I knew that other girls in Aprils past,
Had leaned, like me, from some old tower's room
And watched him clamber up, hand over fist . . .
I knew that I was not the first to twist
Her heartstrings to a rope for him to climb.
I might have known I would not be the last.

'Rapunzel', SARA HENDERSON HAY[1]

This is a story about what it means to be 'woman', which reveals that femininity is a story in itself. The lessons start early, with fairy tales – the eternal childhood favourites that seem so innocuous we rarely question their benign intent:[2] Sleeping Beauty, trapped in her castle, awakened by the kiss of a prince who struggled and fought to find her and takes her as his bride; Cinderella, the poor motherless child bullied by her stepsisters and neglected by her father until her prince seeks her out and saves her; or Rapunzel, the beautiful maiden trapped in her tower, made lonely and sad by her imprisonment, rescued by the knight who climbs up to her window on her unleashed golden tresses.[3]

It doesn't take a crystal ball to read the themes that run through these fairy tales: Beautiful but cruelly treated young woman longs for rescue and salvation, yet endures hardship and misery whilst dreaming her impossible dreams. Her modesty and virtue are without bounds, her kindness and sensitivity matched only by her fairness of face. Eventually, her patience, passivity and tolerance are rewarded – not with untold revenge on her tormentors, but with the attentions and love of a man. These are the rituals of courtly love, transformed into children's fiction. It is the waiting and wanting which are at the centre of the tale; *anticipation* is the name of the game. In fairy stories, courtship is presented as the most important and exciting event in the heroine's life. It is here that she exercises her most important choice – identifying the 'right man' and saying 'yes' to his offer of marriage.[4] We never see what happens to the prince and his heroine after their marriage. It is not of any interest: We already know they 'live happily ever after'.

Fairy tales tell us of the necessity of the transformation of woman from base matter into idealized perfection: Cinderella the scullery maid turns into the belle of the ball; Sleeping Beauty and Snow White are awoken from the death of sleep to life (by a kiss). These innocents are punished for their beauty by other envious women, be they stepmothers, stepsisters, or the archetypal wicked witch. Yet beauty always wins through, and hard work, sacrifice and natural goodness is ultimately rewarded. In fairy stories it is the meek who inherit the earth – at least once they have found their man (and not just *any* man – a prince).[5] Women who silently cope with cruelty and injustice are compensated beyond their wildest dreams. It is the masochistic heroine, the woman in distress, who is the most interesting to the prince, and it is her femininity (and sexuality) that is her major means of redemption. She doesn't have to *do* anything, she just has to *be* – to adopt the feminine masquerade. The narrative device of the beauty contest (Which daughter is the most pretty? Mirror, mirror on the wall, who is the fairest of us all?) makes it clear that the rewards are for the one woman who is fairest of face (placing all others as outsiders). Women are divided by appearance; we are told that beauty is power. To be ugly (or even plain) is the thing to be most feared.

In fairy tales, the ugly sister, the wicked stepmother or the witch, always deserves her punishment; like all active, vicious, ugly women, to be outcast is her rightful fate. This is a celebration of envy and competitiveness between women which perpetuates the suspicion that those who are ugly or old are in fact 'wicked'.[6] This is the eternal conflict between the two archetypal representations of 'woman': the angel and the witch; the Madonna and the whore. So Snow White and her wicked stepmother represent the dilemma between pure passivity and active independent sexuality, a double bind in which no woman wins. As critics Sandra Gilbert and Susan Gubar have argued, Snow White merely exchanges one glass coffin for another. She is saved from a sleeping death to be delivered to the restricted role of goodness, obedience and docility – the mask of femininity which is reflected in her imprisoning mirror. They argue that 'there is, after all, no female model for her in this tale except the "good" (dead) mother and her living avatar the "bad" mother.'[7] This juxtaposition of the good and bad woman reminds the young reader of her dreadful fate, should she stray from the path of perfect femininity – denunciation as wild woman or witch. To be 'good' might be a living death for many women, but it is better than being a monstrous witch. Or so we are told.

Fairy tales offer self-sacrifice and romance as solutions to life's difficulties. Take a tale such as 'Beauty and the Beast', where the father–daughter relationship is the central theme. The young Beauty rejects scores of suitors in order to stay with her widowed father, even when he is made bankrupt and can no longer offer her a life of luxury. She demonstrates the extent of her love by offering herself up in place of her father to satisfy the bargain he made with the Beast. Karen Rowe has interpreted this tale as a symbolic exposition of the 'potent, sometimes problematic oedipal dependency of young girls ... Beauty's three decisions – to stay, to serve, finally, to sacrifice her life – establish her willing subservience to paternal needs'.[8] She obeys the 'law of the father', as all good girls should.

Beauty is initially horrified and disgusted by the ugliness of the Beast, but during her captivity in his palace her aversion turns to affection. She grows to love his inner beauty and goodness, and in a traumatic scene where he is dying (due to his unfulfilled love for her), she agrees to his proposal of marriage, the grief she feels at the thought of his death convincing her that she loves him. Here, romantic commitment replaces revulsion against the sexuality of the Beast. Her reward is that the beast in the bedroom turns into the prince in the palace.[9] This arguably stands as a metaphor for the archetypal feminine existence. The Beast's transformation rewards Beauty for turning sexual reticence into self-sacrifice, for putting his needs before her own. She is a 'good' woman who agrees to a marriage which at the outset looks doomed to failure. But here is the rub: It is in her power to make it succeed, to make *him* into what she wants him to be. This is the ultimate feminine fantasy continuously fed to women and girls – the taming of the (male) beast by the love of a good woman and the redemption or transformation of the beautiful (yet suffering) woman by the love of the 'right' man.

Is this just a trip down memory lane? Or as many critics would argue, do fairy tales inculcate in young girls a restrictive notion of what it is to be 'woman', in which love and romance are the rewards for masochism and beauty? Andrea Dworkin has argued that 'we have taken the fairy tales of childhood with us into maturity, chewed but still lying in the stomach, as real identity. Between Snow White and her heroic prince, our two great fictions, we never stood much of a chance.'[10] In a similar vein, Collette Dowling claims that 'like Cinderella, women today are still waiting for something to "transform their lives"'. She argues that fairy tales feed into a climate of psychological dependency, a desire to be cared for by others, creating a series of impossible wishes and desires which lead to women living life in a 'half-light'.[11]

But is it that simple? Do we simply see and believe? Women aren't all waiting for their prince, passively accepting the narrow restrictions of femininity, as described in traditional fairy tales. Few of us see Cinderella as a useful role model, or still believe that our lives can be transformed by the kiss of a handsome man. We generally assign fairy stories to the category of childish fantasy and claim to be immune to any insidious messages that are conveyed by these tales. Most women take a similar stance when asked about the influence of adult fictions about 'woman': 'I don't believe what I read in women's magazines,' or 'I take no notice of what I see on television,' is perhaps the most common retort when questioned on the subject. It is often mine, too. But few of us *are* immune.

Fairy tales are just the beginning; the message of what it is to be 'woman' is constantly conveyed to women through the mass media. Girls' comics, women's magazines, romantic fiction, advertising, as well as films and television aimed at female audiences, may appear to have moved beyond the narrow romantic script of fairy tales, providing a more sophisticated or complex view of what it is to be 'woman'. But if we look carefully, we can see that the legacy of Cinderella and Snow White lives on.[12] The difficult conflicts women face on a daily basis, juxtaposed with the salvation provided by the glorious phallic prince (or her continued suffering if she doesn't find him), are still dominant themes. Representations of the strong independent woman who survives are very few, very recent, and often derided or dismissed.

Representations of 'woman' are of central importance in the construction of female subjectivity. We learn how to *do* 'woman' through negotiating the warring images and stories about what 'woman' is (or what she should be), amongst the most influential being those scripts of femininity that pervade the mass media. This doesn't mean that women and girls are passive dupes,[13] bombarded with images seething with ideology yet remaining impotent in the face of their regulatory power. Far from it. We are critical readers and viewers, actively negotiating and resisting the various representations of 'woman' which pervade our daily lives. We continuously sift and select from the different scripts we are offered, creating and re-creating the story that is femininity.[14]

The mass media does not merely provide a mirror or a template of what 'woman' is, it provides us with a complex array of contradictory representations,[15] which produces multiple meanings and therefore affords myriad sites for identification. Part of the pleasure (and the pain) is in the very fact of these multiple meanings – in our ability and desire to identify, often simultaneously, with different subject positions within images or texts. It is not possible to predict how any one woman will do this, for there are many potential readings or interpretations in any given image or story, and women will not read or view representations in a simple unified manner.[16] Our interpretations will be partly determined by the conscious and unconscious conflicts, fears and desires which underlie our reading or viewing. It will be partly determined by social context and by our own history – our history as girls and women, and our previous experience with these representations. It will be influenced by the form and content of representations of 'woman', as well as the intentions of those who create them, for to state that we are active readers does not mean that we are immune from persuasion.

Whether we use mass media aimed at women to escape, to wallow pleasurably in fantasy or temporarily to resolve repressed conflicts and desires that are difficult to face in day-to-day life – even if we actively reject the representations of 'woman' that are contained therein – we cannot avoid its influence. Yet these images are not forced upon us. We have a choice in our reading and viewing. So the question is, what is the lure at the heart of these visions of 'woman' that causes us to take up (or resist) femininity, as it is so defined?[17] How, and why, do women take up the script of femininity, and become 'woman'?

Some Day My Prince Will Come: The Fantasy of Romantic Salvation

The Father as Prince: Girls' Comics and Oedipal Resolution

> Girls' comics, because they engage with the production of girls' conscious and unconscious desires, prepare for and proffer a 'happy-ever-after' solution in which the finding of the prince (the knight in shining armour, 'Mr Right') comes to seem like a solution to a set of overwhelming desires and problems.   VALERIE WALKERDINE[18]

Most girls graduate from fairy tales to girls' comics. The characters in the stories are different, but the roles are little changed from the tales of Cinderella, Snow White, or Beauty. Finding, getting and keeping a man is portrayed as the central goal of a girl's existence, a goal which will relieve her of all suffering. The prince may have been transformed, but the underlying message is still the same: Beauty, goodness and passivity are rewarded with the attentions of men.

In girls' comics – aimed primarily at working-class pre-teens – the prince is often represented by the father, and the suffering that girls endure is almost an exact mirror of that described in fairy tales. Except that here the suffering is supposed to be real. It is no coincidence that comics are given girls' names as titles (*Tammy, Mandy, Bunty* or *Judy*); it plays on the belief that they are simple reflections of the lives of real girls. In the early 1980s Valerie Walkerdine analysed eighteen stories in the British comics *Bunty* and *Mandy*. She concluded that the stories 'construct heroines who are the target of wrongdoing and whose fight against private injustice is one of private endurance, which always triumphs in the end'. What we see are bullying cousins, uncaring parents, or, in many cases, no parents at all. The girl is always the victim of undeserved cruelty, but reacts by being tolerant and patient. She is selfless and sensitive, not revengeful and angry: Cinderella transported into the late twentieth century. As with Cinderella, the drama enacted within the stories is centred on the family. Yet here it is not the prince who offers salvation, but the discovery (or fantasy of discovery) of an ideal family, where both the father and mother are loving and caring. As Valerie Walkerdine comments, 'the father simply precedes the prince'.[19]

Whilst there have been some changes in the content of these comics over the last decade, reflecting changes in family life, many of the traditional themes endure. In two comics that have survived into the nineties (many having disappeared in publication wars), *Bunty* and *M&J* (*Mandy and Judy*),[20] the family is still a focus of attention, but there has been a move away from the gothic horror implicit in tales of servant girls and orphans. Today, the 'horrors' are more mundane, and apparently more real. One story depicts a young girl, Geraldine, waiting at home for her two working parents to return from their busy days, observing the quarrel which ensues when it is discovered that there is no food for dinner. While her father moans, 'You're so disorganized these days. You never used to be like this,' her mother replies, 'I never used to work full time.' Later on in the same story both parents present their daughter with a set of encyclopaedias in response to her request for help with her homework. Her sad (but private) response is 'These books must have cost a fortune. Mum and dad have been very generous. But I needed help from *them* – not books. My parents don't mind spending their *money* on me, but they won't spare me their time.' Here the feelings of neglect, of generational conflict and strife, are translated into family dilemmas of the nineties – the family with two working parents. Yet Geraldine, the heroine, is as stoical as a fairy-tale princess. She does not react with anger, but merely wishes to herself that things were like they were in the 'old days', a time when her parents were less obsessed with work and her mother was at home. In another story entitled 'Oh, Mum!' the heroine Karen wistfully gazes at a food mixer in a shop-window embellished with the advert 'The way to a man's heart is through his stomach,' whilst she says to herself, 'Mum's hardly doing any cooking now. It's all burgers and take-aways. Dad must miss her home-made goodies.' These stories stand as an unsubtle criticism of the work-orientated family and of the absent professional mother who is stepping outside her 'proper' feminine role, the one she adopted in the 'old days'. But it is the angst and anguish of the daughter, whose idealized family exists only in fantasy (or memory), that is the focus of this moralistic tale – the perennial passive victim, powerless to intervene in her particular fate. The 'bad' family which is represented here is often restored to an idealized state through the actions of the young heroine: She brings her warring parents together or makes her mother 'see the light'.

The most simple interpretation of these comics is that they reflect the 'real life' concerns of pre-adolescent girls. This would explain why romance is now a frequently occurring theme,[21] replacing hockey, jolly japes with friends and ponies as the focus of the pre-pubertal feminine world; it's what pre-teens now think about (along with honing their consumer skills). These comics also reflect what pre-teens are *allowed* to think about, as these comics tell young girls what their concerns *should* be.[22]

Yet they also work at a deeper level, reflecting fantasies, unconscious conflicts and desires. Valerie Walkerdine sees girls' comics as providing a mirror and outlet for oedipal conflicts – the trauma of the loss of the mother and the transferring of love to the father.[23] The mother provokes anger and hatred because she cannot fulfil all needs – those of either daughter or husband – and the sympathy of the daughter becomes focused on the neglected father (the same figure who sadly wanders through the world of fairy tales). The frustrations inherent in pre-adolescent life – unfulfilled desires for independence accompanied by the overwhelming need to be wanted and loved – are lived out through identification with the comic-story heroine. Her misery and discontent serve to remind unhappy girls that they are not alone, while her successes can restore optimism and hope. It allows girls to live out the fantasy that *they* would do it differently if they were in their mother's role. *They* would feed him, love him and make him content. Psychoanalytic feminists such as Jessica Benjamin[24] have interpreted this overvaluation and idealization of the father, which is accompanied by submission and compromise, as a defensive response to the necessary separation from the mother which underpins heterosexual desire. This is influenced by the social context in which girls' sexuality is developing. As Nancy Chodorow has argued, 'the unavailability of the father as a reliable presence (less available to his daughter than to his son, less available to her than a mother to her son) leads girls, in the normal case, to develop tendencies toward an idealizing love for their fathers that forms the basis of their heterosexuality. Such love pulls towards submission, overvaluation, masochism, and the borrowing of subjectivity from the lover.'[25] Girls' comics both reflect and normalize this process.

In the increasing presence of romance in these comics, they also prepare girls for the transference of their affections from the father to the prince, as we were shown in 'Beauty and the Beast', 'Cinderella' and 'Snow White'. When they graduate to teenage magazines, girls are given the full script.

Dream Boy: Teenage Romance and Unfulfilled Desire

Teenage magazines take as their subject the mysteries of love and sex, how to deal with boys and how a girl should *be*. Up until the nineties the focus was on romance – on expectation and unfulfilled desire. The comic strip or 'photo story' (so much more *real*) told a similar tale week after week. Girl wants boy. Girl worries, feels insecure, makes herself attractive, makes herself available. Sometimes boy notices. Boy approaches girl. Outcome: Romance (short-lived, always threatened by other girls) or heartache (boy is unreliable or unfaithful). Sexuality, while at the heart of the continual pursuit which preoccupies these magazines, was rarely explicit. True love, not lust, was the motivation behind each encounter – at least on the 'good' girl's part. Angela McRobbie carried out an analysis of the dominant representations in the British teenage magazine *Jackie* in the seventies and concluded:

> Romance is the girls' reply to male sexuality. It stands in opposition to their 'just being after one thing', and consequently it makes sex seem dirty, sordid and unattractive. The girls' sexuality is understood and experienced not in terms of a physical need or her own body, but in terms of the romantic attachment.[26]

The major message was 'Play hard to get.' Yet, paradoxically, at the same time being 'got' was supposed to be a girl's main goal. This is the perennial contradiction presented to girls, of being desirable yet unavailable to men. In many teenage magazines today little has changed. Romance is a possibility waiting to occur in any available context. Normal everyday places and events are imbued with a deeper meaning than might initially be apparent as they represent potential arenas for a romantic encounter. A teenage girl's whole world is still geared around the one aim of getting (and keeping) a boy. Take the eleven stories in one edition of '*My Guy and Oh Boy*' in the mid-nineties:

1. Mix and match. 'Is Karen on the right track for love?': Karen meets Duncan in the recording studio after answering an ad for a female vocalist. She gives up her uncaring boyfriend for him.

2. Playing with fire. Ellie meets Sean when he comes to the bank she works in. He seems not to care, leaving her to go home from a party alone. She rows with her mother, who says Sean is no good. Sean comes round to apologize, and both Ellie and her mother agree he is all right.

3. Holiday romance. Gale is at the station and glimpses Dean, who she fell in love with on holiday. She follows him and they are reunited.

4. Biker boyfriend. Kirsty is worried because her boyfriend is a motorbike messenger. After much persuasion he gives up his job for her.

5. No way out. Steve invites Sara to his party. She can't go because it's on a Friday, a Jewish family day. Sara's friend tells Steve and he changes the day of the party.

6. When hate turns to love. Sarah takes a job on a farm, and her attractive colleague Lance initially greets her with sexism. Then he says he's fallen in love with her – and as Sarah doesn't love him, she leaves her job.

7. Best-kept secret. Lynne tells her secret diary how she loves Ian. Two nasty girls steal the diary and send a page of it to Ian. Ian asks Lynne out.

8. Just good friends. Kirsty is bored with her boyfriend Tim – and chucks him. They go out with other people. They both miss each other and then get back together.

9. Er, I love you. Jo is in love with a man at work. She tries to engineer a meeting. Burning with desire, she declares her love for him. But she didn't realize he was wearing headphones, listening to music, so he does not hear her.

10. You got the look. Debbie is going to a party to meet Paul. She spends hours trying on all her clothes and doing her make-up. Paul doesn't turn up but comes to see Debbie the next day. She isn't made-up, so won't see him. Later she gets caught in the rain and Paul bumps into her. He is a mess too, and they go off hand-in-hand.

11. Happy Birthday. Annette thinks that her boyfriend has forgotten her birthday. She sees him in town with her best friend and so she asks another boy out for a date on her birthday. When she takes him home she discovers Sean has organized a surprise party. She is devastated.

This is the entire content of the magazine. Boy meets girl in every conceivable place and space. No other concerns appear in the lives of these photo-story heroines. Work is merely a passport to romance, friends are potential matchmakers or boyfriend-stealers.

This is not an idyllic or idealized world; the dominant emotions running through the stories are fear, insecurity, competitiveness and panic.[27] Capturing a boy isn't easy. Other girls are a constant threat and there is continuous anxiety about keeping him once he is caught. A girl has to get him and keep him by fair means or foul (although if foul, she will move out of the realm of the 'good girl' into the realm of the 'bad', which causes anxiety in itself). Boys are also categorized as good or bad: the bad often exciting and attractive, but impossible to keep; the good initially uninteresting, but more reliable, and often a better bet in the end. The perennial quandary of romantic fiction. Teenage magazines provide us with a detailed script of how to get it right. The first stage is to get him.

How to Get a Boyfriend – Guaranteed

What exactly does a boy go for in a girlfriend? A beautiful face? Feminine charm? Astounding wit? Or just someone they can have a good laugh or natter with? We decided it was time to hear it from the horse's mouth.

Mizz [28]

10 secrets to finding the right guy for you: Don't redo yourself; socialize; take some risks; expect a first date to be awkward; trust your intuition; don't ignore your friends; be enthusiastic; take it slow; don't forget to have fun.

Teen [29]

The very essence of 'woman' is that she is different from 'man', and teenage magazines reinforce this notion. Sexual difference is central to the script of heterosexual desire, yet to be successful in this game of romance a girl must be aware of and negotiate this difference. So the question posed by Freud, 'What do women want?', is turned round and made a focus for girls. It is *their* quest to work out what boys want. A difficult process given the apparent complexities of the male mind.

Teenage magazines tell us that boys and men are a different species, needing careful research and investigation before any approach is made. This is not to say that there are any simple rules that can be given about the methods and motives of male sexuality – far from it. That would make the chase much too easy. What is needed is the careful exercise of cunning feminine wiles in order to uncover the 'real' man behind the mysterious unspeaking façade. God forbid that we might think men are silent because they have nothing to say (to us at least). No – it is because they are thinking 'deep thoughts'. Or because they are 'deeply troubled' and vulnerable underneath the cool façade. The exercise for girls is to work out what these 'deep thoughts' are for themselves.

Magazine features can help us to get inside the minds of men. The American *'Teen* magazine has a regular feature entitled 'Guy Panel'. The opening blurb tells us:

> We know what *you* think of life and love. Clueless about what guys are thinking? Well, we've got their answers to questions you've always wanted to ask. We talked with eight of *'Teen's* favourite guys, who reveal everything![30]

The questions are weighty: 'What do you look for most in a girl? What do you worry about most? Do you like a girl wearing perfume? Where would you be likely to take a girl on a date? Do your 'guy friends' pressure you to have sex with girls you date?' What all girls *really* want to know. On the same lines, a feature in the British *Mizz* magazine quoted earlier entitled 'How to Get a Boyfriend' opens with the confident claim that the article will tell 'us girls' what men simply can't resist, allowing us to 'find out how to attract them, [and] how to hang on to them'. No subtlety here. The feature contains a hornet's nest of contradictory advice and admonition. *Jackie* in the seventies gave a much simpler message: Look good, be good, and good will come to you (unfortunately though, it wasn't that easy). Here's how you apparently have to do it today:

> How can she attract you?
>
> Jason, 18
> With me it's always eye contact, so if a girl sees someone she likes she should keep staring at him – boys love that. I'm not too bothered about what she's

wearing, but then again, if a girl walked into a club wearing shorts and Jesus sandals I'd be off.

Wang, 18
I like a girl who dresses in a way to show off her body – I like to see a bit of flesh – it gets me going!

Lee, 16
She has to be witty and charming.

Tom, 18
She has to have a good sense of humour and must be able to act like one of the lads.

Jamie, 16
I'm always attracted to someone I can have an intelligent conversation with. But she'd also have to enjoy a beer and a good laugh.

Have post-modernism and feminism infected teenage magazines and brought about a rejection of the monolithic advice 'Flatter him, don't interrupt him, and ask him lots of questions about himself', which used to be the recipe for getting and keeping a man?

The modern Mizz has a much harder task ahead of her. Looks are clearly still important, but she also has to have 'personality', a sense of humour and an ability to fit in with 'the lads'. These young men are confident in their assertions – they know what they want. (As did Prince Charming when he sought out Cinderella with the glass slipper.) Implicitly suggesting that they speak for all men ('boys love that'), this feature perpetuates the notion that a girl must moderate her behaviour to fit in with the expectations of boys and that seeking male approval should be the focus of her attention. That she should be herself, or that he should mould himself to fit in with her expectations are concepts that are completely absent. Acting out the script of perfect femininity is the name of the game. It is she who must watch herself,[31] and change. At the same time, she must remember that he's only human. Mizz has a section of the problem page entitled 'Boys Have Problems Too . . .', containing anodyne problems (not getting on with mum, having difficulties at school) which could as easily be reported by a girl as a boy. The function here is to give the impression that boys share the same worries as girls – they are people too. Yet the very fact that there is a special section for boys suggests that there is also something different about their problems.

This necessity of a girl moulding herself for the boy's gaze is never clearer than in the insights of boys on the subject of sexuality. Teenagers in the seventies didn't need *Jackie* to tell them that girls who 'slept around' were slags – everyone already knew this to be 'true'. Stories and features in *Jackie* served as reminders, with tales of girls of easy virtue who were used and abused by boys, then discarded like a piece of trash, while the virtuous girls were asked to be 'serious' girlfriends. 'Sex' was something to be avoided, or engaged in only within a 'steady relationship'. This seems somewhat archaic today, as sexual freedom is celebrated in teenage magazines. Yet despite the apparently open discussion of sex in the nineties – advice on contraception, safer sex and the mechanics of sexual encounters being proffered freely – the traditional Madonna–whore dichotomy is still a dominant theme. Girls are still sent a clear message: Sex is acceptable – but only in certain circumstances. If it takes place on the girl's instigation or outside the confines of serial monogamy, the age-old condemnations still apply. In order to remind girls who might have taken the notion of post-feminism too seriously, *Mizz* continues its insight into the minds of boys with a feature on the subject 'How Should She Approach You?' The answer is simple: Girls should wait . . .

Stephen, 21

In America girls come up and grab you, shouting 'Hi!', and it's too much. I think it's better to wait for the guy to approach you.

Paul, 18

I think it's a good idea to ask a friend to find out if she's interested first. Some girls are just too pushy.

James, 17

I'd be flattered if a girl asked me out but I wouldn't want her to be too confident. What would really impress me is if she gave me a huge present – something she knew I'd like, say tickets to the FA Cup final.

Bradley, 17

I'd like a girl to just come over and say something like 'You look nice,' anything really, and it wouldn't matter if she was nervous because then my part would be to make her feel comfortable.

Jason, 18

I don't think it's a good idea to go straight up to boys and tell them how much you like them because they'll just take the mickey out of you. Be a bit cool.

Jamie, 16

I wouldn't really want a girl to just come up and ask me out straight away because I'd feel like I was put on the spot. You need to find out if you can talk to each other first. Girls are always trying to rush into things, but they should just be really friendly and the rest will happen on its own.

The message hasn't changed much from the fairy tales – the girl should wait to be sought out, she shouldn't take any initiative herself. If she does, she must do it in a meek and mild manner so that the boy will be able to maintain the illusion of control. Don't be 'too confident', be a 'bit nervous'. Yet are girls following these dictates? Clearly not all the time. The boys interviewed by *Mizz* have obviously had experience of 'pushy' girls – and they don't like it. Perhaps confused by the conflicting messages – be fun, one of the lads, but stay passive and acquiescent – girls are taking the initiative and acting out their desires. Yet the consequences for girls can be severe, as 'pushy' girls are often deemed 'slags', and while nice girls may be 'drags', at least their reputations are safe.[32] Confident, openly sexual girls can find themselves completely rejected or condemned. This certainly reflects the views of the majority of the men I interviewed, what follows being a typical response to the question of whether they liked women to 'make the first move'.

'I would just say, "No, thanks", sort of shy away from it . . . It would just be sleazy and cheap, I wouldn't like to feel that. I just would feel that there were too many reasons for it (her approach) . . . It would just reflect that I knew she's likely to do it with everyone else, and just do it with someone she might not even know.'

Even when 'good' girls have 'caught' their man (through *his* efforts and endeavours) they must continue to watch themselves lest they fail to live up to his expectations and lose him. Here is the advice from boys on the matter, having been asked by *Mizz*, 'How Can She Keep You?':

James, 17
I like a girlfriend to be good fun – one of the boys really – and she definitely shouldn't be too clingy.

Jason, 18
It's really exciting when you first go out with someone, but after the first six months it can get boring, so you should keep flirting and make him take an interest in you.

Anthony, 16
My mates have to respect my girlfriend – if they think she's an old tart it's really embarrassing.

Jake, 17
A girlfriend should always be affectionate but never too sloppy.

Danny, 19
She'd have to like the same things as me because I'd expect my girlfriend to get involved with the same things I do – like surfing.

A girl should continue to be sexually interesting (flirtatious), yet still watch her reputation so that his friends don't think her an 'old tart'. She should be affectionate – but not overly, in case it is thought 'clingy' or 'sloppy'. She should fit in with his activities – be an honorary male – yet maintain her femininity by not being too 'pushy'. A tall order for any young woman to fulfil, centred around the expectations and interests of the man. His standards, but her failure if she doesn't succeed in 'keeping him'.

If the directive advice in 'How to Get a Boyfriend' is not explicit enough, *Mizz* also provides a feature on '*How Not to Get a Boyfriend – Guaranteed*'. The message amounts to a list of don'ts: Don't wear too much make-up, flirt with his friends, laugh at his underwear, ignore him, yawn, get drunk, be too loud, too impatient, get too attached, spit, be unfaithful, get in a bad mood, be miserable, be girly, lack confidence, be critical or bitchy, or argue. A wide range of negative stipulations for acceptance. Taking the advice in *Mizz* as a whole, a girl has to be feminine (don't criticize, stray or behave like a boy), but not *too* feminine (don't be girly, or lack confidence). An impossible condition to fulfil, or maintain.

So what do girls make of this? Do they *really* adopt this very traditional script of femininity without any dissent? Some would say 'yes'. Psycho-analytic feminist Susan Contratto has provided clinical accounts of female sexuality which indicate that some women 'spent a great deal of energy trying to figure out what sort of woman the man she is interested in *really* wants so that she can be that sort of woman'. She argues that many women always go with the views of men: 'speaking up in a relationship, even if only to acknowledge difference, carried with it great fears.'[33] In this view, women will accept whatever little they can get from a man in exchange for identification and love. At one level, teenage magazines seem to imply that this is what girls should do.

Yet many women and girls reject or subvert both this archetypal script of femininity and the codes of heterosexual romance. They know what a girl *should* do if she wants to play the game – they have learnt the rules (and know the penalties for transgression). But this doesn't mean that they believe in what they are doing or that the outward appearance of being a 'nice girl' who isn't interested in sex reflects who they are. There is pleasure in the duplicity involved in the very act of *doing* girl, something which is clearly reflected in the texts of teenage magazines, which provides ample opportunities for girls to laugh at the vanity and foolishness of the narcissistic man, and at the ways in which men are so easily fooled by girls' performance of femininity.

Humouring the Conceit of Man

One photo-story in *Mizz*, entitled 'The Male of the Species', draws ironic attention to femininity as masquerade, giving the impression that it is women who are really in control. It starts off with two girls walking down the street, with one commenting, 'You know what, sometimes I think blokes are a completely different species from us.' The two then speculate about what goes on in boys' minds when they look at girls in the street. One girl thinks that boys merely wonder what girls look like with their clothes off, the other believes they think *really* deep thoughts – sometimes. The cynical perspective is confirmed by our insight into the mind of Dale, the hero of the tale, who looks at one of the girls and thinks, 'I wonder what she looks like with her clothes off.' In contrast to the majority of the photo-stories, which are presented from the perspective of the girl, this one is from Dale's point of view.

He is presented as arrogant, confident, and trying very hard – to get his blind date into bed. His anxieties about himself are merely cocky, smug attempts to please: 'She can't fail to be impressed by my new aftershave, Jean Jacques, which I got down the market. £2.50 for a 200 ml bottle . . .' His misogyny and the fact that his primary concern is the opinion of his friends is reflected in his thoughts as he waits for his date:

> Now I'll just go over tonight's excuse if it all goes disastrously wrong. 'Sorry, I've got to go – you're so ugly my face has started to dissolve.' That'll crease the lads up if I actually say it. Not that I will.

Dale's outward appearance contrasts with his thoughts throughout the date (in the manner Woody Allen made memorable in the film *Annie Hall*), as if to underline the duplicity of man (and the message that they cannot be trusted). He greets his 'date' warmly, inwardly congratulating himself for the sexy smile he's practised in the mirror. Throughout the evening he continuously monitors his progress, refraining from forcing his attentions on her only because it will lead to more success in the long run: 'It feels strange walking along without holding hands. Still, everything comes to he who waits and doesn't stick their hand down a bra at the earliest opportunity . . .'

When he is rewarded with a good–night kiss, Dale rubs his hands with glee and thinks to himself, 'Brilliant. You cracked it.' The story ends with an editorial comment on this supposedly archetypal male behaviour: 'Dale, like most guys, had a very high opinion of himself.' As Dale walks off into the sunset his final thoughts are, 'I bet she's thinking of me now. I know what women are like, they're always thinking about love and weddings and sloppy romantic things.' How wrong he is. His date is shown to be *actually* thinking, 'Hmm? I wonder what he looks like with his clothes off?'

This story plays the stereotyped notion that boys are a different species interested only in sex against the acknowledgement that girls are not the romantically obsessed innocents they are expected to be. Teenage magazines here reflect the contradictions inherent in the script of heterosexual romance and comment ironically on girls' solutions to the limitations of the feminine role. Dale's date may have behaved in an appropriate feminine manner (refusing to hold his hand on their first meeting, not asking him in, not seeming too keen) but her intention was the same as his – sex.

This stands in stark contrast to the traditional view of women being interested in love, not sex. It is a view of women which many men still believe. The majority of the men I interviewed told me that women wanted love more than sex, and that men could more easily 'have a fuck'. Many analysts would agree. Ethel Persons, a feminist psychoanalyst who is critical of male dominance nevertheless argues that the power differences which underpin heterosexuality are ineradicable because women long for love and men fear it:

> Women are more at ease with the mutuality implicit in love, as well as the surrender, while men tend to interpret mutuality as dependency and defend against it by separating sex from love, or alternatively, by attempting to dominate the beloved.[34]

Teenage magazines suggest that girls are no longer simply seeking 'love'. Yet they are aware of the need to conceal their intentions from men – man's fear (and his desire to dominate) is no secret. As one woman I interviewed commented:

> 'Women do desire sex as much as men do – but we have to hide it. If you've got the urge and you go out and gratify it, and you do it every time you've got an urge, then you're going to earn yourself a label.'

After over twenty-five years of open feminist critiques of gender relationships[35] there are few women who embrace the traditional feminine position without having serious reservations. So in order to play their part in the romantic script without compromising their sense of being 'equal to men', women position their behaviour as a *choice*; it is something over which they have control. As another woman said, 'If I meet someone I like I'll find a way of talking to them that isn't obvious, and then let them chat me up.' Many women claim to have this down to an art form:

> 'When I'm in the mood I'm so good at it. I can go out and meet someone really easily – and he will always think that it was him that picked me.'

> 'If I'm in a relationship I don't bother with other men. As soon as I'm single again, I put on my "flirting hat" and it's never let me down.'

By covertly taking control of the romantic scenario women are giving themselves permission to 'do femininity' without sacrificing their sense of integrity. There is no doubt in their minds that this mask of femininity does not reflect what they *really* feel – they are merely performing a part. This disparity between inner feelings and outward appearance has always been part of the feminine script: Nineteenth-century conduct manuals emphasized the necessity of female decorum and the danger in showing passion or emotion; Jane Austen's heroines performed this role exceptionally well. In today's interpretation of the script, women allow men to position them as the objects of their desire, while positioning themselves as active subjects. This is the age-old story of the power behind the throne, the woman who controls man through covert manipulation. The fact that men can't see through this perform-ance is used to reinforce women's conception of themselves as powerful – it is they who really know what is going on. Conceiving men as vulnerable, needy, or weak is a concomitant strategy:

'You have to be cool, or they'll get frightened off.'

'Men are intimidated by women whom they think might be better or more experienced in bed than they are.'

'Men pretend they're hard, but when you get them on their own, they're soft. It's nice.'

'All you have to do is flatter them and they'll eat out of your hand. They are so desperate to be liked that they believe everything.'

This can grease the wheels of romance, allowing women to act the part of 'girl' and men to believe that their adoration is true (yet still keeping women in their place – as a foil for men). But it can also act against men, further reducing their power in relation to women, as they can be positioned as 'stupid' or 'foolish' and openly vilified as a result – for failing to live up to their side of the romantic bargain (by acting out the role of 'prince'), or because they believe the woman's performance is authentic. As these young women told me:

'Men still don't have any idea about what's going on and how to behave towards women.'

'They're such suckers – they always fall for the same girly act. You just have to watch men with an attractive woman and they're drooling all over her. Pathetic.'

'All you have to do is flatter their egos and they believe it's all true. It makes me laugh.'

As a *Seventeen* magazine feature declares, 'In your mind, he's perfect: so cool and funny and smart and cute. But then, unfortunately, you really get to know him.' While women might still fantasize about Mr Right, there is also open acknowledgement that outside of dreams, Prince Charming is almost impossible to find. This is most blatantly exposed in the British television programme *Blind Date*, which provides a weekly diet of women's dissatisfaction with the failure of men to live up to their promise. In recent series, during the report-back section with the couple who have returned from their blind date, one of the most common scenarios is an attractive woman expressing vehement disappointment at the lack of sophistication, social skills and general personality in the man she has dated. Here, men are positioned as just not good enough, as not having a clue about women – and as a result are summarily rejected: 'I just didn't fancy him'; 'I thought he was attractive when the screen went back but on the date he was really boring.'[36] These days, it appears that women are prepared to continue with the feminine masquerade only if men keep to their side of the bargain and act out the role of Mr Right. It's an impossible task for most men.

When women or girls do find Mr Right (by definition the current partner), the means of saving him from all the criticism and disdain meted out to other men is by positioning him as different: 'My boyfriend isn't like all the other blokes, he's much more sensitive and understanding,' was a comment I heard from most of the young women I talked to. This process continues into adulthood. In *Our Treacherous Hearts* Ros Coward reports that the majority of the women she interviewed described their partners in such a similar way (as nice, kind, basically different from *other* men) that she thought they were all married to the same man.[37] What they were doing was using the same defensive strategy to reconcile their cynicism about gender relationships with their desire to live with or love a man. So whilst masculinity and femininity may still be positioned as binary opposites, both teenage magazines and the comments of young girls themselves, suggest that taking up the position of 'woman' is not simply a case of taking up a passive, acquiescent position, always secondary and subservient to 'man'. It is a much more complicated scenario.

'Let's Talk about Sex, Baby'

They Saw Us Having Sex

I feel a total slut. I recently went to a party and got drunk. I ended up giving this boy a blow-job and then having full sex with him. The thing was, I thought no one could see us, but there were at least three other people in the room. Now whenever I pass girls from school they call me names. The girls in my class all think I'm a slut. My boyfriend found out and now I'm all alone. The boy I had sex with isn't getting any hassle whatsoever from these girls. It's all so unfair. I wish I had never got drunk, but I did and now everyone is going to hate me forever. I'm so miserable I feel like running away.

Just Seventeen

Ready to Masturbate Him

My boyfriend and I are both 16 and recently he's been asking me if I'll masturbate him. I feel ready to do it as my boyfriend and I love each other but I'm not sure how to. I'm too embarrassed to tell my boyfriend or ask him how to do it, so I just told him I didn't feel like it. Please explain how it's done because I love him and don't want to put him off.

Just Seventeen[38]

Romance isn't the only script girls have to learn. Today, teen magazines 'talk about sex' incessantly. There are no holds barred. The responses to the two problem-page letters in *Just Seventeen* above are devoid of any sense of moral outrage or coyness. In the answer to the first problem the girl is encouraged to hold her head high at school and ignore her class mates, who will soon forget. She is gently admonished about her drunkenness, but reassured that 'everyone makes mistakes.' In the second problem a detailed description of this particular sexual skill is given:

> All that happens is that you clasp your fingers round the shaft of his penis then move your hand up and down in rhythmic strokes. If you're absolutely positive you want to do it, then the best thing is to ask him to get him to show you how to do it.

The reality of fumbling, silent adolescent sex is reflected in the comment, 'It's sad if it has to be done without a word being said and both parties wondering if they're doing the right thing.' As with much adult sex, few teenagers sit down and talk through their sexual preferences or ways of improving their 'sexual technique' with the person they are 'having sex' with. Only in the private, female world of magazines or during conversations with female friends are such subjects broached. The agony aunt is almost like a 'friend' — she has been through all these teenage traumas herself and is always sympathetic, never judgemental (unlike parents, who 'never understand').[39]

Problem pages in teenage magazines used to be more anodyne: How to deal with unsightly spots, how to cope with jealousy over your boyfriend's ex-girlfriend, how to patch up a broken friendship, how to overcome parental pressures. Or the agonies of being incapable of speaking to a boy without blushing so extremely that he turns away and laughs. These problems still appear — the fact that sex is now more openly discussed does not remove all other adolescent anguish. The problem page reflects it all.

The problem page is like a rule book, which defines, navigates and regulates the sexual experience of women and girls.[40] Look at the problem pages in teenage magazines and you will gain insight into the current agonies facing adolescents and the rules they have to follow to find their way out of difficulty. In the fifties the question was 'How far should you go?' (the answer: nowhere before marriage); in the seventies, 'How do you reconcile the new sexual freedom promised by the advent of the Pill with the fact that the old rules still apply?' (the answer: serial monogamy). Today the rule book says that sex (with boys) is normal, natural and open, rather than secret or repressed. Sex is no longer taboo, no one has to wait until marriage (unlike the fairy-tale heroine). It doesn't even have to take place within a 'steady' relationship. Sex is now positioned as a sign of independence, an expression of our inner desires. It's something that every girl should do. The worry is not whether you should 'do it' or not, but how good you are at it. As a recent *Ultimate Sex Guide* produced by *more!* magazine informs girls, 'There's only one essential to being great in bed: enthusiasm, and lots of it. So moan, wriggle, giggle, plead and beg for more.'[41] This assumes that they *want* more. But as sex is now positioned as a skill, a recreational activity with rules to follow and tricks to learn, she only has herself to blame if she doesn't. Women's magazines (avidly read by teenagers) trumpet on their front covers 'Orgasm School' (*Marie Claire*), and 'Be 50% sexier! Your sexuality masterclass starts here!' (*New Woman*), reinforcing this message. Yet the agony aunts still warn girls to be careful, and only to have sex if they want to – the liberal feminist ethos of 'choice' translated for today's teenagers. In a discussion of blow-jobs, the *Ultimate Sex Guide* has the following caustic advice:

> 'But what about deep throating?' you ask. It only exists in movies with full-frontal nudity. But if you insist, here's how you do what porn stars do: Lie with your head thrown back over the edge of the bed so your throat forms a long passage when he thrusts. Now rush to the loo because when you stick anything down your throat, you gag. If he insists you suck, tell him to date a plumber.[42]

So girls can openly have sex, but shouldn't let proceedings slip out of their control (the *Ultimate Sex Guide* tells girls, 'You decide when it's penetration time'). Sex may now be a skill, but it is still associated with 'love' – the sex guide describes fellatio as 'giving pleasure to the man you adore'. There are detailed instructions on 'making sex supersexy', yet girls are told that every man is different – 'Each man and his penis is unique and he's the only one who really knows his heart's (and willy's) desires' – the implication being that she has to learn the rules anew each time. It's not easy navigating these contradictory stories about sex.

Descriptions of fellatio (or blow-jobs) used to be confined to the pages of 'pornography' (it is still a major obsession there; see Chapter Three). It certainly wasn't the subject of polite conversation, or publicly recognized as a desired sexual practice for 'nice girls'. As one interviewee commented:

> 'I remember walking home with my mate Yolanda, and this was when we were still in prep. school, I would have been about ten, and she knew about oral sex, she knew about blow-jobs and was explaining to me about blow-jobs, I think she'd read it somewhere and I was absolutely disgusted [laugh], there was no way anyone was ever going to get me to do that [laugh].'

Today blow-jobs are clearly common practice amongst teenage girls, at least according to British teenage magazines (American teen magazines are more circumspect, with less of a sex-manual style).[43] If knowledge is power, then obtaining explicit information about sex is a necessary part of adolescent development. In the light of AIDS, high rates of date rape and social mores that now position sex as everyone's right it is as essential that girls feel empowered to say 'No' (or 'Use a condom') as it is that they know how to be 'good in bed'. It is disingenuous to suggest that these magazines create the desire for sex in teenagers. Teenage sexual exploration existed long before *Just Seventeen, Sugar,* or *more!* started to describe it in detail. Indeed, as Susan Douglas outlines in her exploration of mass media in the fifties, *Where the Girls are,* sex was a subtext in music, film and comics even in the days when good girls didn't. Banning teenage magazines as 'outraged' parents would have us do would have little impact – adult women's magazines have openly celebrated and described active female sexuality since the 'sexual revolution' was first heralded in the early seventies, *Cosmopolitan* being the archetypal example.[44] The titles of features in a recent selection of women's magazines declare: 'Sex with a Stranger: The Ultimate Turn On' (*Elle*); 'Talking Dirty: Women Who Get Paid to Give Sex on the Phone' (*Options*); 'Orgies: They're Here and They're Happening' (*New Woman*); 'Dirty Sex' and 'Why He Likes You Taking the Lead in Bed' (*Company*); and 'Sexually Assertive Women, How Do Men Feel When You Come on Strong?' (*Cosmopolitan*). (The answer to the last is 'scared', but the magazine doesn't tell us this; it wouldn't fit with their image of emancipated, egalitarian sex.) To censor explicit sex aimed at women when sex pervades mass media aimed at men (see Chapter Two), would be to return to an era of Victorian double standards, when women and girls were the main targets of protection from pornography (See Chapter Three).

These sex-obsessed problem pages do, however, provide a unique narrative about the woes of 'woman'. They are marked out clearly as arenas for the exposure and solution of feminine concerns. Many girls pore over the problem pages together, reading out the sad accounts and ridiculing the agony aunt's replies. This is evidence of the shared, positive function of mass media imagery. The common experience of reading and criticizing, of laughing and grimacing at what we see on the problem page is a reassuring process letting us know that someone else is suffering all the things that we are, or making us feel good about ourselves because we *haven't* got that terrible problem – 'Laughing with my friends distances me from the traumas I read about.' But there is another side to the coin. Many women and girls also read these problems on their own and take them very seriously. Angela McRobbie has argued that teenage problem pages serve to 'initiate girls into a closed world of suffering'.[45] Closed because the problems are individualized, encouraging the girl to focus within herself (or in some cases her family), rather than on the wider social factors which might underlie her difficulties. They also make suffering both normal and private ('We all feel terrible underneath, don't we?') and encourage girls to accept the difficulties they continually face. They may appear to offer an emancipatory script, but in their stories of 'slags' and in the pouring-out of guilt and anxiety they provide a clear indication of what 'normal' girls *should* feel bad about. In the narrow script of concerns they cover, they mark our bodies, and sex, as the centre of female existence – a centre that is positioned as inherently problematic.

Some of this reflects the material reality of girls' lives. Today, many girls *are* having sex; the recent rash of sex surveys tells us so. (See Wellings, Kaye, Field, Julia, Johnson, Anne, M. & Wadsworth, J., *Sexual Behaviour in Britain: The National Survey of Sexual Attitudes and Lifestyles*, London: Penguin, 1994.) Undoubtedly many are expert at giving blow-jobs, but many are not – and what they see and read probably doesn't make them feel any better about themselves. Teenage girls used to worry because they'd never been kissed. Do today's teenagers worry because they've never given a blow-job?

Certainly, many girls do report that they start having sex with boys in order to feel 'normal' and attractive: 'I went out with boys because of pressure from magazines. They pressure you into your sexuality. It makes you feel inadequate.' Many girls said it was because they wanted to find out what all the fuss was about:

> 'Everyone at school was talking about which boys were the best kissers, so I wanted to be able to join in.'

> 'I "did it" for the first time just to get it over and done with. I didn't really fancy the boy very much, but I knew I had to do it some time, and we were on our own in the house, so I thought "Why not?"'

This confirms the findings of large-scale sexual surveys that report 'curiosity' as the main factor which precipitates first sexual intercourse. Romanticism is clearly dying. In the survey mentioned above, whilst over half of women who are now over forty-five report that being 'in love' was what led them to first have intercourse, less than one-third of young women today say the same.

But these early sexual experiences are often very disappointing. They rarely live up to the promised fantasy of the fairy tales:

> 'I liked the thrill and chase, but as soon as they started getting interested it got boring. But I was very conscious of the fact that I was supposed to like it, so I kept practising, trying to kiss boys, because I thought once I'd got used to it I'd probably like it.'

Contrary to essentialist theories of sex (see Chapter Four), there is a large element of learning in sexual behaviour. It doesn't always just 'come naturally'. Most girls persevere with this early sloppy kissing and eventually grow to like it, but it is a common retort that early adolescent experiences are more like kissing a wet puppy than Prince Charming. Equally, few girls find their first experiences of 'sex' (penetration) live up to the romantic myth. Here are some comments on their sexual initiation from North American girls interviewed by Sharon Thompson:

> 'It was just like, psst, one minute here, the next minute it was there. It happened. That was it.'

> 'The pain was like I couldn't stand it.'

> 'It felt like there was a knife going through me.'

> 'It wasn't like I didn't like it. It was just kind of a let-down.'

> 'It wasn't really that good. There was nothing I really liked about it.'

> 'It didn't really hurt. It hurt a little bit. It was uncomfortable. I was pretty bored actually. I didn't see anything nice about it at all.'[46]

The multi-orgasmic sex portrayed in magazines is seemingly not easy to come by, at least not on your first try. Yet not all early sexual experiences are so uncomfortable, painful or boring. Many teenage girls *do* experience sexual desire and arousal, most commonly when they are 'petting'. One woman interviewee reported:

> 'We didn't want to "have sex", but we did everything else but. He used to stroke my legs really slowly, then touch me, and put his fingers inside

me. I used to feel as if I was going to melt. Sometimes it went on for hours.'

In a similar vein, here are two girls who identified as lesbian, again interviewed by Sharon Thompson:

'And then we kissed, and it was the most incredible – I knew I was gay at that minute for the first time, because I had made out before and it never felt like that. And it was just so incredible.'

'This was the first time we ever did anything besides kiss. And I just put her down and then I touched her through her little yellow panties. She was soaked!'[47]

So that which is often dismissed as 'foreplay' or not 'going all the way' is reported by many teenage girls as being amongst their most pleasurable experiences of 'sex'.[48] Many girls limit their sexual activity to foreplay, ostensibly to avoid the label of 'slag' or 'slut', which is still frequently applied if they have penetrative sex outside a committed relationship. For despite the confident proclamations of the new generation of agony aunts, girls who have shed the traditional feminine dictate that they cannot have sex for fun and are as happy as most men purport to be to engage in casual sex or a one-night stand are not greeted with open arms by the majority of men. As one interviewee commented:

'If you were with a girl that loads of men had slept with it would be like really horrible . . . there would be nothing that would be private between the two of you, you know there's nothing intimate, everything is just public.'

The traditional association of female sexuality with 'madness'[49] hasn't disappeared either, as sexually active girls are sometimes seen to have an underlying problem. As one man commented on a girl who 'slept around':

'We thought she was really insecure and tried to do it to make herself accepted. She was messed up . . . I don't know if she enjoyed being like that or not. But I think I sort of felt quite sorry for her.'

This attitude also operates at the level of the law – 'promiscuous' women 'deserve what they get' (see Chapter 5). So girls have to navigate the gap between what boys and society says about girls who have sex and what the more liberal-minded magazine agony aunts say. Apart from abstinence, or careful control of how far they will 'go', the major means by which girls deal with this is through secrecy or discretion. One interviewee said:

> 'There's still that thing where if a woman is sexually active she's a slag, but if she's not she's frigid or something. But that's not so much between individuals, it's more sort of reputation, so I think you can avoid it . . . if you're lucky with your partners and they don't tell anyone about what you're like and everything, you can avoid it that way.'

British girls are notorious in many parts of continental Europe for their lack of sexual inhibitions on 'bonking holidays' – they can go as far as they want without fear of losing their reputation, as long as no one spills the beans at home. The package-holiday company, 18–30s, reinforces this message in its advertising campaigns, which sell sex explicitly; here, women are portrayed as being as sexually voracious as men. One recent cinema advert showed an ecstatic woman standing in a waist-deep pool. A man's head suddenly pops up, suggesting that cunnilingus is the cause of her pleasure. She aggressively pushes his head back down. This view of female sexuality is not a creation of the advertisers (although it reproduces a common male fantasy); it reflects the fact that many girls *are* rejecting the part of the script of femininity which says they should be discreet about their sexual desires and explicitly rejecting the slag– drag dichotomy:

> 'Why shouldn't I have sex if I want to? Boys have always been able to.'

> 'It's just nonsense that girls can't have sex without love. On a Friday night I enjoy a good shag.'

> 'When I want to settle down I'll be more careful about who I go with. At the moment I'm interested in someone who I can have a good time with, and can have good sex.'

In a study of young women in New Jersey, Michael Moffat reported similar findings, with women talking about 'scoring', orgasms without emotional commitment and an enjoyment in heterosexual sex.[50] This is arguably evidence that young women are rewriting the script of femininity in the very act of 'doing girl' – although whether they are as open about their sexual desires when placed face to face with a boy is something I would question. Teenage magazines reflect this change in sexual practices – selling a story of sexual freedom and equality – but also emphasize the need to be 'careful', reinforcing the view that this is 'normal' behaviour for girls and influencing practices. It is a circular process.

Interestingly, the concept of 'slag' has a different meaning for young women who define themselves as lesbian. It is the transgression of the rigid boundaries of heterosexual sex and romance – if you are a woman – which is condemned. As these two lesbians interviewed by Julie Mooney-Somers commented, 'It's a positive word . . . to be a tart you have to have something'; 'I don't use it as something against somebody in a horrible way . . . . It's quite an endearing thing actually . . . like, "you saucy slag".' This is because lesbians who have had a lot of sexual partners, or who enjoy sex, are able to be open about their desires and their sexual history with their sexual partners – not just with their female friends. For many, it is something to be proud of; for others, it is a part of life they take for granted, and if monogamy is a practice which is adopted, it is because of emotional commitment and the realization that more than one sexual partner can lead to feelings of jealousy, envy and insecurity, rather than because of the burden of shame and secrecy which clouds the traditional script of heterosexual sex and romance.

This burden is still felt by many girls in their navigation of the contradictions put forward in teenage magazines (You can have sex, but you shouldn't be pushy; You do have sexual desires that are equal to those of men, but for women sex is associated with love). They may be put off by the undercurrent of guilt still associated with this new version of emanicipated femininity, or by the fact that boys haven't moved on – still categorizing girls who transgress the archetypal script of femininity as 'easy' or 'slags'. Or perhaps they are not so lucky in finding the 'right' man. This leads many teenagers to turn to the fantasy man, the traditional romantic hero. He never condemns, he never disappoints, and in the traditions of courtly love (here reversed, where it is the man who is adored), as he remains in the realm of the imaginary (or at least the unobtainable), he is a source of never-ending desire. Wet knickers and screams in a packed concert hall will not bring the disapprobation and guilt which can follow an encounter with a real-life boy (and will in most cases be more exciting – real-life boys rarely have the sexual and romantic skills of the fantasy man).

Worshipping a Far-off Star . . .

Star quest
Meet Jonathan face to face.
Check out TV's hottest new hunks.
Teen[51]

Luscious crushes
Falling for Keanu, Brad, Jared, Chris, Ethan . . .
Seventeen[52]

Teenage girls do find romantic heroes a bit thin on the ground at school. But fulfilment can be gained from the fantasy world of the male 'star'. From the days of silent film stars such as Rudolph Valentino, peaking with the 'invention' of the teenager in the fifties, adolescent girls have thrilled to the sexualized strutting of a succession of film and pop stars. The longing and desire for the imaginary prince of our childhood fairy tales comes to be channelled in the direction of generations of teen idols who personify male sexuality and heroism, while at the same time stimulating adolescent girls' wet dreams. Teen magazines provide a detailed script for this manifestation of teenage sex and desire.

For example, in a recent edition of the British magazine *Shout*, a fan, 15-year-old Anna Nugent, was interviewed about her devotion to Take That. She is photographed in her bedroom, which is covered wall-to-wall with images of the five-boy pop group. The attraction to the band is unequivocally physical, rather than musical, as Anna explains when asked what first made her notice the band:

> If I'm being honest, it was their looks! When I first saw them half naked on video, I couldn't miss how handsome they were. I think their music's brilliant too, and they're really talented. There's no other band around as nice-looking as them, is there?

There is no pretence here – sex is the issue. Yet in observation of the codes of heterosexual romance, this is discerning sex: Anna has become a fan of Take That after perusing all the other boy bands, concluding that 'there's no other band around as nice-looking as them.' She demonstrates her loyalty now she has made her choice; she is no different from the fairy-story heroine who would never desert her prince: 'I think I'll always stay faithful. If – and it's a big if – they ever lose their popularity, I'll still go after them. There's more chance of meeting them if they're not so famous.' (Like thousands of other Take That fans, no doubt Anna was traumatized when they split up in 1995.)

Monogamy is still the ideal state – young girls can no more be promiscuous with their pop-star heroes than they can with real-life boys. Remnants of the desperate wish that 'one day my prince will come' remain: Meeting these stars could mean being swept off your feet, like Cinderella, Sleeping Beauty, and all the other fairy-tale heroines. Romance is still the name of the game. Anna's explanation for her adoration of Mark, one of the five band members of Take That, is telling: 'I know that he hates being called cute, but that's what he is. Since he looks younger, I feel I've got more of a chance with him, as he looks like a boy, rather than a superstar.'

The boy next door, transformed into icon adorning the bedrooms of legions of hopeful growing girls. The macho 'cock-rock' stars who play out explicit male sexual fantasies and gestures as part of their stage acts are not the stuff of adolescent girls' fantasies (nor those of most adult women, for that matter).[53] They are the unsubtle phallic heroes of heterosexual teenage boys (and heterosexual men who still posture in this unsubtle way). Girls want something more feminine – something more like themselves. Sheryl Garratt, who as a teenager was obsessed with the Bay City Rollers, has commented:

> It is interesting to note that although many of their lyrics tell how girls continuously lust over their irresistible bodies, Rainbow, Whitesnake, or even the more enlightened, younger heavy metal bands just don't get women screaming at them . . . Women seem far more attracted by slim, unthreatening, baby-faced types who act vulnerable and who resemble them. Androgyny is what they want: men they can dress like and identify with, as well as drool over.[54]

While most of us outgrow our teenage fantasies and look back on this adolescent infatuation with a mixture of embarrassment and disbelief, for some women these fantasies continue into adult life. Unsurprisingly, the men who inspire the greatest adoration are those who maintain the image of the vulnerable boy next door well into adulthood (and middle age). Barry Manilow is a prime example – a crooner who provokes almost unrivalled devotion in his female audience. One fan, Joanne, quoted in Fred and Judy Vermorel's *Starlust*, demonstrates the strength of her desires:

> When I make love with my husband I imagine it's Barry Manilow. All the time. And after, when my husband and I have made love and I realize it's not him, I cry to myself. It's usually dark when the tears flow and somehow I manage to conceal them. It happens to a lot of people, too. I didn't realize how many until I got involved with Barry fans. A lot of them are married and around my age and they feel the same way and they do the same thing. It's comforting to know I'm not the only one.[55]

On one level this is a familiar tale: The girl passively (and hopelessly) waiting for Mr Right. Prince Charming and the idolized pop star are stuff of the same fantasies – woman being saved and transformed by the powerful perfect man, who is the only one to realize how wonderful and perfect *she* really is. Pop music perpetuates this process with songs of longing and desire, focusing on the dream of boy meets girl. The romantic wish 'I want to be Bobby's girl' may have been replaced by explicit sex – 'Erotic – put your hands all over my body' – but the subtext is the same. This is not about women achieving power and pleasure for themselves, but finding the right man, who will provide it. It reinforces the belief that someone else will transform our lives and make us happy – and leads to inevitable disappointment when men don't live up to the promise (no one can). Yet there is another side to this. These fans are not simply passive in their desires. They are the ones doing the choosing (and the discarding, if their hero fails to please); in fantasy, they are in control of the relationship. In the same way, the current popularity of women artists who celebrate 'girl power', such as Madonna, Janet Jackson, or the Spice Girls, reflects the fact that teenage girls see themselves as active players in the game of sex and romance. The cynical might claim that these new female role models are merely a marketing ploy – playing on the fact that girls want to be sexy and attractive, as well as independent and strong. Indeed, on the surface, these female icons do still conform to many of the archetypal notions of feminine beauty. But they also act to subvert and parody the traditional feminine script, through being explicit about their own sexual desire, as well as mocking or objectifying men. Equally, whilst they predominantly perpetuate notions of heterosexuality as the norm (with the exception of Madonna during her lesbian phase . . .), it is a version of the script of heterosexuality which has changed drastically since the days when women were told to 'stand by [their] man'.

This channelling of female desire does have another side to it. Adolescent girls attempting to get close to their heroes will buy any product available. They buy records in their millions, keeping the more self-satisfied, supposedly serious groups afloat.[56] Critics such as Angela McRobbie have seen this as a reflection of a trend towards sexuality being simply another product within a consumer-orientated culture, something to buy, or to have, as easily as one buys a new dress or a new 'look'. She argues that 'the insertion of the female teenage subject into an even-more-hectic cycle of consumerism, particularly into the cycle of pop consumerism', is part of a wider process of capitalistic control.[57] The element of consumerism is certainly not hard to find. Take That fan Anna declares that she has spent over £1,000 on merchandise:

> I buy every magazine, one-off specials and posters, I've bought all the jewellery, T-shirts, bags – I think I've got almost everything . . . when I see anything I've not got, I usually try to buy it. I'd pay up to £30 for something if I think it's worth it.

However, this is not to say that girls are simply at the mercy of the music moguls. They do exercise discrimination and choice and will take their buying power elsewhere when they tire of the latest teen hero. Indeed the shelf-life of most teen idols is relatively short – which often leaves the 'investment' of the music industry high and dry. Equally, there is a strong element of solidarity in being a fan, and the paraphernalia that goes with it can act as a visible signifier of group identity, marking them out as experts in this particular arena. Sheryl Garratt describes this eloquently in her analysis of her teenage obsession with the Bay City Rollers, which had less to do with the music, than with her relationship with her female friends:

> We were a gang of girls having fun together, able to identify each other by tartan scarves and badges . . . at the concerts many [of us] were experiencing mass power for the first and last time. Looking back now, I hardly remember the gigs themselves, the songs, or even what the Rollers looked like. What I *do* remember are the bus rides, running home from school together to get to someone's house to watch *Shang-a-Lang* on TV, dancing in lines at the school disco, and sitting in each others'

bedrooms discussing our fantasies and compiling our scrapbooks. Our real obsession was with ourselves; in the end the actual men behind the posters had very little to do with it at all.[58]

Equally, many of the fans quoted by the Vermorels in *Starlust* talk as much about their friendships and feelings of solidarity with other fans as they do about their respective heroes. The same can be said of readers of romantic fiction, where the sense of being part of a 'community of readers' who make similar interpretations of the texts is part of the pleasure of such reading for women.[59]

Romantic Fiction – Passivity and Phallic Fulfilment

If teenage magazines school adolescent girls in the rules of heterosexual femininity, romantic fiction – perhaps the most pervasive and avidly read form of literature aimed at women (millions of books are sold every year) – throws adult women head first into a pit of passion and longing, for the phallic hero who will make her a 'complete woman'. The standard romantic novel – published by Harlequin, or Mills & Boon – has such an established pattern that aspiring authors are sent a template indicating the rights and wrongs of romantic-fiction writing. It is the archetypal script of heterosexual romance, in which being 'woman' is an uncomplicated affair.

Traditionally, sex is implied rather than explicitly described in romantic narratives – fairy-tale princesses don't fuck. Yet today the rules are changing and the heroine is allowed to both express and experience desire for man's 'fiery brand' – but only after appropriate courtship and seduction has taken place and the requisite promises have been made. This isn't realism entering the Harlequin fantasy world. Sexual union is presented in such an idealized manner, that it is a prize *any* woman would wait for:

> Slowly he thrust into her . . . the throb of his heat pulsed within her, a primeval beast, spiralling towards a glorious crescendo, and then she was falling, tumbling down into the vortex, little cries escaping her as the waves of pleasure eddied inside her. His own explosive fulfilment came within seconds . . . He held her, wrapped in his arms, their bodies swathed in the golden glow of love. 'I think,' he said softly, smiling into her eyes, 'you had better marry me very quickly.'   *Flames of Love* [60]

Is this 'real life'? It's certainly never happened to me (nor to any of the women I interviewed). What we have here is the perfect description of the penis as phallic fantasy made flesh, the all-powerful tool that lights woman's passion. Here, penetrative sex is that which leads to woman's greatest ecstasy – everything that comes before this moment is merely a preparation for her flight to heaven on receiving his 'fiery brand' inside her. It is a common fantasy, and the dominant theme in heterosexual pornography (see Chapter Three), as well as an implicit assumption in sex therapy (see Chapter Four). Here it is sold unapologetically to women, who appear to lap up this version of female passivity and male phallic mastery without ever being able to get enough – in their imaginations at least. In romantic fiction the penis is God; it creates 'woman':

> And suddenly through the mist of sleepiness, Kate realized that it was going to happen. It felt exactly as she had read it felt like. Soft, intense waves rather than her excitingly violent, direct clitoral orgasm. It was unmistakably different and it was undoubtedly happening. Kate felt fecund, indescribably female, and earth mother. She felt happy, *she felt at last a complete woman* [my italics].   *Lace*[61]

Within the script of romantic fiction the woman is passive, or at least passive where all outward appearance is concerned. For as with traditional fairy tales, romantic fiction is always about a poor girl marrying a rich man, and the authors must be 'careful to show that the girl never set out to get him and his goods',[62] at least not in an obvious way. The heroine must feign innocence and reticence. She lies to hide her desire and always tries to cover up any signs of sexual interest, upset or indeed any extreme of emotion.[63] She may want sex, but within the codes of romance, she can have it only if she is seduced (the sole means of *true* sexual fulfilment), and that must happen only when she has received his promise of love. As the heroine of the novel *Whirlwind* declares: 'He had offered her desire, a sensual delusion, a sating of the senses – but no love, and she would have starved in the streets rather than accept.'[64]

As a 'good girl', she can't have sex without love, and when she does her desire is always secondary to that of the man. In a manner recalling the nineteenth-century pronouncements of William Acton, who argued that 'there can be no doubt that sexual feeling in the female is in the majority of cases in abeyance, and that it requires positive and considerable excitement to be roused at all; and even if roused (which in many cases it never can be) it is moderate compared with that of the male,'[65] the heroine of romantic fiction experiences her passion only when awakened by his powerful, skilled embrace:

> His hands were tongues of flame as he found her breasts, her thighs, running over her skin as if eager to know every part of her with his touch, and she pulled him ever closer in response, wanting to share the secrets of her body with him. At his persistent touch Laura was suddenly a wild woman, tuned to the wildness in him . . . She shuddered with surprise and ecstasy . . . to feel his fiery brand enter her . . . the heavens and earth exploded in a blaze of white light all about her.   *The Pirate's Lady* [66]

The most extreme version of female passivity in romantic fiction has the heroine unconscious, weak with illness or even close to death. Reminiscent of Sleeping Beauty or Snow White, who lay waiting for the kiss of their prince, this vision presents woman as being *so* inactive she is barely alive. In one Harlequin novel, *Captive*, the heroine Amanda falls from a second-storey window into a snow bank and faints. She is rescued by Jason, the hero, who takes her home and, mistaking her for a boy, removes her clothes. He later declares, 'You were unconscious, but I thought I'd never seen anything so lovely, so desirable.' Tania Modleski's comment on this scene is apposite: 'It's hard to laugh at this near necrophilia, but it does reveal the impossible situation of woman: to be alive and conscious is to be suspect.'[67] Implicit in this scenario is the notion that passive, helpless 'woman' is always at the mercy of strong, determined 'man'. If Jason didn't rape (or 'seduce') Amanda (which he didn't), the fact is, he could have done.

Many men *don't* manage to exert this control, as we know (and as many readers masochistically fantasize), and so the forceable 'seduction' of the heroine while she is powerless to defend herself, is a common theme in romantic fiction – Sleeping Beauty was 'kissed' by the prince as she slept (the kiss symbolizing rape, more explicitly described in older versions of the fairy tale). In the Mills & Boon romance *Whirlwind* the young heroine is wined and dined by the enigmatic (rich, handsome, powerful) hero and, after fainting under the influence of champagne, wakes up to find herself in his bed:

> She shut her eyes again quickly, trying to convince herself that she was dreaming. She tentatively moved her hand next; she explored her hip and felt silky material. It wasn't a dream. She was wide awake in a strange bed wearing just her slip, and there was a man in bed with her . . .[68]

Later she fears that a rape has taken place, with terrible consequences: 'Each time she thought of it she felt a pang of shame . . . there was one possible consequence she hadn't taken into account . . . What if she was pregnant?'[69] In fact, she wasn't raped (her suspected seducer later points out that only a virgin would not know that you could tell whether you had had sex or not – I'm not sure I'd agree, but then, this is fiction), which allows her to marry her hero, as all good girls do. It would be going too far to have the heroine marrying her rapist.

Arguably, the function of these fictionalized 'seductions' is to allow women to experience sex without guilt, and sexual abandonment without the consequences. In this fantasy of forced seduction women can play out their transgressive desires and fears without fear of honour being lost. They can fantasize about sexual power and powerlessness without experiencing the pain, horror and degradation of rape in the real world. That the fantasies played out in romantic fiction are as far from *real* rape as the sun is distant from the moon is evidenced by the following extract from *The Pirate's Lady*:

> She remembered being woken by a man's shadow blocking the moonlight that lay in silver sheets across her head . . . It was the pirate! She had felt her head lifted gently from the pillow . . . she felt the brush of his lips against her forehead, and remembered the incredible warmth that flowed through her. She had reached out to him eagerly and drawn him closer, until at last he lay beside her. His arms met about her, gathering her to him, and she had trembled against him, cradling his head in the hollow of her shoulder. His hands were gentle as they pushed aside the thin cotton of her nightdress and began to caress the swell of her breasts. She recalled the surge of passion that washed over her like a crimson flame as his hands moved across her hips and to the secret places of her body that she yearned for him to claim as his own.[70]

This is a 'rape' that exists only in the world of dreams, where fantasies of being 'taken' or seduced serve as a means of re-enacting our feelings of pre-oedipal dependence and powerlessness, which are so irrevocably tied to sexual awakening and desire. This is a fantasy of masochistic identification; a common part of women's (and men's) inner worlds. Women who read romantic fiction are not unusual in their fantasies. All erotic literature and pornography contains themes of power and seduction (see Chapter Three) – romantic fiction is merely a sanitized version of the more explicit sexual scenarios played out in pornography, where phallic mastery is explored in a more obvious way.[71] What they both have in common is the positioning of 'man' as monstrous brute.

Man as Monstrous Brute

The script of romantic fiction is in many ways misogynistic. In romantic fiction (as in pornography) men punish and control women through sex. In perhaps the most infamous example, in *Gone with the Wind*, Rhett Butler puts Scarlett in her place, and gains her admiration, by raping her – an act which she enjoys. This is a dangerous and invidious message – but one which is in line with rape myths perpetuated in pornography and the law (see Chapters Three & Five). Women are repeatedly fed the message that sexual violence is a sign of passion and love; this might go some way towards providing an explanation why many women stay with violent abusive men.[72] As Tania Modleski has commented, the message is the same one parents sometimes give to little girls that are singled out by bullies: 'he really has a crush on you.'[73]

The pervasive representation of rape in romantic fiction, whether it be graphically described or implied ('he took her forcibly . . .'), normalizes rape. It also dictates the appropriate female response – enjoy (or faint). Fighting back (unless feigned) is inadmissible. Is it any wonder that women don't report rape? That women blame themselves for sexual violence? Is it any wonder that many men still think women want, ask for and deserve rape? That they believe women despise 'new men'? For if the heroine resists the brute, it is only to maintain her honour or to avoid pain, not because she feels no desire. As one heroine is despairingly described: '*She had to protect herself; she had already suffered enough over him, she couldn't bear any more*' [my italics].[74] What the romantic heroine (and by implication all women) wants is a man who is a brute:

Bending suddenly, he swooped to lift her over one broad shoulder. Cassie's breath caught in sharp reaction, her senses raggedly absorbing the unexpected contact. He was all hard-muscled strength; she registered every tough sinew against the softness of her flesh . . . He had taken her by surprise; she had not for a moment thought that he would seize her.

Flames of Love[75]

If the romantic hero doesn't rape, he humiliates. He is unambiguously 'man'; women are putty in his hands. He is hard whilst she is soft; active, whilst she is acquiescent. But as brute, he is desirable, exciting and seemingly all that a woman could want. The strong, dark hero, often tinged with a hint of evil, is juxtaposed with the good, kind, thoughtful man who is pathetic in comparison: Rhett Butler and Ashley Wilkes in *Gone with the Wind*; Heathcliff and Linton Earnshaw in *Wuthering Heights*. Women are won over by passion and darkness: The enigmatic and moody Mr Darcy in *Pride and Prejudice* became a national obsession when the book was televised.

However, the fact that the hero is strong does not inevitably position the woman reader as weak, for in the act of reading romance it is the woman who is in control of his phallic power. Here the woman (as reader) has a choice, as she is not forced to re-enact this scenario and can literally stop it at will, by putting down the book. The woman can also identify with the romantic hero in her reading, and therefore in fantasy take on his power (as well as masochistically share in the delight of his demise). So there are multiple identifications, both sadistic and masochistic positions which can be taken up (many women shift between them at will).

Identification with the heroine is not inevitably masochistic as the heroine is often in (covert) control of the scene. Here again, femininity is very much a masquerade – the heroine sticks to the rules and plays the game very effectively, but underneath her simpering smile is a welter of ambition and emotion.[76] As Tania Modleski has argued, 'a great deal of satisfaction comes . . . from the elements of revenge fantasy, from our conviction that the woman is bringing the man to his knees and that all the while he is being so hateful, he is internally grovelling, grovelling, grovelling.'[77] So whilst the heroine may have to *appear* to sacrifice herself at the altar of femininity she ensures that she exacts her rewards. Romantic fiction gives the woman much more than the fairy-tale endings of childhood. The hero is reduced to her level – literally if not metaphorically – as he worships the heroine at the altar of love. For it is always the moment when his true feelings are revealed – his deep unsettling love for her, and her vulnerability and hurt – that is her chosen moment of conquest:

> He hadn't offered her love because he had none to give; he had once been hurt and he was determined never to love anyone again. Laird must be very lonely and emotionally in deep freeze; he wouldn't want her pity, but he had it.
>
> *Whirlwind*[78]

We could interpret this as evidence that authors of romantic fiction are acting to emasculate men, castrating the hero by having him brought down to a level that is lower than that of 'woman'. But the heroine does not want him castrated – symbolically or literally – she wants him to be 'all man', yet still be beholden to her: prostrate but not quite passive; desperate, but not destitute. There is no fun for her in conquering a weak, hopeless creature, but immense pleasure in belittling a strong brute. Rhett Butler feigns indifference for Scarlett, as does Mr Darcy for Elizabeth Bennet, yet the romantic hero's brutality is demonstrated to be simply a mask, concealing his hurt at having been rejected before. In *Whirlwind* Laird exposes his weakness immediately prior to the final seduction scene:

> Without looking at her, Laird said huskily, 'I'll never marry again, I couldn't risk it. I got too mauled last time, she chewed me up and it took me years to recover. No, that's not even the truth. You never *do* recover from something like that, especially if it follows on from a traumatic childhood' . . . she picked up his suffering and hated the two women [his mother and his wife] who had caused it.[79]

This is the classic fairy-tale myth of the *other* woman who cause men pain – the wicked witch, the stepsister or the whore. When Laird later relents and asks for the heroine's hand in marriage the story comes full circle: Beautiful princess redeems wounded man. ' "I've changed a hell of a lot," he said ruefully, "since I met you." ' Only the good woman can save his soul. So, ultimately, the final seduction is positioned as testimony to *her* power, not to his. Or she may exact revenge by rejecting him, encouraging him to express his desire and then casting him aside.

These are all fantasies far removed from the reality of most women's lives. But the anger expressed by the heroine of romantic fiction may closely resemble the anger of the woman reader. The heroine fights the male authority figure with a vengeance not permissible within the strict boundaries of femininity. This may provide a safety-valve for those women denied the opportunity of such open conflict (at least without cost) in their daily lives, as does identification with the hero himself, who experiences no such boundaries to his behaviour at all. Yet whilst romantic fiction arouses anger, it also acts to neutralize it, as it is contained within the tightly structured narrative (and always resolved).

Whether this acts as catharsis, or as a form of inoculation which prevents women's rebellion,[80] is debatable. If fantasies of power or revenge can be acted out in fantasy, is action less likely to be undertaken in 'real life'? Does the romantic myth serve to keep women down? Does it keep women with misogynistic, brutal men? This is the question continually addressed by those documenting the effects of television violence or pornography. Some say exposure to such fantasies increases the desire for living them out; others that such desire is reduced. We know that many women are filled with a sense of disappointment and despondency by the failure of men to live up to the romantic myth; it provides us with an image of 'man' which is ultimately destructive for men, as it is for women, as it sets up an ideal which is impossible for most men to match. Women are also made despondent by their inability to make men cower or quiver with passion or declare undying love, by not being able to transform themselves into the fairy-tale princess. Romantic fiction may thus be seen not as a celebration of love and romance but as a reflection on women's dissatisfaction with the options open to them. As Alison Light has argued, romance-reading is 'as much a measure of [women's] deep dissatisfaction with heterosexual options as of any desire to be fully identified with the submissive versions of femininity which the texts endorse. Romance imagines peace, security and ease precisely because there is dissension, insecurity and difficulty.'[81]

Janice Radway carried out a succession of interviews with readers of romantic fiction and found that the majority of women used reading as a direct escape from the continuous demands made by their husbands and families.[82] It is a disappearing act not dissimilar to that of the romantic heroine who conceals her true feelings in order to maintain her masquerade and fulfil the desires of man. Women readers escape from the disappointments in their relationships with men, from a world of dissension and strife into a world where there is perfect resolution of conflict. The act of reading serves to erect a barrier between women and their families, the women 'declaring themselves temporarily off limits'.[83] Women I interviewed about romantic fiction challenged this interpretation. One woman claimed, 'I'm not escaping from anything, just doing something else. Not going into a dream world'; another commented, 'I read to relax, not to be escapist – it's a form of brain relief.' All the women distanced themselves from the 'average reader':

> 'If I'm being honest, I distance myself from other women . . . It's about quality of life – I see myself as a strong individual, able to effect change in my life. For a lot of women who read romantic fiction it is an escape from the reality of the economic trap of marriage, a housewife, with no recognition. This is not my everyday life. For women like us it's about being able to have another experience, an alternative stimulus.'

By positioning romance-reading as an 'alternative stimulus' or 'brain relief' women can legitimately escape into this fantasy world without compromising their sense of themselves as 'strong'. They claim to be aware of what they are doing in the act of escape.

Radway interprets women's escape into romantic fiction as an act of 'individual resistance' to the confines and constraints of a narrow feminine role. A fair comment, but a depressing thought, as it is a passive protest of the powerless, which arguably stifles a more effective form of resistance (such as actually changing your life). Escaping into a romantic novel is a limited form of escape, if it is escape at all. It may be seen as a voyage into a more restrictive version of femininity, where the eternal fairy-tale rules still apply. This voyage may also make matters worse for the woman who wishes to escape from daily life and strife. For romantic fiction might be seen as a key player in maintaining phallocentric power because it actively reconciles women to the necessity of the feminine masquerade: Woman's escape is contingent on beauty, and is still into the arms of a man. For as Janice Radway urges, in reading romance 'women are repetitively asserting to be true what their still unfulfilled desire demonstrates to be false, that is, that heterosexuality can create a fully coherent, fully satisfied, female subjectivity.'[84] The impossibility of romance parallels the impossibility of life and assures us that dissatisfaction is a central aspect of the traditional script of femininity.

The Transformation of Woman Through the Mask of Beauty

She's Got the Look: 'Doing Girl' in Teenage Magazines

> There's no doubting the brilliance of the new foundation/powder compacts. The effect is flawless skin without looking made-up, and the low oil content makes them great for absorbing shine on greasy and combination skins . . .
>
> *Mizz*[85]

Cinderella was transformed by her fairy godmother, Sleeping Beauty by a kiss. In real life, woman is transformed from base matter into beauty through the artifice of make-up and fashion. Indoctrination into the secrets of beauty starts early. Teenage magazines provide adolescent girls with detailed instruction on make-up, clothes and the current regimes necessary for maintaining the 'perfect figure'. Today the secret of make-up is often to look 'natural', with girls being allowed to 'choose' to wear as much or as little make-up as they want. But the underlying message of the fairy story that beauty is essential for romantic fulfilment is unchanged: Two recent American magazines, *'Teen* and *Seventeen,* boast front covers which show the smiling winner of a teenage 'model' contest, each entwined in the arms of a sexy man:

> *Super Star and Super Model:* Jonathan Brandis and *'TEEN'S* Great Model Search winner, Michelle Holgate.[86]

> *She's the one!* Carol wins our cover model contest (and a hug from Jamie).[87]

Don't we all want to be her? We just have to take on the appropriate mask of beauty, which is easy, as long as you know how. Twenty years ago, before the welcomed eclecticism of post modernism, fashion dictated that there was only one look to follow (at least for working-class girls – middle-class girls have always adopted a more 'natural' look), and it was outlined in exact detail. Girls would copy the horrendous layers of coloured eye-shadow described in the beauty pages of *Jackie* as they desperately tried to 'do girl' properly. What was taught was the importance of developing 'beauty skills'. So eyebrows were chiselled to the appropriate degree, eye-liner just so; lips glossy one month, matt the next; all blemishes and imperfections banished. The hope, or desire, was that by looking the part, one could really *be* 'woman'. It is a fragile, shallow mask. Yet a mask, we are led to believe, all women should wear.

The myth that *any* girl can be transformed into the idealized state of glamour and beauty through perfect make-up is perpetuated through the before-and-after features, where a number of women are shown in their 'natural' state and then transformed by the expert hands of make-up artists and hairdressers. The message we are given here is that it is not an easy process; becoming a beautiful woman takes effort and skill. The comments of the girls transformed in a before-and-after feature in an issue of *Just Seventeen*[88] published as recently as 1986 are no different from those I remember from my own youth: Girls consumed with fears of incompetence in the 'art' of perfect make-up, which prompts their desperate desire for help in the mystifying, difficult rituals of feminine beauty:

Julia, 14

I always stick to the same make-up . . . but I can never get the foundation right. It always looks cloggy on me.

Philippa, 18

I don't like my eyes so I'd like to be shown how to make the most of them with eye-shadow.

Vicki, 14

I hate my face and my legs are like tree-trunks . . . I just want to look different and learn how to put on make-up properly.

Lorna, 14

(Lorna wears make-up occasionally . . . but gets into a muddle when it comes to applying it properly.) It always looks too heavy and I can never get my eyes to match, so I don't bother with it every day.

Debbie, 14

I hate my hair! . . . I haven't got much of a clue with make-up either. I try out loads of colours but I never like the result.

These features serve to reinforce the view that in their natural state, young women are unattractive and unappealing and that they must conceal themselves in order to appeal to men. We are led to believe that it is understandable that these girls are unhappy with their looks (their legs, hair or complexion) – what woman isn't? This inadequacy – presented as the natural adolescent state – is not a problem; it can be remedied simply by the regular purchase of cosmetic products and the absorption of expert advice. Not advice on self-esteem, or on the means of attaining a positive identity, but advice on how to put on perfect make-up, which all the girls gratefully absorb. So the 'after' pictures show a more confident gaze, flawless skin, redesigned hair and bright new make-up. How could we not be convinced? The girls themselves all proclaim their delight with their 'new look', while bowing down to the expert who transformed them:

> Julie, 14
>
> The make-up's really nice, not too heavy or anything. I'd never thought an orange lipstick would suit me.

> Philippa, 18
>
> I really like the look – it makes me feel more confident. But I doubt if it'll turn out the same when I try it for myself.

> Vicki, 14
>
> I really like it! The problem is I'll never manage to get my make-up as good as this.

> Lorna, 14
>
> I'd like to look like this all the time, but I don't think I'll be able to do my hair or make-up like this. I haven't really got the time to spend on it.

> Debbie, 14
>
> I can't believe it, I feel so much better. I looked so ill in the first picture! My hair's actually in a style now. I wonder what my boyfriend's going to think?[89]

That this transformation is almost as magical as the fairy-tale kiss is reinforced by the repeated refrain, 'I won't be able to do it myself.' Is this because the girls witnessed the lengths to which the make-up artist had to go in order to produce the 'smooth', 'even' or 'warm' complexion and the 'evenly balanced' eyes? Have they witnessed firsthand the con that is concealed in the supposedly natural images of beauty we see in advertisements and in women's magazines – where models have to spend hours under the make-up brush to look 'perfect'. The message in many of these teenage magazines – the message I grew up with – is that to get it right, beauty must become a constant preoccupation, as the rules and regulations and the 'right' colours to wear are always changing. So you can never rest on your laurels: there's always a new skill, or new fashion to learn. Some girls have little chance of success – their anatomy may work against them. As one black woman commented:

> 'A couple of years ago when all this shit was coming out about Lady Di and how shy and pretty she was and all that, I wished I could look like her. I started straightening my hair and trying to sort of flip it up and all that. But it wouldn't go that way. I remember crying . . . wishing that my hair would fall out and grow back in again straight and smooth like they have on TV.'[90]

If women do not resist these narrow representations of 'beauty', it's not surprising that many experience a deep sense of inadequacy as a result.

Post-Feminism and Individual 'Choice' of Beauty Mask

Be comfortable

If your face feels like it's set in plaster when you wear anything more than a bit of lippy and mascara, then don't invest in any other make-up than a bit of lippy and mascara . . . Then again, if you don't feel dressed without full slap then let loose to your heart's content.[91]

With feminism, post-modernism and the rise of the 'thinking' woman, the edicts of the beauty editors have had to be subtly recast. Today make-up is not presented as a necessity – it is a *choice* (like sex). Girls are told they can choose to wear the 'full slap' or just a bit of 'lippy'. Or the 'natural look' can be achieved with subtle use of cosmetics that appear invisible to the unknowing (i.e. male) eye. Yet the fact that girls will want some make-up is accepted without question – their flawed complexions, their naked faces, cannot face the world just as they are (the dreaded combination skin needs to be tackled and treated regardless of fashion trends). The grunge look of the early nineties was short-lived, and even it did not result in a move away from the tradition of cosmetic adjustment in the name of feminine beauty – it merely led to a greater degree of artifice and duplicity. If boys don't like make-up, as many magazine features clearly declare, this doesn't mean a releasing of girls from the need to conceal and contrive. It merely means more effort and pretence.

The impact of feminism and the notion of 'choice' is evident in many of the beauty features which exhort girls to 'be themselves' and, paradoxically, tell them not to take too much notice of expert advice. For example, in a feature entitled 'Me', with the caption opening 'Don't Feel Bullied into Making-Up Like the Next Kate Moss,'[92] it's *your* face, do with it as you please . . . Adele gives you a few pointers,' girls are advised to make up their own minds. On the subject of lipstick:

> OK, so you know berry shades are fashionable, but if you can't live without chocolate-brown lippy then go with it. Think about how you want to look, not just about what fashion dictates.[93]

So have the fashion editors taken on board the critiques of their magazines from feminists such as Naomi Wolf? Or is it that their readers now talk freely about the 'beauty myth', and as a result are critical of the exhortation that putting on 'slap' will lead to beauty and happiness? In *Just Seventeen* in the nineties, the message of the beauty editors appears to have moved on, now getting girls to re-evaluate themselves. So one article opens with the question 'What do you like best about your face? (Nothing isn't an option).' So far so good – this seems to suggest that girls should stop focusing on their bad points and try to see what is good about their appearance. Yet is the message really any different? The next sentence is meant to reassure, but it drives home the eternal message: 'Making up is about making the most of your best features and playing down the ones that aren't much to write home about.' Girls are reminded that they have 'features' to be ashamed of and hide, something most women need no reminding of:

> 'I've got a terrible nose, it's lopsided.'

> 'My hair is too frizzy. I can't ever do anything about it.'

> 'My skin is really patchy, and spotty.'

That woman's imperfection is irrevocably linked to sexuality and to the fear of men's reactions if the 'real' girl is inadvertently revealed is demonstrated by the scenarios in photo-stories which accompany the features on cosmetics. In one story a mother admonishes her daughter as she elaborately prepares herself with make-up for her date: 'You're digging your own grave. If he gets used to you looking perfect, what happens when you *do* take it off?' The extreme reaction to this fear is women having their make-up tattooed on.

So girls are taught that concealment, ritual display and beauty are 'essential' aspects of being 'woman' and at the same time that these rituals must be kept private, a secret shared between women, or at least conducted far away from the prying eyes of men. Angela McRobbie has claimed that 'underpinning this is a sense of shame and humiliation that women and girls have to resort to official aids . . . which stems from an open acknowledgement that the subject does not "naturally" measure up to these beauty standards'.[94] It is a message that is repeated, and reinforced, in adult women's magazines.

Youth and Beauty – at a Price

> Younger looking skin than you ever thought possible in *eight days*: primoriale Visibly Revitalizing Solution . . .

> A desire. A suggestion. Acqua di Gio . . .

> Time is on your side with chronologix line minimizing make-up. This time-fighting make-up creates a soft-focus look that helps put visible signs of aging under cover. Quickly. Easily . . .

> nobody is perfect (well, almost nobody). ok, so you're not a model. that's why we make flawless finish foundation in six different formulas. one is right for you. elizabeth arden.

The extracts above are a selection of the advertisers' promises from the glossy American women's monthly *Harpers Bazaar*,[95] all juxtaposed with the faces of extraordinarily beautiful women (hence the ironic comment, *almost* nobody is perfect). What may have been an exciting adventure, or an option, at fourteen (that first experimentation with the magical world of make-up . . .), is a serious business, and a necessity – we are told – at forty. The art of artifice is still alive, yet the aim to be achieved is reversed. The teenager desperately wants to look older – embracing adult sexuality at an age when it is unacceptable within the law – whilst the older woman wants to look younger, her hours of cosmetic ritual attempting to accomplish the impossible, the achievement of immortal youth. Is she simply trying, as many sociobiologists tell us, to mimic fertility in order to attract the biologically driven man who is interested in women only for reproductive purposes (see Chapter Four)? Or is she annihilating herself through a mask of perfection, turning herself into a fetish object and thereby ensuring she poses no threat to man? Whatever our explanation, as Jennifer Craik has argued, make-up is central to many women's secret projection of their desired self-image[96] – the perfect models photographed in advertisements and magazines represent the image many women would themselves like to present. These visions of beauty partly work through perpetuating fear – the fear of getting old, and therefore being unattractive (as beauty equals youth), but also the fear of 'getting it wrong'. As one 'beauty expert' comments:

> I know women who were absolutely devastating at 17 – vamps with bedroom hair and tiny dresses. Now, 20 years later, they dress exactly the same. It's not that their figures have changed, but their faces have, and it looks all wrong . . . In the 1970s they were dollybirds; now they look like blow-up dolls.[97]

'Getting it right' differs across social classes, and so there are a number of different beauty messages sold to women in magazines reflecting this. In the mass-market women's weeklies sold in Britain (*Woman, Woman's Own, Woman's Realm*) the message is not so much the fantasy of youth as a fantasy of attraction. The readers' make-over is still a common feature: The busy mum shown that a quick and careful application of make-up skills can give her a lift in a hectic day; the pleasures of a thirty-minute soak in the bath after the children have gone to bed. Beauty is still a necessity, but is fitted in around more pressing chores.

In the up-market glossies the message is markedly different. Here, beauty is an activity which consumes woman: Not only does she disappear beneath the mask of perfection, but in the amount of time, effort and energy devoted to it – if she follows all the advice literally, that is – she would have to sacrifice all else in her life. The implicit message is that a woman who does not engage in this charade is not only misguided but clearly missing out. Beauty is presented here as something a woman does for herself; no woman today is simply doing it to attract a man (or so women protest). To underline this post-feminist message, magazines such as *Marie Claire* regularly present features which show a range of differently styled women, who are rated for attractiveness by a group of men. Unsurprisingly, the men differ in who they judge 'best'. Presumably this is meant to suggest that there is no point in trying to please 'man' – so please yourself. What it actually does is reinforce the point that men judge women on the basis of their looks, and that they also feel qualified to make character assessments of women on the basis of their style of dress ('she looks boring'; 'she looks exciting'; 'I bet she'd be a bit of a goer').

Fashioning the Body

New looks for night: black lace, sheer and shiny, the heels to have . . .

Fall wrap-up: From the hippest tweeds and the hot short coat to the season's sexiest dresses . . .

Vogue magazine, in the same season (October, 1995), but on either side of the Atlantic two versions of what to wear, how to be seen. Fashion is one of the core components of the feminine masquerade, for through constructing our clothed image we construct ourselves. Fashion emphasizes sexuality and femininity, and in its ever-changing nature mirrors the transitory and fragmented nature of female subjectivity. Fashion also emphasizes display, and through a series of codes intelligible only to the cognizant acts to communicate subtle information about women. Whether it is the latest couture collection or the street styles of shifting subcultures fashion acts as a visible symbol of both individual and group identity. We are what we wear, whether we like it or not.

Knowing the rituals of fashion shows we know what it is to be 'woman' at a particular point in time. Readers of *Jackie* in the seventies learned about platform shoes, maxi and midi skirts, and long pointed collars, and felt confident that they were being 'grown-up'. Today fashion codes are less strict – there is a genuine post-modern mix (choose which Spice Girl to emulate . . .) But the process has undergone little change, and the training in the subtle nuances of fashion constitutes one of the central training grounds for femininity. As Baudelaire argued, 'All the things that adorn woman, all the things that go to enhance her beauty, are part of herself . . . making . . . the woman and her dress an indivisible whole.'[98]

Fashion is a commodity which arguably transforms woman *into* commodity, our sexuality simultaneously concealed and emphasized in a ritualistic way. Jennifer Craik has argued that 'fashion constitutes an effective and pervasive means through which women become objects of the gaze and of male sexual desire.'[99] Techniques of fashion – codes of dress, instructions on appropriate display – serve to create a unified image of femininity in which women are instructed. In creating her fashionable self she is fixing herself within the boundaries of the feminine masquerade. Or she rejects fashion and places herself outside the boundaries of archetypal femininity (as many self-avowed feminists have done). Yet she is still attending to the codes of fashion in her very rejection of its rules and regulations. So to examine fashion and clothes is to examine what it is to be (or to reject) 'woman', in a specific cultural sphere.

It is only since the eighteenth century that women *en masse* have been instructed in the art of femininity through dress.[100] After the industrial revolution, with the increasing economic strength of the middle classes, having an attractive, fashionable wife became a sign of man's status and power. This was a wifely duty, but women were also encouraged to view the task of learning and rehearsing appropriate feminine demeanour and dress, as a pleasure, an act of leisure. In the nineteenth century fashion designers and milliners exercised an almost autocratic authority in determining the details of feminine dress; at all levels of the social class hierarchy women learned the changing codes which marked them out as acceptable (and respectable) by reading clothing catalogues and popular magazines.[101] Today, whether training manuals for the masses or appeals to the aspirations and snobbery of those who would be queen, magazines and advertisers still play a key role in convincing women that clothes and fashion are worthy obsessions and that the body as a whole is an arena which deserves careful attention and disguise despite our 'post-feminist' protestations.

The codes of fashion also vary across age groups. 'Style' in teenage magazines is invariably tied to the notion of individuality, of identity and youth culture. Designer fashion is often emulated, the latest trends mirroring those in adult magazines, but there is a sense of irreverence in the mixing and matching of styles. The message pervading teenage magazines is to cock a snook at couture fashion, a process which

McRobbie identifies as poking fun at the high-minded tones of fashion journalism.[102] Many of the young women I interviewed took up this position of critical individuality, claiming not to want to follow the crowd:

> 'I wear clothes because I like them. I want to look different.'

> 'I like to think I can put things together in an individual way – not be a clone, you know?'

In the monthly women's magazines fashion is presented as both a pleasure and a pain. The emphasis of the pages and pages of fashion advertising is on the latest style (regardless of cost, which is mostly exorbitant); the fashion features are as likely to focus on practical aspects of 'building a wardrobe' or on fashion as disguise (wide-hipped women shouldn't wear horizontal stripes; large-bottomed women shouldn't wear leggings . . .). It is a minefield of possible flaws and mistakes, through which the careful navigator can only find her way by studying the form. So features give advice on what is currently 'in' or 'out', serve to remind us that what was acceptable last season might provoke ridicule in the next. Take these 'pressing problems' sent in by readers to the fashion doyens at *Vogue*:

> Can you suggest what jewellery I should wear this winter? The high sixties necklines leave no room for any more elaborate baubles?

> Can I wear hipsters even if my legs are not of Nadja proportions?

> My eyes look like slits when I wear the new Sixties style eye-liner. How can I avoid this?

More pain than pleasure here. Fashion journalism perpetuating the notion that women are somehow 'not right'?

Supermodels: The Ideal Woman?

> Fashion models epitomize the objectification of the female body – being 'used as a piece of flesh' as one top model put it.[103]

Fashion is as much about the body as it is about clothes. Fashions in shape clearly change over time: The flat-chested flapper of the twenties, the hourglass woman of the fifties, the muscled supermodel of the eighties, the prepubescent anorexic of the nineties – each has represented the ideal in vogue. The clothes and body shapes change with the whims of designers, fashion editors and photographers, not with the desires of women or because of a genuine change in female physiognomy. As the emancipated flapper of the twenties personified the move to modernity rather than the reality of women's lives,[104] the supermodels of the nineties are no more representative of real women, than the creations the couture designers present as realistic possibilities for women to wear. Each image presents a fantasy which women are supposed to aspire to fulfil, with satisfaction for many remaining an impossible dream.

The supermodels are impossibly beautiful, impossibly proportioned, impossibly thin. They are not 'perfect women' but genetic aberrations – rare stalking beauties with long lean legs, extremely attractive faces and often (disproportionately) ample breasts. They may represent the archetype of beauty, yet the irony is that these icons are themselves dissatisfied with their appearance; even the women who are objects of such envy do not achieve that elusive sense of self which the fashion myth promises. One model, Elle Macpherson, who has been described as having 'the body of our time' by *Time* magazine, comments:

> I don't particularly like the way I look, to tell you the truth . . . When you're trying to sell how beautiful you are and you don't think that you're that beautiful, it's a bit scary.[105]

Jean Shrimpton, a fashion icon of the sixties, describes a similar sensation of dissatisfaction and insecurity:

> We were so vain that we continued to dress ourselves up and go out to be looked at . . . I was so insecure that I was always fiddling in the bathroom or running to the ladies to check my appearance. It was pathetic! Here I was at the height of my fame behaving like this. I was just an accessory.[106]

These supermodels are similar to the sleeping princess or the unconscious romantic heroine – they are beautiful women who are unspeaking and *still*. Their essence is in their appearance; their skill is in their silent, effortless beauty. That they have starved and surgically altered themselves in their quest for perfection is concealed under the illusion of 'natural' glamour and beauty. They perpetuate the dangerous myth that woman does not have to act, she just has to appear. The fact that they are idols is insidious in that they are not deemed to have any intellect or ability for independent thought. As Lauren Hutton, a model whose career spans the seventies, eighties and nineties comments: 'I've met people who apparently felt that by virtue of being attractive, I was dumb. It's still a prevalent cliché.' Social psychological research shows that attractive women are expected to be unintelligent, the stereotype of the 'dumb blonde' acting to categorize beautiful women as objects, not subjects. Many women and girls maintain this illusion by disguising their intellect under the veneer of flirtatious femininity.[107] They learn that to be beautiful is more desirable than to be clever, and certainly less threatening to men. That the icons of the late twentieth century are not women who have achieved power through their brains but those who have achieved power and fame through their looks says it all.

Fashion and beauty act as body disciplines, producing self-regulating female subjects who aim to demonstrate control over the physical body.[108] Fashion provides boundaries for the body, for the expression of self and sexuality. It provides a visible signifier of who we are (or who we would like to be). Yet the body is not only regulated through clothes and make-up. For as fashion dictates, the body itself must be closely managed.

The Sculpted Body

In order to achieve the wasp waist which was necessary to fit into the crinolines of the nineteenth century women wore restrictive corsetry or, in some cases, had their lower ribs removed. In the twenties, to achieve the flat chest of the flapper the breasts had to be strapped down. Today the ideal female body is both thin and sculpted. The slender, toned body has come to represent the feminine ideal – stripped of fat, desire and all uncontrolled appetites. Body management for women has to go deep within – to the dangerous fat cells which threaten the very boundaries of what it is to be 'woman'. The control of cellulite – the dreaded 'orange-peel' fat that afflicts thighs and bottoms (and if not controlled, beyond) – has become the obsession of the modern woman.[109]

The emphasis today is not just on weight loss, but on achieving a tight, taut boundary to the body. 'Even thin women can have cellulite,' the magazines declare. Starvation is no longer enough. Women are entreated to monitor continuously the intake to their bodies through cutting out certain types of food and counting calories, but also to be fit and healthy and strong. What has been described as a 'tyranny of slenderness'[110] has been transformed into a tyranny of fitness and firmness. Feminism has impacted upon the world of magazines, moving them away from notions of a frail or passive femininity and from starvation as a means of sexual success to images of an ideal woman who is powerful, lean and strong. She is in control of her health and her body and, by implication, in control of her life. This is fitness for herself, not simply for man. So women can 'eat healthily' (not diet), work out in the gym and pay continuous attention to the boundaries of their flesh without feeling that they are giving up on the 'post-feminist' principles they are supposed to aspire to. As one woman interviewed for a British newspaper which was celebrating the birth of the 'sports model' commented:

> When you start to get fit, you feel sexy, because you have this really powerful body – it gives you a new appreciation for this fantastic machine that your body is. I think women want to feel sexy for themselves, not to look sexy for men, because some men find it intimidating.[111]

Here we are told – in the words of a woman, so it must be true – that women 'work out', pay attention to the contours of their flesh, 'for themselves'. It's hard work, though. Muscles and tone (that obsession of the post-modern woman) are not easily achieved. It requires hours in the gym, as well as the now accepted attention to food. If the aspiring woman can't achieve this look the 'natural' way, she can turn to the knife. Or the liposuction tube. As one magazine tells us:

> Liposuction. Developed in the 70s, this was the pioneering fat-removal technique and is still the most widely performed. During the procedure, small incisions are made in the skin and a cannula – a fine hollow tube – is then inserted. A machine extracts fat from below the skin surface through the tube and into a suction jar. Anything up to a safe limit of 2.5 litres is sucked out at a time ... This is the standard operation if you want to remove 'jodhpur' thighs.[112]

The reader is warned that the side-effects of this treatment may include 'lumps and hollows', crinkling of the skin's surface and damage to the nerve endings. Yet despite this, thousands of women every year undergo this extreme form of fat removal in search of the perfectly regulated frame. Articles on more invasive cosmetic surgery for the breasts, the face or the torso perpetuate the belief that women must change – post-surgery swelling, scars and infections seem to be a price worth paying for beauty. Female 'stars' who turn to the surgeon to tuck and trim or to add to the size of their breasts are rewarded with greater fame and fortune – Pamela Anderson, Demi Moore, Cher, to name but a few. There is no attempt to disguise the artifice in their appearance – they position themselves as independent women merely improving upon nature. Paula Yates was quoted as saying after her breast enlargement, 'Now I feel I'm a woman.'

Researchers have repeatedly shown that up to 80 per cent of women wish to change their body shape or size. The majority want to be thinner and leaner. Dieting is now described by psychologists as 'the pathology of the norm'. Eating disorders such as anorexia nervosa and bulimia are rife, particularly in adolescent girls. Adult woman regulate and restrain their food intake to an extreme, which results in complete distortion of normal eating patterns. Women ban food, restrict intake below that which is needed to sustain energy and then become obsessed with the very foods which are denied.

In this context food and eating are nothing to do with the sustenance of the body – food is synonymous with desire. The juxtaposition of advertisements and features is designed to produce desire, a desire that women must resist. Food is seductively displayed in cookery articles, whilst women are encouraged to be hungry and thin. The need to regulate food signifies the need to control desire. Being able to resist desire is the goal to which women aspire: Supermodels starve themselves – but look how successful they are. Yet this denial of desire (or hunger) cannot be maintained for ever and most women eventually fail. They turn to the desired object – the cakes, the biscuits, the forbidden calorific fruit – and consume. In anger, or in misery, food is the obvious solace, leading to a vicious spiral of guilt, and then to further deprivation.

This obsession with food, with shape, with firm-fleshed thighs, is not just about health – it is about control of female sexuality. Control of female *sexual* desire. Susan Bordo has argued that the images of unwanted bulges and fleshy round stomachs that pervade women's magazines and the talk of young girls are metaphors for anxiety about internal processes which are out of control: 'uncontained desire, unrestrained hunger, uncontrolled impulse'.[113] The emphasis on the need to control and regulate the boundaries of the female body which pervades the pages of magazines is irrevocably connected to fears of the terrible consequences of unleashed sexuality, of the body without boundaries. It is not *fat* that is frightening but a female body without clear, firm boundaries. It is not weight that is disgusting, but the feminine form. The curves which signify femininity and fecundity are trimmed to attain a muscular, masculine form. The ideal goal is to make them disappear altogether, as Susan Bordo has shown in her discussion of diet advertising, 'now [a typical ad] runs . . . Have a nice shape with no tummy.'[114] Women who diet try to achieve this goal. One woman interviewed by Helen Malson who was asked what slimness meant to her replied 'having no tummies or no great bottoms . . . and having nice thighs, thin thighs'.[115] Like the romantic heroine who makes herself disappear, the extremely thin woman is hardly woman at all. She is in control of all that base, female flesh. By demonstrating control over her body she demonstrates control over her life. As one woman commented:

> There are a lot of characteristics that I admire, like being slim . . . it's the kind of idea of being in control of your life doing all your work and sticking to deadlines and . . . being competent, sort of perfection, yeah, the perfect ideal.

Women who *can't* exert this (impossible) control can be positioned as failures:

> I felt such a loser because I felt like I couldn't control my weight because I was overweight . . . so there must be something wrong with me because . . . I didn't have enough self control.[116]

But as she focuses on her flesh instead of other means of gaining power or control, is the woman not being conned? This is now a familiar refrain. From Susie Orbach's *Fat is a Feminist Issue*, published in 1978, to Naomi Wolf's *The Beauty Myth*, published in 1990, popular feminism has unleashed a never-ending tirade on the combined forces which present us with an image of the ideal woman as thin and beautiful. Now everyone from tabloid journalists to health professionals appears to blame the media for eating disorders and for women's obsession with their bodies and with beauty. The conclusion seems to be that we should change the images of women which currently pervade and we will rid ourselves of the scourge of the 'beauty myth'. It isn't so simple, and neither are women.

Negotiating the Beauty Myth

Women are not passive recipients of the myriad messages in magazines. They are not unaware of the critiques that can be levied against these visions of what it is to be 'woman'. In fact, the readers of these magazines are perhaps their greatest critics. In interviews carried out with groups of teenage girls,[117] the most common responses were that magazines were a waste of time or trash; they make you feel bad about yourself; they make you feel angry because of the focus on beauty, on being seductive or slim; they present a narrow model of sexuality; the media has too much power. So the act of reading magazines is not seen as unequivocally positive:

'I come away feeling fat, ugly, unattractive.'

'I feel depressed because I can't afford the clothes.'

'It makes me more aware of not being in a relationship.'

Yet at the same time these girls said that they enjoyed reading magazines and used them as a treat; that they were amusing and informative; that they enjoyed the voyeuristic elements; they helped them to feel not alone; they are a form of escapism; and they could enjoy looking at beautiful women without feeling bad about themselves. Adult women hold similarly contradictory views:

'You have this myth that being so beautiful, so chic, and all the rest of these things is important. It's bullshit.'

'You can learn a lot from magazines. The tips are useful.'

'I do enjoy looking at the women – it's a joy to look at, and the fashion spreads are an inspiration.'

'I get fed up with all the focus on men and sex. There's more to life.'

The range of comments demonstrates that there is no one fixed reading of magazines, no one correct interpretation. They can bring pleasure and pain, incite interest and irritation. We know the theory – that no one can look as beautiful as the models and that it is a waste of your life to try – yet try we do (often secretly). Women distance themselves from magazines, describing 'other women' as the ones that are influenced: 'I just flick through them and take no notice' is what *all* women say. But as sales of the cosmetics on which the magazines base their advertising revenue are in the millions (both dollars and pounds sterling), and as each month thousands of copies are sold, *someone* is reading them carefully. Women may distance themselves from the archetypal images of 'woman' which pervade magazines and say that they can see through the mask of feminine perfection that is peddled there. But that doesn't mean that they no longer want to 'do femininity'. As one woman I interviewed said of her experience at an up-market cosmetics counter:

> 'I was at a Lancôme counter and the assistant was telling me that if I didn't follow the proper cleanse, tone and moisturize routine, using their products, my face would eventually crumble. She actually said it was like a brick wall which was crumbling inside. I know it's all rubbish, because I've got good skin, but I bought a whole load of skin-care products. It cost a fortune, but it does make me feel more confident when I use it.'

Women can both be critical of the 'beauty myth', and still get pleasure from 'doing femininity'. Reading the magazines is part of the process: Women sink into a glossy magazine as they would into a luxurious bath (often doing both at the same time). As Susan Douglas comments, 'I don't read *Vogue* or *Glamour* . . . I enter them. I escape into them, into a world where I have nothing more stressful to do than smooth on some skin cream, polish my toenails, and lie on the beach.'[118] In a post-feminist world, where women are supposed to reject traditional models of femininity and be independent and strong, this is transgression (and therefore pleasurable), indeed.

Women who act out these regimes of beauty are not simply indoctrinated or brainwashed, but position themselves as expert performers of this complicated masquerade. They have both knowledge and skill about how to look and what to wear and can exercise this skill in transforming themselves into *their* version of 'woman': 'I know what I like and what suits me; I don't take any notice of the latest craze.'

Sharing such knowledge with friends, or dissecting the contradictory advice together, can add to the pleasure as well as provide a sense of community:

> 'Getting ready with my mates is the best part of the evening. We have a laugh and try on lots of different things. Sometimes we make each other up. I got a new Mac lipstick last week and everyone wanted to try it.'

Angela McRobbie interviewed a group of working-class teenage girls and found that the process of 'doing girl' through wearing the latest fashions and acquiring make-up skills provided them with a means of asserting their independence from authority. It also marked them as different from the despised middle-class girls at school: 'They wear horrible clothes. I mean they do not know what fashion is. They're not like us at all.'[119] Fashion was the only area where these girls were 'experts'. It is ostensibly a world from which men are excluded (unless they are designers or models) and so is a sphere in which women reign supreme.

So mass media imagery can't simply be damned. Equally, the message that the thin, beautiful girl is the one who achieves her goal is not an invention of women's magazines or the fault of the supermodels. They are merely the new scapegoats, the ones who can conveniently take the blame because they currently carry the age-old message that a woman is defined by her looks. We should not merely kill the messenger, but instead look far deeper for the reasons the message is still conveyed. Most importantly, we should examine why women still buy it – if they do.

Being (and becoming) 'woman' is not an unequivocally positive process. There is much about femininity that is difficult, contradictory and impossible to achieve. Arguably, for many women, the body has become the repository of all that we hate and despise about ourselves, all that we find difficult about being 'woman'. Who can blame us? Are we not told repeatedly, from the cradle to the grave, that to be 'woman' is to be 'other', to be second-rate, the second sex? Yet simultaneously we are offered the hope of salvation, of rising above the drudgery and exploitation that is many women's lot, through our bodies, through our beauty, our divine goodness, which will be recognized by a knowing prince. When this doesn't happen (or when the fairy story goes wrong and the prince leaves us broken-hearted or disappointed), is it surprising that so many women blame their bodies, rather than questioning the romantic dream? If we give up on the dream, where else will our salvation come from?

> I thought if I lost some weight I would look much nicer and attractive . . . and then I would be more happier because then I would have confidence in myself . . . I would be able to do things I've never dreamed of doing because I was ashamed of the way I *was* altogether. So I thought that if I could change the way I look I might be better able to do things that I want to and I'm afraid to do.[120]

This is a pervasive view, and one that runs deep. I have found examples of women blaming their bodies and hating themselves as a result within all the research I have carried out over the last fifteen years – when working with women experiencing PMS, women with anorexia nervosa, women who have been sexually abused and women who weren't presenting any particular problem or history of psychological difficulty at all. The striking thing is the similarity between them: A wish to be different and a blaming of problems on the body not being right.

This isn't a trivial issue, simply about vanity or narcissism. Women who worry about their bodies worry about their sexuality. The woman who believes she is not perfect (most women) is unlikely to want to reveal her body to others. Women I interviewed repeatedly talked about the fact that they often refrained from sex for fear of rejection, for fear of being compared to a woman more beautiful than they. It effectively stops many women from going out to find their 'prince' – and again puts the blame for his absence on the woman herself.

> 'My thighs are too big. No one could possibly fancy me . . .'

> 'Men like girls with big tits and thin bodies. It's just a fantasy, I know, but if you don't look like that you just feel inadequate.'

Not being 'picked' by the proverbial prince is increasingly blamed on the body, which is punished (by severe dieting) as a result. As these anorexic women commented:

> 'I felt like . . . guys didn't like me or guys never paid any attention to me as much as they did to, like, my room-mates who were, like, gorgeous.

And I, and I just felt ignored, like, no, like they didn't look at me because I was fat.'

'It's all tied up with the image that it was good to be slim and you'd attract the boys if you were slim.'[121]

Even when they are in relationships many women feel inhibited and embarrassed about their bodies, going to inordinate lengths to avoid being seen.

'I used to make him pin these blankets over the windows so there was no light in the room, I was embarrassed about him seeing me, I used to get in the bed and lie under these thick blankets and it was the middle of summer and he used to slip off me because we were both absolutely soaked in sweat, and this went on for about a year, I mean I wouldn't let him see me I was so uptight.'

'I'm still a bit uncomfortable about my body, I mean not my genitals or breasts or anything, but just like my figure and whatever, just like walking around the room and stuff like that . . . it takes me ten years to come around to doing that and I haven't been with anyone ten years yet so, I've slept with people and I still couldn't walk around the room naked.'

The very bodily differences at the centre of heterosexual desire may be women's worst enemy. The mass media encourages heterosexual women to desire masculine bodies, which are hard, lean and slim – at least in their ideal state. It is this that many women measure themselves against (and are certainly measured against in the media – those cellulite-free thighs are very like those of boys; we may wonder whose fantasy is at play here, given that it is largely men who create this imagery). Women who desire women perhaps find it easier to appreciate that they can be desired themselves, regardless of the contours of their thighs (although lesbians are not immune from anxiety about weight or fitness). We can all learn a lot from this:

'I've always worried about not having a perfect bottom, or flat thighs or whatever. When I realized how irrelevant all of this is to my own desire, I felt really different about myself. The first woman I slept with was much bigger than me – fatter, I suppose – and she was gorgeous.'

Lesbians don't have a monopoly on appreciation of the female body. Realizing that a woman's body is beautiful in its natural state, with all its imperfections and curves, is a revelation many heterosexual women also talk about.

> 'P. is a sports place and there are women there doing keep fit and stuff and I thought . . . there were women there in their leotards, you know, and they look fantastic and, you know, when they take their leotards and leggings off I think they still look fantastic but in a different sort of way, you know, everything is much softer and there's cellulite and there's scars and, you know, there's boobs that droop, and that was one of the first times I decided I would take my clothes off, too . . . I realized that I wasn't that different, you know, I'm not saying that I'm beautiful because that's far from it, but, you know, I'm not that different.'

Other women resist the 'beauty myth' by explicitly rejecting the boundaries of appropriate feminine appearance:

> 'I never wear make-up, and I just wear my hair really short. I can't stand all that fuss about looks and things.'

> 'I deliberately eat a lot so that I'm overweight and then men don't look at me. They treat me as a person, not as a woman.'

> 'I've always hung around with boys, so I didn't do all the make-up things at school. Men don't like all of that anyway, so I don't know why women bother.'

These women are actively choosing not to 'do girl', either to mark themselves outside of the masculine sexual gaze (to be treated 'as a person'), or to mark out their rejection of the passivity and subservience associated with archetypal femininity. It is not just 'beauty' that these women are rejecting, but the notion that 'beauty' is what defines a woman and that her main interest in life should be making herself attractive to men. This is one of the reasons why many lesbians explicitly reject feminine modes of appearance – in order visibly to signify their different sexuality and identity,[122] as well as their rejection of heterosexual hegemony. At the same time, lesbians who look 'femme' have for decades been subjected to criticism for not looking 'authentic' and questioned about their lesbian status.[123] As one woman I interviewed commented, 'It's much easier if you cut off your hair and act butch. It feels more powerful. With long hair I was always being asked when I went out if I knew this was a gay club.' Things are changing, though. 'Lesbian chic' – the celebration of 'lipstick lesbians' in the media in North America and Britain during the nineties – is not just a media fantasy. Many lesbians now want to enjoy being 'woman', as well as being lesbian (implicitly rejecting Monique Wittig's claim that 'lesbians are not women because woman has meaning only in heterosexual systems of thought and within heterosexual economies'[124]) – and are now 'doing femininity'.[125] This is 'doing girl' with a very different meaning from that prescribed within the script of heterosexual romance: taking up the position of 'woman' outside the sexual gaze of man; a performance by women who are able knowingly to enjoy (and subvert or parody) the very notion of femininity as masquerade. Yet lesbians are not the only women who know that 'doing girl' at the same time as rejecting the traditional position of 'woman' within the script of heterosexual romance is possible.

As femininity has traditionally signified passivity and subordination to men, at the beginning of the second wave of feminism in the seventies many women explicitly rejected archetypal modes of feminine appearance as a means of signifying their rejection of patriarchal authority: Wearing no make-up and not removing body hair stood for something far deeper – the rejection of objectification.[126] In contrast, at the close of the century, many self-avowed feminists wear make-up and sexy clothes to signify that they can be *both* feminine and strong, Madonna being the most-oft discussed example. Women claim that they don't want to compromise their pleasure in femininity and sexuality in order to be equal to men – the much reviled 'power suit' of the eighties, which downplayed femininity, was a short-lived affair. Today, many women want to have it all:

'I can do my job as well as any man. I don't have to look like one as well.'

'I enjoy clothes and making myself look good. If men think I'm a bimbo because of that, I soon put them right. I enjoy that even more.'

'I don't mind if men think I'm a "babe". I'm flattered. The fact that I like to look sexy doesn't mean I'm not intelligent, though.'

Women's magazines, such as *Cosmopolitan*, reinforce this view of 'woman'. The cover of a recent magazine proclaimed:

Psst! Want to lose weight and meet SEXY men? Turn to page 101 for the catch.

Party confidence! You'll need our attention-grabbing gambits and foolproof chat-up lines.

Love and insecurity. When he likes you a little and you like him a lot.

NOT sleeping with the enemy. How to get the best from a womaniser.

SEX and the pregnant girl. (Forget it! Three's a crowd).

Yet we shouldn't judge a book by its cover, for inside there are features on 'positive action', encouraging women to take a more active role in public life. A caption reads 'Positive action is a floodgate that could regenerate our inefficient country and bring in the many talents of women,' and a ten-point checklist tells women how to institute such practices. Yet turn the page from an affirmative feature on career networking, women entrepreneurs and the dangers of workaholism, and the opening text to the feature proclaims 'Who Doesn't Long for Perfect Skin? Whilst for Some it Comes Naturally, Others Have to Create it for Themselves.'

On the same lines, an article in an edition of *Elle* magazine published in the mid nineties proclaimed 'The Return of The Real Girl'. It espoused 'girl pride', bemoaning the fact that the fight for equality has left woman 'stripped of certain vital assets'. The power-dressing, iron-pumping, sister-bashing behaviour of previous decades is castigated as 'playing men's games by men's rules', causing women to 'throw out their baby selves with the bathwater'. The assets we are encouraged to reclaim as we label ourselves 'girls' are those 'silly frilly things' cast aside in the serious seventies and eighties, for we are told that 'only now can women . . . afford to be girly without compromising their feminist principles.' This means that it's now OK to wear lipstick, little skirts and bows in your hair. It's OK to say 'I like to shop.' It's good to 'hang out with the girls'. And lest we think that this is a slide back into a form of fifties femininity exemplified by Doris Day in her sugary, hausfrau roles, the article ends with the confident pronouncement on nineties girlishness, 'this time it is not helpless and childish, but brazen, strong-armed and liberating.'

It's an interesting notion. That a short-skirted, made-up, bow-bedecked woman can indulge her love to shop yet receive respect from and equality with men. The pictures of 'girls' that accompany the article are predominantly of models and actresses (the two exceptions being a powerful TV executive and a well-known designer), the implication being that success and power can be achieved without sacrifice of femininity. This is a laudable wish, but we still have some way to go. Many people cannot read these subtle codes, and both men and 'other' women still see 'sexy' clothes and 'girly' behaviour as a sign of availability, of 'bimbo' status, focusing attention on a woman's appearance rather than her ability or her mind. The women that I interviewed were able to provide critical analyses of their own following of fashion, or wearing of sexy clothes: 'It's my choice'; 'I do it for myself, not for men'; 'Women should be able to be sexy and enjoy themselves without being seen as slags.' Yet in nearly every case 'other women' were seen as 'too obvious', 'easy' or 'tarts' if they dressed in an overtly sexual way. Double standards are clearly not just applied by men.

We shouldn't be surprised. For as Cinderella was ill-treated by her stepmother, who favoured her 'ugly' daughters, and the heroine of romantic fiction fought off or derided her competitors for the strong, seductive man, the message that women should compare themselves with other women and that other women are often the cause of conflict and strife rather than being allies or a source of support, pervades mass media aimed at women. It invades relationships between women, maintaining envy and competitiveness, ensuring that it is women who are often the main culprits in putting other women down, in identifying imperfections or categorizing other women as slags and whores.

Life as Strife: The Other Side of Women's Roles

Fighting off the Enemy: Woman against Woman

Women are best friends, but potential enemies; a source of fun and intimacy, yet the ones who may let you down the most. The contradictions in female relationships are played out in fairy tales, girls' comics and in magazines. Underneath it all there is a strong current of envy, of competition, and the message that no woman should stand in the way of a girl's aim to get the man. This is one of the most unpleasant lessons of womanhood: Femininity entails every girl fighting for herself.

In young girls' comics, such as *Mandy* or *Bunty*, the issue of friendship between girls dominates, both in the comic-strip stories and in the 'real life' sections where readers (aged seven to twelve), send in their photographs and resumés of their lives. The friend is always another girl; boys never fit into this category. *Bunty* has a section, 'Girl Talk', where letters give snippets of readers' lives, concerns about animals and friends being of primary consideration. Yet friendship is presented as an arena of insecurity, risk and deception. For example, in a recent edition of the comic stories depict a girl upset because her best friend has apparently forgotten to send her a postcard from holiday; two friends rowing over a boyfriend; an argument over a table-tennis game; and an eavesdropped conversation where a 'friend' is overheard criticizing the heroine, resulting in the defiant response: 'So! Silly and childish am I? And to think I was going to apologize to her – no way!' Other stories concern jealousy and rivalry between cousins, with one manipulating events to cause trouble with the other's parents, or jealousy at school, when one girl is voted 'Miss Popularity', resulting in secret attempts at sabotage by others.

In teenage magazines girls compete over boys. If the heroine can manage to steal the boy that every other girl wants, the conquest will have extra allure – like Cinderella stealing the prince from her stepsisters. So photo-stories tell of girls desperately trying to gain the attention of a boy in the face of competition from other girls. Or of so-called friends stealing their 'guy'. No wonder life is an ongoing war of maintaining beauty and feminine perfection – we are continuously reminded that there is always some other woman waiting in the wings. That boys should come before friends is an implicit message in many of the teenage magazines. Take this 'problem page' in *'Teen* magazine, where we are promised 'advice on friends, fights and fixes'. Suzanne tells us:

> I started going out with Dave a few months ago. I didn't want it to interfere with my friendship with Erin, but she was always acting as if I was intentionally shutting her out of my life. When something good happened between me and Dave, I didn't feel I could talk to her about it . . . instead of talking to me about how she was feeling, she found someone else to hang around with. If our friendship really meant anything to her, this could have been worked out.[127]

This is presented as a recurring problem between girls, and it undoubtedly is. The underlying message is that a true friend should take pleasure in another girl's achievement of the romantic dream and should want to talk for hours about 'him'. Only envy could stop her from doing so. The notion that a relationship with a man is always more important than a relationship with a woman (unless your man dumps you, when you are supposed to congratulate yourself on having kept in contact with your women friends) is instilled at a young age.

Friends might be a cause of problems, but they are not seen as the solution. Strange, given that research shows us support from friends is one of the factors that protects both girls and women from depression and anxiety more effectively than anything else.[128] In comics and magazines the focus of features is invariably on the individual; there is little room for notions of common interests (or woes) between women. Take this photo-story, which opens with the diary-writing heroine commenting: 'I can tell my diary anything I want. It's much better than people. They call themselves friends, then bitch about you the moment you're gone.' This epitomizes the dominant view of female friendship in much of the mass media. The girl is beset with problems, distressed and alone; the only person you can ultimately rely on is yourself.

Every second feature in teenage magazines seems to be about the *perils* of life, love and romance, which a girl must face alone. For every feature on getting a boy or worshipping a star there is one on 'How to Survive being Dumped' or 'I Tried to Commit Suicide When My Boyfriend Broke up with Me' (two articles in recent editions of US teen magazines). They remind us that the path of love isn't easy. Next time she must try harder, be nicer, be more beautiful, and she might *keep* her man.

In adult magazines the constant emphasis on beauty and fashion and on maintaining the boundaries of sexual etiquette is as much about warding off other women as it is about attracting a man. How many men understand the nuances of fashion anyway? It is only the *cognoscenti* (other women) who will recognize the designer bag, shoes, dress . . . the latest make-up style (or, horror of horrors, the inability to attain the current image). An effective means of ensuring that those who strive to maintain the illusion of perfect femininity won't be thinking or talking of anything more meaty than the latest fashion ensemble, and a good way of dealing with the perennial fear directed at women gathered (and talking) together: There is no fear if they are all talking about clothes. All through the magazines women are encouraged to compete against and to beat each other.

These themes, again, reflect and reinforce many of the anxieties which women report: fear of other women being better, fear of not being good enough, envy and jealousy towards the girl who seems to 'have it all', or who ignores the rules and 'has a good time'. Yet it doesn't stop girls or women being friends, and the importance of female friendship *is* a subtext in comics and magazines even if it is implicitly placed in a position secondary to romance. The main arena where women *are* shown together is in the domestic sphere, where we see the fairy-tale script of domestic subordination ('Cinderella', 'Snow White' . . .) transformed into 'gritty realism' in women's magazines and television soaps.

Domestic Bliss in Women's Weeklies

From their early evolvement at the end of the nineteenth century women's magazines have functioned as purveyors of domestic advice. How to cook, how to clean, how to manage a growing family. How to design the perfect home. How to amaze and surprise family and friends with wonderful recipes, yet still appear cool, calm and collected when the food is placed on the table. The glossy fashion monthlies may eschew such direct involvement in the mundane running of the home, focusing almost exclusively on pleasure and leisure (only condescending to examine 'designer' homes). Yet the women's weeklies and the more home-orientated monthlies still manage to continue the tradition of domestic advice to women, maintaining the illusion that such concerns are close to a woman's heart, whilst presenting them under the veneer of pleasure and accomplishment.

Janice Winship has commented in her analysis of the development of women's magazines that the earliest versions, such as *The Englishwoman's Domestic Magazine*, published in the nineteenth century, presented fashion and home-making as signs of both wealth and feminine accomplishment. This continued into the twentieth century and was perhaps most marked in the fifties, when the boom in consumer spending presented the housewife for the first time with *choice*. Making the right choice between the bewildering array of goods became the route to feminine success.[129]

> Make your choice from this wide array of *Bachelor's* Wonder soups (*Woman*, 1957)

> Mum, you're wonderful (for providing Bisto) (*Woman*, 1957)[130]

Here, what it is to be 'woman' is defined by choice of household product – buying the right product buys her happiness, success and the love of a good man. Take the example of a frozen peas ad, where the logo reads, 'Birds Eye peas will do anything to attract your husband's attention.' As Judith Williamson has commented, this clearly informs women that if they buy the product, they will get their husband's attention:

> Presumably *you* would do anything to attract your husband's attention. A woman and Birds Eye peas are made interchangeable; the peas represent what a woman can't do, they have the same aim: to make her husband notice something at dinner. She must buy the peas and let them buy love for her. They are thus interchangeable both with love and with her: they mean, and they make her mean.[131]

The ultimate cupboard love. Editorials have traditionally conveyed a similar message, perhaps with less subtlety. Janice Winship describes an article in *Woman* from 1958, on the subject of 'New Home-Makers', which begins:

> All over the country new brides are coming back from Honeymoon to a house that's one of a row. Edith Blair visited three clever brides who show how beautifully individual a room, same size, same shape as the neighbours' can be.[132]

Here the woman is challenged to show her feminine skills in turning an anonymous box (the standard fifties new house) into the palace of her dreams. Her fulfilment is unquestioningly in the home, through her clever consumption and, implicitly, through beating her competitors – other women: Like the 'housewives' who compete with each other in the TV advertisements for cleaning products, all trying to get their floors washed quicker, and more effectively, than each other. This is what a woman really wants: the cleanest, shiniest floor.

Few women today are persuaded that the achievement of a gleaming floor is at the centre of their heart's desire. Housework is mostly fitted in around a busy schedule of work or childcare rather than being the sole activity of the day. The majority of women in Europe and in North America work in paid employment outside of the home. Yet surveys show that women still carry out the majority of the cooking, cleaning and decorating within the home. So whilst magazines may still contain 'tips' on housekeeping and cooking, there is less attempt to make this work a vocation or joy, with the possible exception of gourmet recipes and up-market interior design, aimed at those few whose main leisure is the pursuit of a beautiful home and garden (or fantasizing about the homes of others), or those who view ideal homes, or read recipes for escapism and pleasure ('pornography for women'). For most women the domestic sphere is not one of leisure and pleasure, it is one of hard work, conflict and strife, as epitomized in that most ubiquitous form of mass media entertainment – the soap opera, where misery and strength go hand-in-hand, to the apparent delight and pleasure of the viewer.

Soap Opera: Mirror of Woman's Misery?

> Soap operas invest exquisite pleasure in the central condition of a woman's life: waiting.[133]

> The open-ended, slow-paced, multi-climaxed [structure of soap operas is] in tune with patterns of female sexuality.[134]

Tania Modleski has described soap opera as providing a 'unique narrative pleasure'.[135] Whether through the glamorous fantasy-world of *Dallas* and *Dynasty* (the American blockbuster soaps of the seventies and eighties) or the gritty realism of *Coronation Street*, *EastEnders* and *Roseanne* (all presented as 'social realism'), soap operas in many ways play out in minute detail concerns which are central to women's lives. They also present us with a vision of 'woman' in far more complex roles than is the case in most other forms of mass media aimed at women.

In soap opera there are many conflicting narratives, but identification is primarily with women and with 'the family'.[136] The soap opera focuses on women in the home, and so in many ways is very traditional. Whether the home be palatial and decadent (*Dallas* and *Dynasty*), a crumbling terraced house (*Coronation Street* and *EastEnders*) or a thin-walled modern house (*Brookside* and *Neighbours*), the central drama takes place around and within it. Story-lines which focus on the local pub or shop are merely a distraction from the 'real life' going on within the family, merely a different stage for the central concerns about men and children, love, death and family strife, played out in miniature again and again.

Kathryn Weibel has identified a number of common themes in soap opera: the evil woman, the great sacrifice, the winning back of an estranged lover or spouse, the issue of marrying for money or respectability, the unwed mother, deceptions about paternity of children, career versus home; the alcoholic woman (and occasionally man).[137] To these we might add the tragic death, domestic violence, lesbianism and the primacy of the mother.

The woman as mother is central to the narrative of the soap opera. Yet this is not the traditional myth of sublime motherhood, but motherhood as source of conflict, consternation and worry. Motherhood may be presented as an ideal state, but women in soap operas suffer for it. Equally, love and marriage are not presented as the idyllic states we see in romantic fiction, but as states of antagonism and sources of anxiety and pain. The characters in soap opera are more like those of tragedy than those of romance. The core message is that life is hard. As Ien Ang has argued in her analysis of *Dallas*:

> In soap opera it is by definition impossible for the characters to remain happy. A utopian moment is totally absent in soap opera narratives: circumstances and events continually throwing up barriers to prevent the capture of that little scrap of happiness for which the characters are none the less searching. Life is presented as inherently problematic. Unhappiness is the norm, the rule and not the exception . . . As a consequence, women in soap opera can never be simply happy with the positions they occupy.[138]

This mirrors the reality of many women's complex lives, where little is easy. The personal dramas of life are played out here in exacting detail, providing women with the knowledge that they are not alone in their own despair and misery. Yet as was the case with the problem page, misery is seen primarily as a problem of the individual woman or her family, rather than invoking suggestions of more societal causes of women's distress, or of a more collective response. Tensions between women are openly played out – most notoriously (and enjoyably) in the fights between Crystal Carrington and Alexis Colby in *Dynasty*, or the tensions between Pam and Sue Ellen in *Dallas*. The message is that other women are not to be trusted: In *EastEnders*, *Coronation Street*, *Brookside* and the up-market US soaps, they are frequently shown stealing or seducing another woman's man.

Tania Modleski sees soaps as a parallel to women's lives, the fact of a life where there are too many jobs to be done simultaneously being reflected in the fragmented existence of women in soaps. Soaps, she says, act as training for adult femininity, for what she describes as the 'art of being off centre':

> The housewife . . . is perpetually employed – her work, like a soap opera, is never done . . . her duties are split among a variety of domestic and familial tasks, and her television programmes keep her from desiring a focused existence by involving her in the pleasures of a fragmented life.[139]

This is a view of soap opera as social control – not distracting a woman from the tasks of home and family but encouraging her in her rightful role by reassuring her of their primary importance. Even if the woman is temporarily distracted by her viewing habits, a cynic might argue that this is functional. For as Modleski comments, 'a distracted or distractible frame of mind is crucial to the housewife's efficient functioning *in* her real situation.'[140]

On the other hand, soap operas are one of the few forms of mass media which shows the gritty side of women's lives: exploring themes of rape, incest and domestic violence. The British soap *Brookside* notoriously portrayed family violence in the Jordache family during the mid nineties, with teenage daughter Beth sexually abused by her father, her mother Mandy repeatedly beaten, and both women eventually fighting back – Mandy by killing her husband; Beth by helping her. In an earlier story another major character, Sheila Corkhill, was shown being raped on the street and then going through post-rape trauma (including a court case). In *Dallas* the domestic turmoils of J. R. Ewing and Sue Ellen and their effects on Sue Ellen's mental health were minutely dissected in discussions between the Southfork women (and by their millions of viewers). This is domestic trauma from the woman's point of view, exposing the tension between the traditional notion of what it is to be 'woman', and the aspirations of a post-feminist generation: Women are trapped in relationships with unthinking, uncaring men, but are no longer prepared to take it lying down. The increasing appearance of women living outside the control of men in soaps –

single mothers and lesbians have appeared in the British soaps *Brookside*, *EastEnders* and *Emmerdale* (as well as in *Roseanne*) – is a challenge to the traditional orthodoxy that a woman must live her life through 'her man' (although these characters are rarely presented as happy or fulfilled – and they often come to an untimely end – Beth, the lesbian character in *Brookside*, died of a heart attack in her late teens).

Identification with the problematic lives of women in soaps may lead to feelings of fatalism and resignation, encouraging women to seek their happiness in the eternal cycle of home and love. For as Ien Ang has commented, 'in spite of all miseries [women in soaps] continue to believe in the ideals of patriarchal ideology . . . the patriarchal state is non-viable but remains intact.'[141] Equally, soaps can fulfil a fantasy of community, of family, of drama in life and love. A fantasy of a strong, self-sufficient woman who rises above all adversity. They may act as escape, allaying anxieties (other women feel like me), fulfilling desires (the fantasy of home and hearth). That they are so popular with women suggests a pleasure in pain as well as in romantic escape. Yet in the increasing appearance of strong women in soaps, they also suggest a pleasure in resistance and retribution. In this they share many features with a very different genre of television, the audience-discussion programme, where women's problems are at the centre of every scene.

Talking on Television

> Audience discussion programmes are a forum in which people can speak in their own voice, which as Gilligan (1982) emphasizes, is vital for a construction of a gendered or cultural identity.[142]

Audience participation programmes are as central to daytime 'women's television' as the ubiquitous soaps. In Britain, *Kilroy* and *The Time . . . The Place . . .* are broadcast every weekday morning. In the US, the *Oprah Winfrey Show* and *Donahue* (as well as *Ricki Lake*, the eponymous presenter being a recent challenger for the chat-show-queen crown) play a similar role in airing controversial and often extremely personal issues within the forum of a studio debate. Aimed predominantly at women,[143] they have received little critical attention, probably for the same reasons that soaps were ignored by media critics for decades – as 'women's TV' they are cheap and trashy and positioned as the lowest form of the television art (in fact, as not deserving of the title 'art' at all, and therefore not deserving of any serious deconstruction). Yet a glance at the position of women in such programmes and of their meaning to female viewers provides a further insight into what the mass media says about 'woman'.

These audience-discussion programmes all have a similar format. An invited audience interacts with a host in discussing a specific question or theme. Particular members of the audience are invited because of their experience of this issue or problem and usually primed as to their specific contribution. There are usually a number of invited 'experts' who act as a foil for both the host and the audience, providing a voice of authority that can be disagreed with, as well as emphasizing the serious nature of the topic under discussion. So a programme on sexual violence might include women who have been victims of rape or sexual abuse, men who have committed such acts, and psychologists or rape counsellors who work in this area. Ideally there are a number of experts, who are pitted against each other so that disagreements between them can be aired.

These programmes have been described as a forum of the construction of identity through talk.[144] For example, *Donahue* has been described as reinforcing and reproducing the notion of the American self as individual, with 'being honest' and 'sharing feelings' positioned as a core part of individual identity.[145] It has been claimed that 'to read America . . . we first need to learn how to read talk shows.'[146] Perhaps this should say 'to read American woman', for it is women's concerns (or those concerns positioned as feminine) which dominate these programmes. For these talk shows air women's concerns; again, like the soap opera, the personal becomes public. But this time it is presented as overtly political, not concealed within the narratives of the soap. Women publicly air grievances about men, relationships and their general lot in life.

Women's talk has for centuries been positioned as trivial, as gossip, as superficial. Juxtaposed with the serious talk on the news, audience-discussion programmes could be said to reinforce this notion of women's talk as inconsequential. However, it can also be argued that talk shows act as a forum to give women a voice. Oprah Winfrey is overt about this; she has claimed on camera that 'we do program these shows to empower women.'[147] Winfrey herself positions her own 'womanhood' in terms of her oppression as a black woman, a working-class woman, and as a woman who has experienced abuse. She provides a powerful role model with whom the viewing public can identify – one who has stood up against the many forces which oppress her and insists on speaking out. This has led to the claim that the talk shows 'afford women the political gesture of overcoming their alienation through talking about their particular experience as women in society.'[148] But at the same time, they reinforce the notion of *difference* between women and men. Winfrey emphasizes women's communication skills and emotional qualities in contrast to the strengths (and weaknesses) of men.[149] As Corrine Squire has argued, 'the show's woman-centred talk is always, silently, about men'[150] – like all traditional stories about 'woman', there *is* no story without a man in the frame.

Women who are isolated in the home use the forum of 'talk television' in the same way that they use soaps – to gain an illusion of access to a public domain, engaging in dialogue with the debates on the set. Yet the genre of talk television is potentially more powerful than that of soaps as the participants are seen as 'real'. One respondent interviewed by Sonia Livingstone and Peter Lunt in their study of viewers of such programmes commented, 'one of the things about this is that it's real, and it is real people and different to the normal reality of television.'[151]

This dialogue with the television (or radio – talk radio can have the same function) is an interesting facet of increasingly alienated and isolated lives which many women (and men) lead. Is it a means of giving an illusion of community, of access to the public sphere, whilst maintaining the position of the public, in the words of Habermass, as a 'mindless mass'? For this isn't 'real' engagement or debate – it is an illusion, a fantasy. The woman at home doing her housework or caring for her children who is watching the talk shows or soaps may talk back to the television, but she is no less isolated than the woman of the 1950s towards whom the first 'women's programmes' were directed.[152] Early programmes focused on such clearly feminine concerns as fashion and cookery or on gentle exercises 'to lighten the housework' (not dissimilar from the format of day-time magazine programmes aimed at women today). The talk shows may present more contentious issues, but are they really serving a very different function?

Sonia Livingstone and Peter Lunt have claimed that 'in significant ways, the genre resembles a romance, with the romantic hero, constructing identities as real, authentic.'[153] As the hero of romantic fiction brings the heroine alive through his very presence, through his kiss, the host of the television talk show is the hero who discloses the problem and sets out to solve it, striding through the mythical world of the television studio where he or she is king. Alternatively, we could see the studio-audience members as heroes, confessing their sorrows and then publicly claiming redemption or almost miraculous solutions.[154] Here the programmes move away from the powerful hero of literature, who is impossible to emulate, towards the realism of ordinary lives, allowing closer identification:[155] We are all heroes now.

Talk shows ostensibly empower the people; the expert is invariably there to be dethroned. Expert knowledge is traditionally positioned as objective and rational; however, in the talk show this 'expert' knowledge is revealed to be alienated from experience and unhelpful. It is with lay knowledge, subjective and emotional, grounded in experience and helpful, that true expert knowledge lies.[156]

As it is 'man' who is traditionally positioned as expert, and 'woman' as inexpert,[157] this reversal explicitly valorizes the feminine position. In this way it can be seen to be truly subversive. However, as hosts such as Kilroy address women members of the audience in an intimate, sympathetic manner ('Go on, love') – which Livingstone and Lunt deem 'courteous' but I would read as patronizing – in contrast to the 'experts', who get treated more harshly (but respectfully), this authentic lay narrative produced by women could still be seen to be devalued as 'emotional'.

In allowing expression of emotion, the talk shows act as public therapy, airing women's woes and offering solutions for all to share – analogous to both problem pages in women's magazines and the problems aired in soaps. The programmes present a façade of intimacy, where the host encourages participants to disclose personal suffering and trauma in an explicit and emotional way. If participants break down in tears, all the better. Oprah Winfrey is particularly skilled at asking questions of such a personal (and often confrontational) nature, that they would not seem out of place in a therapy setting – they would certainly seem out of place in most 'ordinary' conversation. The talk show is a ritualized forum in which personal testimonials are elevated to truth – the experts can say little in the face of such heart-rending declarations of misery, the stories of abuse, neglect and personal adversity. Emotions such as anger or bitterness, which are usually deemed unfeminine and therefore inappropriate for women to express publicly, are here encouraged. In talk shows women are shown actively talking back, actively resisting the notion that to be 'woman' is to be silent and acquiescent. The anger, the self-disclosure, and the notion of intimacy may thus be cathartic – for both participants and viewers – as critics have suggested.[158]

Alternatively, talk shows may be offering a therapeutic promise which cannot be fulfilled, a false notion of intimacy, as the end of the programme brings the end of the intimate contact (for neither participants nor viewers are offered any continuity of the 'therapeutic' relationship or any follow-up for difficult issues aired). The women's lives which are exposed on the television talk shows are only briefly examined, offering the mythical fifteen minutes of fame, but little else. Perhaps this is the most important lesson for female viewers: Air your troubles but don't expect much of a response beyond an initial voyeuristic interest and a simulation of sympathy. Ultimately, women's woes are their own, to be sorted out at home, not really part of the public domain.

When Princess Diana availed herself of the world media to present her marital strife on *Panorama* in November 1995, she was merely following in the tradition of the talk-show hosts and audiences who had gone before. But she achieved the same aim: Sympathy from the British public, the majority of whom came out in support of this poor, lonely figure, telling us how badly she had been treated by the Palace. People felt that they 'really' knew her because of her disclosures: Something so personal and so painful must be the 'truth'. It was an archetypally feminine act – disclosure of romantic hurt and pain, presented with doe eyes, flirtatious smiles and downtrodden demeanour. It worked: She was only acting as a 'real' princess should. Just like in the fairy tales (which she reminded us of, in her allusion to her fairy-tale wedding). But here fact is really stranger than fiction – for we have a real princess who is treated badly by (male) palace officials and by her real-life prince, who refuses to live up to his allotted role. Like Cinderella before her, she has to be strong and beautiful in order to overcome her pain. Except that in this modern tale the princess claims not to want a man – her work, and her boys are all she says she needs for happiness and contentment. Is this a new reading of the romantic fairy tale? Or was it merely yet another example of archetypal feminine subterfuge, a misleading statement to focus attention on the other villain of the piece, the 'other woman' who had stolen the prince from the poor maiden's arms. The wicked witch made flesh in the late twentieth century, in the person of Camilla Parker Bowles.

The Silent Spaces

The representations of 'woman' in mass media aimed at women are limited. But that which we don't see is as significant as that which we do. In romantic fiction, comics and magazines we see a surplus of sexuality, but little mention of sexual violence or abuse which we know is a pervasive aspect of women's lives. We see little about sexual problems or difficulties, about sexual boredom or despair. We see little about the difficulties women face in shoring up men's egos and dealing with their sexual anxieties and fears. It was the most pervasive comment from women I interviewed about sex: Men want to be strong, to be 'man', and so women allow them to think that this is what they are.

We see little of the 'serious' side of women's lives and achievements. We see little about the reality of mothering or child care, except in the soaps, or in specialist women's magazines. We see little of lesbian relationships, of discussions of class, race or age (outside of the context of 'beauty' being synonymous with being heterosexual, white and young). We rarely see 'woman' in the traditional 'masculine' position of serious, speaking subject. When we do, the woman is notable because of this 'reversal of roles', as it is termed (as if woman usurps man by her very presence in a moving, speaking role). Take the 1970s furore over women as serious TV broadcasters, as newsreaders. It prompted comment that 'a good reporter needs a pair of balls.'[159]

> Angela is forceful, even dominant. In how many secret viewers' dreams does she deliver the *Nine O'Clock News* in black leather. Anna has a twinkle in her eye, a tease in her manner. Together they achieve much for women's equality without loss of – indeed with enhancement of – femininity.   *Sunday Telegraph*, 30 April 1978[160]

This was the analysis of women in 'serious' media roles I grew up with. Women in serious television broadcasting have in the past evoked such fascination and discussion that it is easy to imagine that they are more prevalent than they actually are. It is also easy to dismiss these women as ornamental, as more attention is paid to their appearance than to their journalistic skills. In the seventies in Britain there was almost a national obsession with Angela Rippon's legs, the female newscaster provoking such a level of sexual fantasy in the nation's males that she became as famous for her legs as she did for her skills as a journalist or broadcaster. She appeared on a Christmas entertainment show in 1976 (with the comedy duo, Morecombe and Wise), scantily clad, revealing her much discussed body in a dance routine. Women's talent effectively trivialized. The notion that this charade could have taken place with a male newscaster is clearly ridiculous. What man in this position would have subjected himself to such treatment, even if there were such interest in his body (which there rarely is)? Angela Rippon may have been attempting to show a sense of humour in gamely joining in with the interest in her sexuality, but she reinforced the notion that women, underneath it all, are not to be taken seriously. A reminder that whatever a woman aspires to, she is essentially a sexual body, to be scrutinized and admired; that shapely legs are as (if not more) important than a good brain. As Patricia Holland has commented 'women are about sexuality, the news is not'.[161] Angela Rippon no longer presents the news; she was for a time the front person for *Come Dancing*, a ballroom-dancing programme where the contestants reveal as much of their bodies as she revealed of hers on the 1979 show. Her 'rival', Anna Ford, the second female newsreader to achieve prominence in Britain, in 1978, still presents serious news programmes on television and on the radio. She has always refused to show her legs.

Women may now present news and documentaries without the same level of tabloid comment, but they have by no means been absorbed into the mainstream. In the early nineties, there was a furore in Britain over the presence of a female reporter, Kate Adie, reporting the events of the Tiananmen Square student protest in China. Adie was only present because she had coincidentally been in China prior to the riots. Yet her apparently fearless reporting of the violent and dangerous riots caught the attention of the nation – to the annoyance and chagrin of many of her male colleagues who would otherwise have been in this prestigious media spotlight. She appeared tired and dishevelled in flak jacket and army fatigues – her sexuality was a source of fascination because she was *not* emphasizing it, because she *wasn't* 'doing girl'.

Here, as with Angela Rippon almost two decades earlier, the fact of the journalist being 'woman', rather than her skills, was the focus of attention. Women can't seem to win. Equally, Hilary Rodham Clinton has been vilified by the press either for looking unattractive (her early hairstyle and spectacles), or for being too glamorous; Marcia Clark, the prosecutor in the infamous O. J. Simpson trial, received far more attention for her changing hairstyle and mode of dress than for her legal skills. To reduce a woman to her appearance is an effective means of ignoring what she has to say.

Over the last twenty years there has been some effort to bring more visibility to women in serious slots on television. In Britain, women present the serious BBC2 programme *Newsnight* and are frequent presenters of the daily news. In the USA, in 1970, there were no female anchorwomen on the national news. Today, most national and local news programmes are presented by a male–female team[162] and the president's spokesperson is often a woman. This is an advance to be commended. But is it merely window-dressing?[163] Women still form a minority of reporters (frequently being relegated to 'family issues') and are rarely invited to act as 'experts'.[164] The women who do appear are still likely to be relatively young and attractive (something which was wittily parodied in the recent film *To Die For*, where Nicole Kidman played a scheming TV anchorwoman). Age and appearance are not basic criteria for the selection of men in such roles.[165] Equally, as there are few changes in the basic hierarchies of power in the television world (or the world of politics for that matter) does not the token serious woman on the small screen merely act to pacify those who might otherwise comment on women's invisibility? Act to salve the conscience of those who pay lip-service to notions of equal opportunities? The fact that there are now a few more women taking up serious roles in the media gives a misleading impression of the reality of women's position. Again, there is evidence of inoculation – providing a token response to feminist critics who bemoan the absence of women in broadcasting, and heading off widespread dissatisfaction, without seriously addressing the issue. For the *content* of the news is still strikingly free of women; indeed female under-representation in this arena of life has been described as a 'symbolic annihilation'.[166]

In many ways 'woman' as newsreader will always be a contradiction because, as Patricia Holland has argued, the newsreader's image is subordinate to their speech – it is what they say rather than how they look which is of significance. The authoritative newsreader presents himself (sic) as a confident presence infused with authority and power. He is formal, serious, and his unchecked gaze puts him in a position of control: He is looking, rather than being looked at. For 'woman' to be represented as looking, as anything other than object of the masculine gaze, is unusual to say the least (see Chapter Two). Equally, for women to be presented in the rigid, formal head and shoulder position of the newscaster, with focus on her words rather than on her body, is a subversion of normal representation of 'woman' in the media.

Yet this subversion *is* starting to take place, as representations of the strong, agentic woman are becoming more common in television. The early seventies gave us the *Mary Tyler Moore Show*, a single woman working in a man's world;[167] in the nineties we have *Ellen* and Agent Scully in *The X-Files*. The family in *Roseanne*, one of the most highly rated shows in both the US and Britain, is hardly 'ideal' – this is no passive, acquiescent woman, pandering to the needs of her man. The real-life power and riches of Roseanne Barr – like those of talk-show host Oprah Winfrey – are equally celebrated, and symbolize the move away from the little woman controlled by her man. In series such as *Kate and Allie* or *The Golden Girls*, the focus is on the maintenance and development of relationships, not on the acquisition or proving of power.[168] We are shown solidarity (and pleasure) between women (whose lives are not centred on men). 'Personalities' such as Ruby Wax, Joan Rivers, Jo Brand, French and Saunders, or Lois Lane in the *New Adventures of Superman* present models of 'doing girl' within a different mould; women who are strong, challenging and sexy – and not afraid to show it. *Dyke TV* and *Out on Tuesday* show lesbians as they really are.

Yet strong women don't always win: In *LA Law* we saw independent women winning in court, yet often losing in life (and having to fight each other to get on); in *Prime Suspect* the female detective, Jane Tennison, can handle both the sexism of her police colleagues and the difficult crimes she has to solve, but leads a lonely life the rest of the time, the contents of her shopping basket – single TV dinners and whiskey – signifying her status as unloved woman. One of the most popular TV shows of the eighties among many women was *Cagney and Lacey* – the US detective series which showed two strong women who could fight, win and still keep their mascara in place. They worked together, got on with each other, and took no nonsense from any man. But as Susan Douglas has asked, 'did the unmarried, childless one really have to be an alcoholic, especially since the mother of three had a lot more reason to drink?'[169] Two recent British TV series, *The Governor*, which depicts the stressful life of a female governor in a male prison, and *Silent Witness*, which dramatizes the work of a female forensic scientist, show women achieving success (against all odds) in a man's world. Both women live alone and are constantly reminded of that (sad) fact by family and friends. It seems that the mass media still finds it difficult to show women *really* having it all. These women might have 'success', but they don't have a man. The daytime television programmes hosted by the 'couple' presenters – *Anne and Nick* or *Richard and Judy* (the latter a real-life couple) – redress the balance, showing how woman should be.

The development of *The Girlie Show* and *The Pyjama Party* in the late nineties in Britain – late-night magazine programmes hosted by 'laddette' girls who have 'outrageous' fun, are strong, stroppy and openly joke about sex – is an interesting shift. Here we see women taking up an overtly sexualized position, which at first glance appears to contradict all the rules of femininity. The 'girls' are bawdy, sexy, assertive and won't take any nonsense from anyone. They are rude and crude – one of the features of *The Girlie Show* is 'Wanker of the Week', where a man or woman is pilloried (Hillary Rodham Clinton was one example). They brag about sex in a 'laddish' manner – here is Katie Puckrick, host of *The Pyjama Party*, interviewed by *Loaded* magazine:

> I like a firm mattress and a wild sex life that's filthy, dirty and creative. I have to admit that I like sex a lot ... I'll do it just about anywhere – bus-stops, theatres, open fields. I'm up for just about anything.[170]

The interviewer's interest in this subject is in no way disguised. He tells us:

> In an interview last year she confessed with disarming frankness to a liking for the sexual delicacy known in some circles as The Hungarian Method – more familiar to the rest of us as 'going it up the arse like a good 'un'.

The sexual proclivities of the hosts of *The Girlie Show* are given extra spice by the knowledge (first disclosed in *Vanity Fair*) that supermodel host Rachel Williams is in a lesbian relationship. We are informed that she has also slept with 'lots of men', and in a recent show, Rachel was shown fondling plaster casts of penises in an interview feature with a New York artist. Is this to reassure us that this attractive lesbian is 'really' interested in men? (The fact that her girlfriend is beautiful and famous also helps – *anyone* would desire her.) These programmes may seem to celebrate female equality; women now have the freedom to be as crude and rude as men. On the surface they do. Yet they are hosted by extremely attractive women, adorned with the usual mask of beauty, whose sex lives are paraded in a voyeuristic manner. Women may claim to read this as 'We can be strong and sexy, too'. Men may read it as 'What an old slapper', and gain great pleasure from the titillation of seeing a long-legged 'lesbian' stroke a penis – an image which is more usually seen in pornography. These shows may be advertised as being emancipatory for women, but they are little more than the age-old fantasy of sexualized 'woman' in the eyes of men. It is an interesting example of men and women viewing the same representations with a completely different gaze, and therefore making very different interpretations. As these programmes are made by men, I'm not sure that the joke is on them.

Reading the Mass Media: Woman Duped, or Actively Resisting?

The myriad mass media representations aimed at women – fairy tales, girls' comics, women's magazines, romantic fiction and 'women's television' – provide us with a script of ideal femininity to follow. They form the instruction manual for the neophyte follower of the feminine masquerade – everything you needed to know about 'woman' but were too afraid (or confused) to ask. Follow the script and 'do girl' correctly and you will become an object of male desire. Femininity, as it is currently constructed, is still defined in terms of sexual difference: To be 'woman' is to be the antithesis of 'man'. It is to be consumed with (heterosexual) sex, romance and beauty. Yet as we have seen, women are not passive dupes. We negotiate and resist the narrow boundaries of femininity presented to us in the mass media; we can actively reframe what it is to be 'woman' within a female gaze, and can reinterpret or resist much of what we see. We can play at femininity (and enjoy it) without believing it to be 'true' and enjoy representations of strong independent women as much as those of the romantic heroine consumed with desire for man. We shape the representations of 'woman' which circulate. In a market-led economy (which the mass media is), public demand will shape the products produced. This is why the fifties image of 'mom' has been replaced by the nineties working woman, and the passive 'girl' by the sexual siren (who *tries* to have it all), and heterosexual hegemony by a greater acceptance of lesbian and gay sexuality.

In the closing years of the twentieth century the traditional script of femininity that Cinderella followed so well is followed to the letter by only a few women. It is perhaps only male drag queens who now do it to perfection, and to them it is clearly a show or a sham. When they take off the mask of make-up, 'woman' is left behind. Trying to *be* the fairy-tale princess is impossible (even for 'Princess Di'); to follow the feminine masquerade to the letter, to accept dominant representations of 'woman' as *true* is to become an illusory figure. Like the 'lady' who fills the mind of her suitor in the traditional narrative of courtly love, the ideal feminine 'woman' is not real. She is acting a part – and the essence of her role is her unavailability, her perfection and her status as idealized object of man's desire. Like all idealized objects, once taken down from her pedestal and examined in the light, she rarely lives up to the fantasy. She can approach it only by constantly acting out a part, never being subject, but always object. No wonder women are disappointed, distressed and dismayed – they cannot be an agentic person and 'woman' within this script. Perfect femininity as it is defined is an impossibility, a dangerous, invidious trap. To resist is to survive – through parody, rejection or negotiating a way of living with it (as most women do; see Chapter 6). The survivors are those who can perform the role of 'woman' without becoming the second, subservient sex. Those who believe the script is true and try to be the ideal woman may live a life as empty and ineffectual as that of the princess waiting for her prince. In real life, the prince rarely comes.

NOTES

1. In Zipes, J., *Don't Bet on the Prince. Contemporary Fairy Tales in North America and England*, Hants: Gower, 1986, pp. 186–208.

2. Barthes has argued that myths are presented as 'natural' as a means of

disguising their historical origins and social meaning. Barthes, Roland, *Mythologies*, New York: Hilt & Wang, 1972, p. 11.

3. In an analysis of the tales of the Brothers Grimm, Ruth Bottigheimer points out that what we consider to be the archetypal fairy tale is only one example of the genre, and that the nature of the tales is a reflection of the culture of nineteenth-century Germany in which the Grimm brothers produced their now legendary stories. Bottigheimer claims that the humbling of women, the denial of female voice, the castigating of women's speech, the prohibitions and punishments meted out to women in the tales, are not typical of traditional myths and fairy stories, but reflective of the deeply engrained values held by the authors of these tales, and their immediate society – the image of woman as Eve, needing to be controlled and punished. Bottigheimer, Ruth, *Grimms' Bad Girls and Bold Boys. The Moral and Social Vision of the Tales*, Newhaven: Yale University Press, 1987.

4. Leiberman, M. K., 'Some Day My Prince Will Come: Female Acculturation through the Fairy Tale', in Zipes J., 1986, pp. 186–208.

5. The heroine never marries a man less powerful than herself – she may fall in love with a poor man, but invariably discovers that he is a prince in disguise, or a prince unbeknownst to himself. The pairing of a powerful woman with a powerless man upsets too many notions of appropriate hierarchies.

6. This perpetuates both sexist and racist stereotypes through the rewarding of passivity and obedience in the 'good' princesses, the perpetuation of the notion that the best woman is a housewife, that stepmothers are evil, that men are shrewd, strong and aggressive, and that good is white whilst bad is black. See Moore, R., *From Rags to Riches: Stereotypes, Distortion and Anti-Humanism in Fairy Tales*, Interracial Books for Children, 6, 1975, pp. 1–3.

7. Gilbert, S. & Gubar, S., *The Madwoman in the Attic: The Woman Writer and the Nineteenth-Century Imagination*, New Haven: Yale University Press, 1979, p. 42.

8. Rowe, K., 'Feminism and Fairy Tale', in Zipes, J., 1986, pp. 209–26, p. 215.

9. Ibid., p. 216.

10. Dworkin, A., *Woman Hating*, New York: Dutton, 1972, p. 34.

11. Dowling, C., *The Cinderella Complex*, New York: Summit, 1981.

12. See Douglas, Susan, *Where the Girls are: Growing up Female with the Mass*

Media, London: Penguin, 1995, for an analysis of this process 1950–90.

13. See Hall, S., 'Encoding/Coding', in Hall, S., Hobson, D., Lowe, A. & Willis, P., *Culture, Media and Language*, London: Hutchinson, 1980, pp. 128–38, where women are presented as 'cultural dupes'.

14. See Smith, D. E., 'Femininity as Discourse', in Roman, L., & Christian Smith, L. K., *Becoming Feminine: The Politics of Popular Culture*, Sussex: Falmer Press, 1988.

15. Deemed 'warring forms of signification'. Hall, S., 1980, pp. 128–38.

16. The notion of contradictory representations allows for a movement away from the notion of a unitary reading subject dominant in early cultural theory.

17. Ros Coward has begged the question: 'What is the Lure in the Heart of These Discourses which Causes Us to Take up and Inhabit the Feminine Position?' (Coward R., 'Female Desire and Sexual Identity'; in *Women, Feminist Identity and Society in the 1980s*, M. Diaz-Diocavetz & I. Zavala, Amsterdam: John Benjamins.) Quoted by Threadgold, Terry, in Threadgold, Terry & Cranny Smith, Anne, *Feminine and Masculine Representation*, Sydney: Allen & Unwin, 1990.

18. Walkerdine, Valerie, *Schoolgirl Fictions*, London: Verso, 1990, p. 88.

19. Ibid., p. 91.

20. The two comics used here were *M&J* no. 132, 20 November 1993; and *Bunty* no. 1817, 20 November 1993.

21. For example, in *Bunty* and *M&J*.

22. In this way they work in the same manner as the 'conduct manuals' of the late nineteenth and early twentieth centuries.

23. See Walkerdine, Valerie, 1990, for development of these arguments.

24. Benjamin, Jessica, *Bonds of Love: Psychoanalysis, Feminism and the Problem of Domination*, New York: Pantheon, 1988.

25. Chodorow, Nancy J., *Femininities, Masculinities, Sexualities. Freud and Beyond*, London: Free Association Books, 1994, p. 59.

26. McRobbie, Angela, *Feminism and Youth Culture*, Basingstoke: Macmillan Education, 1989, p. 101.

27. Ibid., p. 84.

28. *Mizz*, 23 November 1993, p. 10.

29. *'Teen*, October 1995, pp. 46–7.

30. Ibid., pp. 82–3.

31. See Berger, John, *Ways of Seeing*, London: Penguin, 1972, for an analysis of woman watching herself.

32. Lees, Sue, *Sugar and Spice*, London: Penguin, 1993.

33. Contratto, Susan, 'Father Presence in Women's Psychological Development', in *Advances in Psychoanalytic Sociology*, Gerald M. Platt, Jerome Rabow & Marion Goldman (eds.), Malaber: Krieger, 1987, pp. 138–57, p. 143.

34. Persons, Ethel S., *Dreams of Love and Fateful Encounters: The Power of Romantic Passion*, New York: Norton, 1988, p. 265.

35. I am talking here about the 'second wave' of feminism, which overturned a lot of the notions of femininity current in the fifties. See Douglas, 1995, for an exploration of this contrast.

36. Men are also often shown to be critical or disinterested in their date – but this is a more familiar form of 'family entertainment', having been the subject of jokes and sitcoms for decades.

37. Coward, Ros, *Our Treacherous Hearts. Why Women Let Men Get Their Way*, London: Faber and Faber, 1992.

38. Both letters are from *Just Seventeen*, 10 November 1993.

39. The contrast between parental and agony-aunt positions was made the subject of parliamentary debate in England in 1995 when an 'outraged parent' discovered detailed instructions on 'lying back and enjoying' oral sex in his ten-year-old daughter's teenage magazine, *TV Hits*. The magazine was removed from the shelves. The publicity surrounding this story shocked many parents, as they hadn't inspected what their teenage daughters were reading. Their daughters didn't know what the fuss was about – reading about oral sex was clearly familiar (and unshocking) stuff to them.

40. McRobbie, 1989, p. 161. Other critics have made similar arguments, examining problem pages in other cultural contexts. For example, Erica Carter has examined problem-page letters in the context of the construction of femininity in Germany in the 1950s, in Carter, E., 'Intimate Outscapes: Problem Page Letters and the Remaking of the 1950s West German Family' in Roman and Christian Smith, 1988.

41. Sussman, Lisa, *The Ultimate Sex Guide: A Bedside Book for Lovers*, BPCC Paperbacks, distributed free with *more!*, 1993, p. 27.

42. Ibid., p. 29.

43. In continental Europe explicit information about sex has been aimed at teenagers for decades.

44. McMahon, Kathryn, 'The Cosmopolitan Ideology and the Management of Desire', *The Journal of Sex Research*, 27 (3), 1990, pp. 381–96, p. 391.

45. McRobbie, 1989, p. 160.

46. Thompson, Sharon, 'Putting a Big Thing in a Small Hole: Teenage Girls' Accounts of Sexual Initiation', *The Journal of Sex Research*, 27 (3), 1990, pp. 341–61.

47. Ibid., p. 353.

48. It's not surprising; the focus is often on the girl's pleasure, on anticipation and on unfulfilled desire (with a heavy dose of transgression to add spice and excitement, as this is invariably a forbidden activity).

49. Ussher, Jane M., *Women's Madness: Misogyny or Mental Illness?*, Hemel Hempstead: Harvester Wheatsheaf, 1991.

50. Moffat, Michael, *Coming of Age in New Jersey*, New Brunswick: Rutgers University Press, 1989.

51. October 1995.

52. October 1995.

53. For an analysis of cock-rock versus teenybop rock, see Frith, S. & McRobbie, A., 1978, 'Rock and Sexuality', in *Screen Education*, 29; reprinted in Frith, S. & Goodwin, A., *On Record. Rock, Pop and the Written Word*, London: Routledge, 1990, pp. 371–89.

54. Garratt, S., 'Teenage Dreams', 1984; reprinted in Frith & Goodwin, 1990, pp. 399–409. See also Steward, Sue and Garrett, Sheryl, *Signed, Sealed and Delivered. True Life Stories of Women in Pop*, London: Pluto, 1984.

55. Vermorel, F. & Vermorel, J., quoted in Frith & Goodwin, 1990, p. 481.

56. See Frith & Goodwin, 1990, for an analysis of this. Garratt, 1984, p. 400, makes this point explicitly.

57. McRobbie, 1989, p. 145. With Simon Frith, she has also argued that 'music is a means of sexual expression and as such is important as a mode of social control.' Frith & McRobbie, 1978, p. 387.

58. Garratt, 1984, p. 402.

59. Radway, Janice, *Reading the Romance: Women, Patriarchy and Popular Literature*, London: Verso, 1987, p. 8.

60. Neil, J., *Flame of Love*, London: Mills & Boon, 1993, pp. 188–9.

61. Conran, Shirley, *Lace*, London: Penguin, 1979.

62. Modleski, Tania, *Loving with a Vengeance. Mass-Produced Fantasies for Women*, London: Routledge, 1990, p. 48.

63. Snitow, Anne Barr, 'Mass-Market Romance: Pornography for Women is Different', in *Desire: The Politics of Sexuality*, A. Snitow, C. Stansell & S. Thompson (eds.), London: Virago, 1984, p. 263.

64. Lamb, C. *Whirlwind*, London: Mills & Boon, 1987, p. 34.

65. Acton, W., (1870). Quoted by Jeffreys, *The Sexuality Debates*, London: Routledge & Kegan Paul, 1987.
66. Janney, K., *The Pirate's Lady*, London: Mills & Boon, 1988, p. 64.
67. Modleski, 1984, p. 52.
68. Lamb, 1987, pp. 39–40.
69. Ibid., p. 53.
70. Janney, 1988, pp. 33–34.
71. Snitow, Stansell & Thompson, 1983.
72. See Dobash, R. E., & Dobash, R., *Violence Against Wives: A Case against the Patriarchy*, London: Open Books, 1979, for a discussion of male violence and women staying in violent relationships, and Browne, E., *When Battered Women Kill*, London: The Free Press, 1980, for a discussion of women who react with violence themselves.
73. Modleski, 1984, p. 43.
74. Lamb, 1987, p. 166.
75. Neil, J., 1993, p. 15.
76. Cora Kaplan has described Scarlett O'Hara in this way, in Kaplan, C., 'The Thorn Birds: Fiction, Fantasy, Femininity', in *Formations of Fantasy*, Victor Burgin, James Donald, & Cora Kaplan (eds.), London: Routledge, 1989.
77. Modleski, 1984, p. 45.
78. Lamb, 1987, p. 103.
79. Ibid., p. 160.
80. Barthes, 1972, talks of inoculation in this way.
81. Light, Alison, *Feminist Review*, 16, 1984, pp. 7–25.
82. See also Taylor, Helen, *Scarlett's Women: Gone with the Wind and Its Female Fans*, London: Virago, 1989, for accounts of women on *GWTW*.
83. Radway, 1987, p. 12.
84. Ibid., p. 14.
85. *Mizz*, October 1995, p. 35.
86. *'Teen*, October 1995.
87. *Seventeen*, October 1995.
88. *Just Seventeen*, 2 April 1986.
89. All quotes from *Just Seventeen*, 2 April 1986, pp. 50–1.
90. Lakoff, R. T. & Scherr, R. L., *Face Value: The Politics of Beauty*, London: Routledge & Kegan Paul, 1984, p. 252.
91. *Just Seventeen*, 10 November 1993, p. 40.
92. A 'supermodel' renowned in the early nineties.

93. *Just Seventeen*, 10 November 1993, p. 40.

94. McRobbie, 1989, p. 121.

95. *Harpers Bazaar*, October 1995.

96. Craik, Jennifer, *The Face of Fashion. Cultural Studies in Fashion*, London: Routledge, 1993, p. 158.

97. MacSweeny, Eve, 'Don't Do the Time Warp Again', in *Observer Review*, 10 March 1996, p. 8.

98. Baudelaire, C., 'The Painter of Modern Life', in Baudelaire, *Selected Writings on Art and Artists*, P. E. Charvet (trans.), Cambridge: Cambridge University Press, 1972, pp. 423–4.

99. Craik, 1993, p. 46.

100. Weibel, K., *Mirror, Mirror: Images of Women Reflected in Popular Culture*, New York: Anchor Books, 1977.

101. Steele, V., *Fashion and Eroticism: Ideals of Feminine Beauty from the Victorian Era to the Jazz Age*, Oxford: Oxford University Press, 1985, p. 79.

102. McRobbie, 1989, p. 179.

103. Craik, 1993, p. 76.

104. Pumphrey, M., 'The Flapper, the Housewife and the Making of Modernity', *Cultural Studies*, 1(2), 1987, pp. 179–94.

105. Quoted in Craik, 1993, p. 88.

106. Shrimpton, J., *Jean Shrimpton: An Autobiography*, London: Ebury Press, 1990, quoted in Craik, 1993, p. 88.

107. See Walkerdine, 1990.

108. Bartky, S., 'Foucault, Femininity and the Modernization of Patriarchal Power', in *Feminism and Foucault: Reflections on Resistance*, I. Diamond and L. Quinby (eds.), Boston: Northeastern University Press, 1988.

109. See Douglas, 1995, Ch. 11, for a discussion of the significance of the obsession with thigh control.

110. Chernin, Kim, *The Obsession: Reflections on the Tyranny of Slenderness*, New York: Harper and Row, 1981.

111. Lacey, H., 'Real Life', *Independent on Sunday*, 26 November 1995, p. 3.

112. *Top Santé Health & Beauty*, March 1994, p. 63.

113. Bordo, S., 'Reading the Slender Body', in *Body Politics: Women and the Discourses of Science*, M. Jacobus, E. Fox Keller & S. Shuttleworth (eds.), London: Routledge, 1990, pp. 83–112, p. 89.

114. Bordo, 1990, pp. 89–90.

115. Malson, Helen, *The Thin Body*, London: Routledge, 1996, p. 253.

116. Ibid., p. 229.

117. Teenage interviews carried out by Deborah Picker (unpublished manuscript); adult interviews by Fahimeli Shanghai.

118. Douglas, 1995, p. 251.

119. McRobbie, A., 'Working-Class Girls and the Culture of Femininity', in: *Women Take Issue*, Women's Studies Group, Centre for Contemporary Cultural Studies (ed.)., London: Hutchinson, 1978, p. 103.

120. Malson, 1996, p. 195.

121. Malson, 1996, p. 199.

122. It is arguable that the notion of women taking on an androgynous or masculine appearance has become more 'mainstream', which has led to the growth of 'drag kings' (women dressing as men, with beards and packing). These women (usually lesbians) mark out their rejection of the feminine masquerade in the most blatant manner – as well as still managing to transgress (something a short haircut or 'butch' appearance no longer serves to do).

123. See Faderman, L., *Odd Girls and Twilight Lovers*, London: Penguin, 1993.

124. Wittig, Monique, *The Straight Mind and Other Essays*, Hemel Hempstead: Harvester Wheatsheaf, 1992, p. 32.

125. The media can't decide whether this is a good thing (they look more 'normal' and contradict the media stereotype of an 'ugly dyke') or not (they can pass as straight – so could be anywhere!) See Ainsley, R., *What is She Like? Lesbian Identity from the Fifties to the Nineties*, London: Cassell, 1996.

126. Susan Douglas (1995) explores the negative reactions to this in the mass media, in the vilification of feminists as 'ugly' – most notably the case of Kate Millett, who was described by *Time* as 'unwashed'.

127. *'Teen*, October 1995, p. 52.

128. Brown, G. & Harris, T., *Social Origins of Depression*, London: Tavistock, 1978.

129. Winship, Janice, *Inside Women's Magazines*, London: Pandora, 1987, p. 60.

130. Ibid., p. 60.

131. Williamson, Judith, *Decoding Advertisements. Ideology and Meaning in Advertising*, London: Marion Boyars, 1978, p. 38.

132. Winship, 1987, p. 60.

133. Modleski, 1984, p. 88.

134. Kinder, Marcha, 'Review of Scenes from a Marriage by Ingmar Bergman', *Film Quarterly*, 28 (2), 1974–5, pp. 48–53.

135. Modleski, 1984, p. 87.

136. Ibid.

137. Weibel, 1977.

138. Ang, Ien, *Watching Dallas. Soap Opera and the Melodramatic Imagination*, London: Routledge, 1985, p. 122.

139. Modleski, 1984, p. 101.

140. Ibid., p. 103.

141. Ang, 1985, p. 123.

142. Livingstone, S. & Lunt, P., *Talk on Television. Audience Participation and Public Debate*, London: Routledge, 1994, p. 31.

143. Ibid., for an analysis of the viewing figures for these programmes.

144. Ibid., and Carbaugh, D., *Talking American: Cultural Discourses on Donahue*, Norwood, NJ: ABlex, 1988, p. 2.

145. Carbaugh, 1988.

146. Fogel, A., 'Talk Shows: On Reading Television', in *Emerson and His Legacy: Essays in Honour of Quentin Anderson*, in S. Donadio, S. Railton & O. Seavey (eds.), Carbondale: Southern Illinois University Press, 1986.

147. Quoted by Corrine Squire, in 'Empowering Women? The *Oprah Winfrey Show*', *Feminism and Psychology*, 4 (1), 1994, pp. 63–79.

148. Masciarotte, G. J., 'C'mon Girl: Oprah Winfrey and the Discourse of Feminine Talk', *Genders*, 11, 1991, pp. 81–110.

149. Squire, 1994, p. 67.

150. Ibid., p. 67.

151. Livingstone & Lunt, 1988, p. 59.

152. Leman, J., 'Programmes for Women in 1950s British Television', in Baehr, Helen & Dyer, G., *Boxed in: Women and Television*, London: Pandora, 1987.

153. Ibid., p. 59.

154. Squire, C., 'Is the Oprah Winfrey Show Feminist Television?' Paper presented at the *International Women Studies Congress*, New York, 1991.

155. See Chesebro, J. W., 'Communication, Values, and Popular Television Series – A Four-Year Assessment', in *Television: The Critical View*, Oxford: Oxford University Press, 1982.

156. Livingstone & Lunt, 1988, p. 102.

157. Keller, Evlyn Fox, *Reflections on Gender and Science*, New Haven, Connecticut: Yale University Press, 1985.

158. Livingstone & Lunt, 1988; Carpignano, P., Andersen, R., Aronowitz, S. & Difazio, W., 'Chatter in the Age of Electronic Reproduction: Talk

Television and the Public Mind', *Social Text* 25/26, pp. 33–55.; Habermas, J., *The Structural Transformation of the Public Sphere: An Inquiry into a Category of Bourgeois Society*, T. Burger with F. Lawrence (trans.), Cambridge, MA: MIT Press.

159. A comment by a senior newsroom official. Quoted by Holland, P., in 'When a Woman Reads the News', in Baehr & Dyer, 1987, pp. 133–50, p. 133.

160. Ibid., p. 135.

161. Holland, P., 'The Page Three Girl Speaks to Women', in R. Betherton (ed.), *Looking On: Images of Femininity in the Visual Arts and Media*, London: Pandora, 1987.

162. Douglas, 1995, p. 277.

163. Baehr & Dyer, 1987, p. 11.

164. Douglas reports that in 1988 10.3 per cent of guests on the US programme *Nightline* were women, and in a survey carried out in 1988, only 15 per cent of correspondents were female. Douglas, 1995, p. 277.

165. Douglas reports that Christine Craft was sacked from reading the news in 1983, at the age of thirty-six, for being 'too old, too unattractive and not deferential to men'. Ibid., p. 278.

166. Butcher, H., Coward, R., Evaristi, M., Garber, J., Harrison, R. & Winship, J., *Images of Women in the Media*, Birmingham: CCCS, 1974; Eddings, B. M., 'Women in Broadcasting (US) de jure, de facto', in *Women in Media*, Helen Baehr (ed.), Oxford: Oxford University Press, 1996.

167. Susan Douglas (1995) discusses the development of Mary Tyler Moore from an apologetic, feminine character, to an independent, strong woman.

168. Byers, Jackie, 'Gazes/Voices/Power: Expanding Psychoanalysis for Feminist Film and Television Theory', in *Female Spectators. Looking at Film and Television*, Deirdre Pribram (ed.), London: Verso, 1988.

169. Douglas, 1995, p. 274. And despite high ratings, as Susan Faludi, *Backlash: The Undeclared War against American Women*, London: Vintage, 1992, has argued, the male network chiefs continually tried to drop the programme from their schedules.

170. *Loaded*, March 1996, p. 38.

CHAPTER TWO

The Masculine Gaze: Framing 'Woman' in Art and Film

Men act and *women appear*. Men look at women. Women watch themselves being looked at. This determines not only most relations between men and women but also the relation of women to themselves. The surveyor of woman in herself is male: the surveyed female. Thus she turns herself into an object – and most particularly an object of vision: a sight . . . the 'ideal' spectator is always assumed to be male and the image of woman is designed to flatter him.   JOHN BERGER[1]

[The image of woman] stands in patriarchal culture as the signifier of the male other, bound by the symbolic in which man can live out his fantasies and obsession through linguistic command by imposing them on the silent image of woman still tied to her place as bearer and not maker of meanings.   LAURA MULVEY[2]

Mass media aimed at women does not exist in a vacuum. The script of femininity it presents is repeated again and again in many other contexts – in art, film and literature; in pornography; in the law; and in psychological and medical treatises on sexuality. What is unique about the story we have examined so far is that women are the target audience for the myths. If we look to representations produced for the consumption of men we see a different image of 'woman'.

Disentangling the lure at the heart of the representations of 'woman' in the masculine gaze is a necessary part of any analysis of femininity or female sexuality. If, as John Berger has argued, 'men look at women' and 'women watch themselves being looked at,' the way in which 'woman' is framed in the gaze of 'man' will influence how women come to see themselves. Equally, if femininity is a performance which takes place primarily within the theatre of heterosexual sex and romance, 'woman' is inevitably situated in relation to 'man'. For in the archetypal masculine gaze, there is no question about the order of these positions: 'Woman' stands as other, against which men define themselves as one – as 'man'. She appears as a creature to be worshipped or an object to be denigrated; her very essence is irrevocably linked to sexuality in all its myriad forms.

In order to unravel these particular visions of 'woman' I will focus primarily on art and film[3] (looking at pornography separately in Chapter Three). These are spheres of visual representation that are available to all, and whose power rests in their simplicity; no apparent effort or skill is needed on the part of the spectator – we only have to be able to *see*. These are also powerful and influential media, often designated as 'high culture'[4] by academics and critics who inhabit them (in contrast to 'popular culture', which is often dismissed as 'trash').[5] The pervasive nature and status accorded to 'high culture' affords the representations of 'woman' created therein a smokescreen of authenticity. The reverence with which the genius of the 'old master' or the 'director' is celebrated bestows upon these agents of artistic creation a power to define reality we lesser mortals can never hope to achieve. Yet they are not neutral observers of the female form. For as feminist critics have consistently and persuasively argued, it is the masculine gaze which has, historically, dominated the world of art and film.

This was a view first voiced in a now classic paper by feminist film critic Laura Mulvey,[6] who drew upon Lacanian psychoanalytic theory in arguing that the 'gaze' in film is male. This gaze operates in three ways. Man is filming, controlling the voyeuristic gaze of the camera;[7] the gaze of the man within the narrative of the film, the actor, is structured so that the woman actor is positioned as object – man gazes at woman, woman is looked at; and the spectator, the person watching the film, is assumed to be male, imitating the voyeurism of the camera and the actor within the film. So at a number of levels, 'man' is positioned as active, whilst 'woman' is passive, and therefore captivated, controlled and contained 'as erotic object for the characters within the screen story, and as erotic object for the spectator within the auditorium'.[8] Similar arguments have been made about art,[9] and could also be made about mass media imagery (and pornography) aimed at men.

Today, critics talk about the gaze as 'masculine', for it is the socially constructed position of phallocentric masculinity, rather than biological maleness that is at issue here. So it isn't inevitable that art or film produced by men will frame 'woman' in a masculine gaze; it is not irrevocably tied to the sex we are born with, but rather reflects and reinforces the relative cultural and psychological positions of 'woman' and 'man'. In this context, to speak of the masculine gaze is to speak of imagery which reifies the social position of 'man' within the traditional script of heterosexuality – the position of power, authority and sexualized control over 'woman'. It is the flip side of what we see portrayed in romantic fiction or fairy tales – the vision of 'woman' from the position of the prince or the strong romantic hero, who is unquestionably in control. As was the case with mass media imagery aimed at women, these are representations which circulate meanings about masculinity and femininity, providing a script for our relations with each other – and a script for the construction of heterosexual desire.

This analysis of the masculine gaze is not necessarily the depressing tale of 'woman as victim', that it might at first appear. For as women have resisted the myths at the heart of fairy tales, they have reformulated and resisted the archetypal 'masculine gaze'. This has taken the form of feminist criticism, the development of feminist representations or a 'female gaze', censorship, and re-readings of these 'images of "woman"'. After two decades of such critiques there are few representations of 'woman' as 'other' or object that survive unscathed, or at least un-criticized. It is arguable that it is only in the transgressive world of pornography that the unfettered masculine gaze is given free rein today; indeed, the very attraction of pornography lies partly in the subversive celebration of this sexualized, morally and politically incorrect, positioning of 'woman'.

But regardless of the remarkable impact of feminist critiques, we cannot afford to be complacent. We cannot afford to simply dismiss or disregard the representations of 'woman' framed within the masculine gaze. There is a lure at the heart of this particular sexualized vision of 'woman' – particularly for men – and we need to ask why.

Exploring Art and Film: Exposing the Fears and Fantasies of 'Man'

The Idealization and Overvaluation of 'Woman'

> If men could see us as we really are, they would be a little amazed; but
> the cleverest, the acutest men are often under an illusion about women:
> they do not read them in a true light: they misapprehend them, both for
> good and evil: their good Woman is a queer thing, half doll, half angel;
> their bad Woman almost always a fiend.
>
> CHARLOTTE BRONTË, *Shirley*[10]

Visual representations of 'woman' framed in the masculine gaze reflect
a fantasy of perfection. Woman as ideal, worshipped, revered and held
up as an icon. Here, 'woman' is flawless; beauty personified, the 'angel
in the house',[11] an apparent role model for all women who see. In
pre-Renaissance European art, this idealization took the form of the
Madonna. In countless religious and secular paintings the image of
woman as beatific mother was repeated, both allegorically as the Virgin
Mary and baby Jesus, and simply as a depiction of a mother nursing her
child in her home. It was the only image of 'woman' produced for
centuries.[12] In the nineteenth century these representations of the
feminine ideal reflected the fantasy and fiction of happy domesticity, a
domesticity which centred on woman. George Elghar Hick's triptych
Woman's Mission (1863) is a typical example of this genre. It depicts
'woman' in the approved feminine roles, as mother, wife and daughter,
always proper, always pure. In three separate guises which implicitly
define what it is to be feminine, we see 'woman' worshipping, serving,
obeying.[13] As Lynda Nead has commented, ' "woman" is offered as a
unified and coherent category through the fulfilment of her domestic
duties and mission.'[14]

It was also in the mid nineteenth century that 'woman' came to stand
for 'beauty' in the world of art; a connection seen most notably in the
paintings of the Pre-Raphaelites, particularly in the work of Dante
Gabriel Rossetti. These were images of visual perfection, combining
physical loveliness and a non-threatening remote gaze,[15] an appropriate
feminine look: 'Woman' never directly challenging by looking directly
at the spectator, but gazing obliquely to the side, lowering her eyes and

her face in the archetypal expression of feminine passivity. This is an expression of 'natural' feminine beauty which continues in advertising imagery a century later,[16] or is taken on by women as part of the masquerade of 'doing girl'.

The 'angel in the house', the irrevocable connection between femininity and passivity, was also a dominant theme in nineteenth-century literature. The image of the 'eternal feminine' – the ideal of feminine purity and goodness – was prevalent in both poetry and prose. Milton had already typified this idealization of 'woman' in his homage to his 'saintly' wife, who had died. She

> Came vested all in white, pure as her mind.
> Her face was veiled, yet to my fancied sight,
> Love sweetness goodness in her person shined
> So clear, as no face with more delight.[17]

Like the eternal image of Ophelia – the perfect woman who is frozen in death as a vision of beauty, and so never shatters the illusion of loveliness. Goethe's Faust has a similar vision of 'woman' as the 'eternal feminine' in her role as symbol of contemplative beauty and purity, in contrast to man as 'ideal of significant action'. The age-old dichotomy. One of Goethe's translators describes his representations of 'noblest femininity' in the novel *Wilhelm Meister's Travels*:[18]

> She . . . leads a life of almost pure contemplation . . . in considerable isolation on a country estate . . . a life without external events – a life whose story cannot be told as there is no story. Her existence is not useless. On the contrary . . . she shines like a beacon in the dark world, like a motionless lighthouse by which others, the travellers whose lives do have a story, can set their course. When those involved in feeling and action turn to her in their need, they are never dismissed without advice and consolation. She is an ideal, a model of selflessness and of purity of heart.[19]

In this fantasy of femininity, 'woman' is an inspiration, always sacrificing herself to others, a 'model of selflessness'. In Goethe's words, 'woman lifts us up.'

A similar process continued into the world of film. From the first stars of the silent movies, through to the mass-market Hollywood blockbusters of today, women have been transformed into goddesses through their overvaluation in film:[20] Greta Garbo, Marlene Dietrich, Marilyn Monroe, Betty Grable, Brigitte Bardot . . . the list goes on. These women are icons, ideals – air-brushed fantasies of sublime perfection frozen in photographic stills and magnified and exalted in their projection on to the cinema screen. It is beautiful women who are most likely to be elevated to the status of 'star'. Others, however excellent their acting skills, are generally relegated to 'character parts'. In cinema, we can also see the continuation of the myth of the Madonna, the same story of motherhood as idealized bliss, with romance and domestic harmony central to women's happiness. There is simply a variation on the traditional imagery, bleached hair and perfect make-up replacing the beatific beauty of the religious icon. This is perhaps epitomized in the sugary films of the fifties, in which the likes of Doris Day were shown as glorified housewives, perfect femininity resulting in the attraction of a 'real' man. A lesson for all women watching.

The 'film-star' is the idealized image of perfection made 'real'. We are as fascinated with the mystery of the private life of the star, her changing styles, her moods and marriages, as we are with her performance on the screen. Shifting fashions may determine which style the latest icon will adopt – thin or very thin, 'made-up' or 'natural' – but the process is the same. She is fantasy incarnate, a vision of perfection who inspires desire. In her romantic union with a handsome man, the fairy tale is (temporarily, at least) made to come true (if it doesn't work out in the Hollywood version of life, she merely swaps her prince). And as was the case with fairy tales, this Hollywood princess is always young, white and heterosexual.[21] In every way she signifies feminine perfection.

These myriad representations of the idealized 'woman' may on the surface seem to be a positive process, a glorification of feminine grace. It is how 'art' has for centuries been presented – a demonstration of men's adoration of female beauty – and film-makers are merely carrying the 'old masters'' mantle through to the twenty-first century. If we accept this line of argument, the worst we could accuse them of is marginalizing or making invisible the ugly or the plain (as well as the old, the black, the lesbian . . .). But if we scratch beneath the surface and ask what the *meaning* behind these narrow images of 'woman' is, we see a very different story altogether – a story we might not really want to see. For as feminist psychoanalyst Karen Horney percipiently observed:

> Is it remarkable . . . when one considers the overwhelming mass of the transparent material, that so little recognition and attention are paid to men's secret dread of women? It is almost more remarkable that women themselves have so long been able to overlook it . . . The man . . . has in the first place very obvious strategic reasons for keeping his dread quiet. But he also tries by every means to deny it even to himself. This is the purpose of the efforts to 'objectify' it in artistic and scientific creative works . . . his glorification of women has its source not only in his cravings for love, but also in the desire to conceal his dread. A similar relief . . . is also sought and found in the disparagement of women that men often display ostentatiously in their attitudes.[22]

In this view the glorification of 'woman' we see in the masculine gaze is not worship but a reflection of unconscious anxiety, envy and fear. As Horney argues, this apparent adoration signifies 'there is no need for me to dread a creature so wonderful, so beautiful, nay so saintly'; in raising 'woman' on to the pedestal, she is not elevated into a deity but reduced to the status of object.

In Karen Horney's view, man's dread of woman is irrevocably connected with sex – a fear of not being good enough or 'man enough' within the script of heterosexual sex. Within dominant constructions of masculinity 'man' is expected to be sexual, powerful and in control (the opposite of 'woman'); any failure to live up to these expectations might suggest that men are not 'man'. As Horney explains, man's 'original dread of women is not castration anxiety at all, but a reaction to the menace to his self respect.'[23] Or as Margaret Atwood has commented, women fear that men will rape them; men fear that women will laugh at them. His dread also reflects a fear of rejection; as Horney comments, 'the dread of being rejected and derided is a typical ingredient in the analysis of every man.'[24] This is associated with a fear of vulnerability and of the potential loss of autonomy in the face of desire. To return to Ethel Persons' argument in the previous chapter, 'men tend to interpret mutuality as dependency and separate sex and love';[25] and so, the merger or mutuality which is central to sexual relationships can act as a potential source of anxiety or dread.[26] The idealized image of 'woman' on a pedestal poses no threat; there is no opportunity for merger here. There is no possibility of rejection, or even of sex, for she is 'too good', too untouchable, to even look at man, like the 'lady' within the ritual of courtly love. In this way, representations of 'woman' in the masculine gaze 'reflect the male search for self definition',[27] rather than being part of any attempt on the part of women to negotiate femininity.

The idealization of 'woman' as mother/Madonna is equally deceptive. This is a representation of 'woman' as mother where the reality of fecundity is denied or dismissed. There are few images in art and film of pregnant women. The sexual connotations of breast-feeding are overtly repressed. This stands, arguably, as a defence against envy of women's reproductive power and of the relationship between mother and child. As Horney has argued:

> from the biological point of view woman has in motherhood, or in the
> capacity for motherhood, a quite indisputable and by no means negligible
> biological superiority. This is most clearly reflected in the unconscious
> of the male psyche in the boy's intense envy of motherhood . . . of
> pregnancy, childbirth . . . as well as of the breasts and of the act of
> suckling.[28]

This is an envy which is repressed, rarely spoken of. Yet idealizing or worshipping the figure of woman as mother is not the only means of dealing with these deep-rooted feelings. We also see evidence of it in the denigration of female reproduction, in its being positioned as illness or weakness in both medical and scientific accounts (see Chapter Four).[29] We see evidence in the systematic exclusion and discrimination against women who become pregnant and bear children in the world of work, and in the theological and common laws which legitimize this process and conceal female reproduction within moral codes (such as those positioning abortion or contraception as 'crime' or 'sin'). This disparagement of the power of female fecundity allows man to defend himself against the terrible fear that the penis, even when raised to mythical proportions in the phallus, can never match up to the power and potential of woman's womb.

This process of detraction is not confined to motherhood, and the idealization of 'woman' is not the only means of dealing with the conflict between desire and dread. The feminist analyst Jessica Benjamin[30] has argued that in order to take up a position of heterosexual masculinity, men have to develop a 'false differentiation' from their mothers (and subsequently other women), which involves objectification and a denial of her subjectivity, in order to counter their own feelings of dependency. In order to be able to relate to and gain recognition from women, yet not be made dependent themselves, Benjamin argues that men seek to dominate women, which leads to both the eroticization of dominance in the normal case, and erotic violence in the abnormal.[31] This is why representations of the whore are almost as ubiquitous as those of the Madonna.

If we look at the nineteenth century again we find that representations of the 'angel in the house' were juxtaposed with those of the 'fallen woman' or the prostitute – the woman who *wouldn't* obey. In the late nineteenth century the prostitute was seen as a scourge on society, a folk devil, a moral imbecile, and representative of the supposed animalistic nature of 'woman'. It was feared that prostitution was spreading like a disease and that no man was safe from desires for the fallen woman. She was positioned as both temptress and avenger (see Chapter Five). As one nineteenth-century commentator declared: 'Who can tell the influence exercised on society by one single, fallen woman? Woman waylaid, tempted, deceived, becomes in turn the terrible avenger of her sex.'[32]

As the British parliament passed laws to control and contain this devil woman (in the form of the 1860 Contagious Diseases Act), artists depicted her fearful form, to fascinate and warn the watching women and men. So art stands both as a product of its time and as a reflection of unconscious fantasies and fears.

Rossetti's unfinished work *Found*, which literally depicts a woman fallen to her knees in front of an upstanding (in every sense of the word) man, epitomizes this genre in its fascination with and condemnation of the 'fallen' woman who was sexual outside the confines of marriage. Rossetti himself described the painting thus:

> He had just come up with her and she, recognizing him, has sunk under her shame upon her knees . . . while he stands holding her hands as he seized them, half in bewilderment and half guarding her from doing herself a hurt.[33]

The fallen woman stands (or lies) in stark contrast to the angel in the house. The latter is represented in nineteenth-century art as upright

and true, whilst her counterpart is literally bent down and bowed. Lynda
Nochlin juxtaposed Rossetti's *Found* with a contemporary painting by
William Holman Hunt, *The Awakening Conscience*, which depicts an
angelic, contained woman, looking upwards and outwards. Nochlin
has described the two paintings as 'opposing visions of a single moral
issue: rising versus falling, salvation versus damnation'.[34] One woman
without hope and one woman filled with faith. One closed off, falling;
the other rising out and up, saved.

But not all representations of the sexual woman show her shamed
or saved. A dominant representation of 'woman' in the masculine gaze
is of the exposure and denigration of the female body and of the
irrevocable connection between 'woman' and 'sex'.

Desire and Repulsion . . . Containing Her Danger through Framing Her Form

> Woman is a temple built over a sewer. Tertullian, pp. 160–225

> Turn thy face from a woman dressed up: and gaze not upon another's
> beauty. For many have perished by the beauty of a woman, and hereby
> lust is enkindled as a fire. Ecclesiasticus, *Holy Bible*

These public pronouncements on the duplicitous nature of 'woman' –
a beautiful façade concealing loathsome sexuality and fecundity – are
possibly the most blatant examples one could find of the conflict between
fear and desire, or lust and disgust. For whilst the image of 'woman' as
perfect, whole and unthreatening might satisfy and reassure, the image
of 'woman' as different, dangerous and uncontained can evoke anxiety
and fear. This is fear of the physical difference which 'woman' represents
– her corporeality, her mess, the 'filth' she is feared to contain within.
Through looking at perfection and beauty, the fear and anxiety aroused
by the knowledge of this difference can be contained. As Françette
Pacteau comments in *The Symptom of Beauty*:

> The beautiful woman, a fleeting image caught in a glance, surrenders for
> an instant, but completely, to the man's desire to annihilate the wounding
> difference. This is an image which has been exorcized of its disquieting
> meaning, and confined to the 'purely visual'; it is an insignificant image,

which is also a screen, a protective veil against the intolerable, the unthinkable.[35]

The 'unthinkable' is that 'man' takes up the position of 'woman', that he becomes the 'second sex'. The unthinkable is also that 'man' is consumed by the voracious sexuality of woman – the sexuality which is denied or refused in representations of the Madonna or the pure, ascetic angel in the house. This threat can be denied or annihilated through literally stripping 'woman' of all defences and depicting her in a naked form. This is why one of the most common images in art is that of the female nude – the art form that has come to act as a shorthand for 'art' itself.[36]

The 'celebration' of the female nude can be traced back to the Renaissance, when the erotic reappeared as a central preoccupation of art. Botticelli's *The Birth of Venus* (1478) is an early example. Initially, these representations of sexuality, and in particular the sexual woman, were all contained within the realm of myth or allegory, thus distancing the artist and the spectator from the sexual fantasies and desires which they reflected. Yet, mythical or not, Botticelli's work stands as an archetypal example of the female nude – that transformation of the unclothed woman from being naked to being 'nude' which has been seen as one of the 'achievements' of high art.[37] As Lynda Nead has argued, it acts to transmute 'the base matter of nature into the elevated forms of culture and the spirit';[38] analogous to the way in which women themselves contain and transform their bodies within the regimes of beauty which are central to the feminine masquerade.

In the archetypal female nude 'woman' is painted lying resplendent and exposed in a formalized, languid pose. She is beautiful and calm as well as passive and sexually available. She is thus disarmed, her danger diluted, her body sanitized. Desire for her can be measured, mastered, but is always in the control of the spectator. He can turn away, and thereby control what he sees. Or he can look for as long as he wants. Unlike the capricious woman in the material world who will not always play out the masquerade, in the sphere of representation she cannot escape his gaze or decide she does not want to be seen. Man can calm himself with her surface beauty and suppress his fear of the horrors that rage within. It maintains the divide between order and chaos, between man and his desire for that which is so dangerous: 'woman'.

The idealized nature of the female nude embodies this process. It frames 'woman' in a way that cancels any intrusions from reality. Her genitals are reduced to a slit, if that. Her body is hairless, innocuous, clean. Both her power and his fear of failure are diminished. This is a transformation of base flesh into idealized beauty which must be repeated again and again. For as Lynda Nead has argued:

> If the female body is defined as lacking containment and issuing filth and pollution from its faltering outlines and broken surfaces, then the classical forms of art perform a kind of magical regulation of the female body, containing it and momentarily repairing the orifices and tears. This can, however, only be a fleeting success; the margins are dangerous and will need to be subjected to the discipline of art again . . . and again.[39]

As with all mechanisms of defence against deep-seated fantasies and fears, the repetition serves temporarily to ward off anxiety, yet at the same time fixes the need for this 'cure' (it is a process we see most blatantly in pornography, as outlined in Chapter Three).

To illustrate the role of art in transforming 'woman' from nature into culture, from chaos into order, a number of critics have turned to a painting produced by Albrecht Dürer in 1538, entitled *Draughtsman Drawing a Nude*.[40] Dürer depicted a draughtsman and his model, the man separated from his muse by a screen divided into squared sections – a symbol of both order and distance. He looks at her through his screen and transposes her image on to his carefully sectioned paper. She is divided, dissected, her blurred boundaries and physicality are transformed through his gaze into order and precision. She represents nature, he represents culture. He is the agent of control; she allows herself to be drawn. Dürer depicts 'woman' as languid, passive, exposed and sexualized (both through the suggestion of masturbation in placing her hand over her vagina and the semi-gynaecological nature of her stance). In contrast 'man' as artist is absorbed and alert, seriously attending to his art. 'Man' sees 'woman', he tames her threat. She is an object to be dissected, not a person to be feared. And in his transformation of her, she becomes an ideal image to be admired and worshipped. It is a picture which stands as a symbol of the regulatory power of art.

In the late twentieth century the female nude is no longer such a powerful cultural icon in art. Modern art has moved away from iconic to abstract representation. Decades of feminist art criticism, post-

modernism and the awareness of artists concerning the mythical significance of their work have taken their toll. The early avant-garde
twentieth-century painters moved away from idealizing the sexual
woman and no longer focused on the nude. Today, when 'woman' is
displayed, either as sexual object or as ideal, the image is as likely to
refute these earlier mythical themes as it is to confirm them. There is
often a knowing irony or a playing with these themes. For example,
in *Laura I* (1984) by Chuck Close we see a blown-up photograph of a
reclining female nude, her body segmented in the manner of Dürer's
nude by the five separate photographic images that make up the whole
frame. Yet this is a vision of 'woman' gazing out openly at the spectator,
a woman who is not shameful or attempting to conceal her exposure.
As we see no artist within the frame, she could be gazing at a woman
or a man. Or take the work of Stephen Spender, who presents the
sexual woman in an apparently realist form, not air-brushed fantasy,
but human flesh. Pendulous breasts and genital hair are not ignored but
luxuriously described. This is more woman as she is rather than how
man might wish her to be.

However, many artists continue in the traditional vein: David Salle,
one of the most celebrated American artists of the eighties, has produced
many images of 'woman' sexually humiliated, naked, bending over
exposing the vulva or anus; Eric Fischel's *Bad Boy* (1981) – a painting
of a naked woman exposing her genitalia to her young son, whilst he
reaches into her purse, a traditional symbol of female genitalia[41] – has
been said to have made his career; Jeff Koons gained notoriety as well
as serious critical attention with garish porcelain sculptures of fragmented
women juxtaposed with pigs in, for example, *Fait d'hiver* (1989), and
then went on to produce multimedia images of himself and his ex-porn-
star wife La Cicciolina in a series of overtly sexual poses. Outside the
hallowed world of 'art' this process of exposure and dissection of woman
continues in pin-ups and page-three girls in British tabloid newspapers
(as well as in pornography). It is also evident in representations of
'woman' on advertising hoardings and in women's magazines, for
women do not have to be naked to be dissected and exposed. Equally,
in film, it is rare for the female star not to expose her body at some
point in the film, regardless of the plot. Those women that *don't* are
notable (often having it written into their contracts). The question is,
why does this process continue, regardless of vociferous critiques?

This turning of 'woman' into a sexualized object has been seen by many psychoanalytically orientated feminist critics as the transformation of 'woman' into a fetish – in Freudian terms, an object on to which sexual anxiety and the fear evoked by the knowledge of woman's difference is displaced by men. Griselda Pollock has argued that 'fetishism as an avenue of escape and a defence mechanism is imposed upon an earlier pre-Oedipal organization of the drives, the component instincts of sexuality, the prime one of which is scopophilia, love of looking.'[42] Freud described the 'love of looking' as a pleasure central to the experience of the infant, who is literally immobile and powerless and can only imagine power and control over others through submitting them to a controlling gaze. And given the gendered segregation of child care, scopophilia would be a pleasure derived from looking at the mother.[43] In adulthood, these fantasies come to be projected on to woman,[44] who stands in the realm of the symbolic as repository of early infantile fears and desires.[45]

The fragmentation of 'woman' into part object rather than whole object in visual representation is a more obvious example of fetishization. In both art and film (as well as popular culture) the vision of 'woman' as idealized beauty is not always seen in her full form. She is often represented as a face or a head; as lips, breasts or legs. She may be literally split into parts, as in the work of Jeff Koons, where truncated portions of the female body are celebrated as art. In a less obviously sexualized manner, artists have for centuries focused their attentions on the face, the worshipped woman incarnated in a smile or an enigmatic gaze. That Leonardo da Vinci's *Mona Lisa* has captured the minds of generations of men is testimony to the power of such an image (her smile also suggesting hidden sexuality or desire). The Hollywood film stills of the forties and fifties continued this tradition. Today, the major focus of worship is more likely to be the breasts:[46] 'Woman' made manageable through reducing her to her most sexually evocative body part, that which is most likely to have been the focus of infantile 'looking' and consequent defensive fetishization.[47] The celebration of female stars with exaggerated breasts perpetuates the notion that body part is all that 'woman' is: Marilyn Monroe in the fifties and sixties; Raquel Welch in the seventies; Pamela Anderson in the nineties.

Depictions of the fetishized female can also act as concrete representations of imaginary phallic trophies, symbolizing masculine power (or

warding off fears that 'man' is powerless). One of the most crude examples in film in recent years was the disembodied woman as fetish shown in the film *Boxing Helena*, in which a woman whose arms and legs have been removed following an accident is literally kept in a box by her possessive lover. Her limbless torso is eroticized: Her sexuality, and therefore her power and danger, are contained within the box, to be taken out at his pleasure. She is both infantile, because helpless, but adult, because sexual and beautiful.[48] Do the men (or women) who enjoy such films realize what fantasies are being played out here?

Deriding the Witch in Woman

> From a male point of view, women who reject the submissive silences of domesticity have been seen as terrible objects – Gorgons, Sirens, Scyllas, serpent-Lamias, Mothers of death or Goddesses of the night. But from a female point of view the monster woman is simply a woman who seeks the power of self-articulation.[49]

> The witch is portrayed in myth as having ferocious sexual energy . . . she is impelled by sexual envy; and she seeks power. She takes the treasure all to herself, and hoards it, giving out nothing to anyone else. She stands for all the worst of the feminine.[50]

The witch is the antithesis of the Madonna. She is 'woman' so imbued with sexuality that her very existence stands as threat to 'man'. She may be seen as a monster or a whore, she may be seen as mad, but her essence is daring to challenge masculine authority, attempting to have a voice of her own.

The myth of Lileth, described in Jewish lore as Adam's first wife, has stood as a metaphor for the witch in woman for centuries, in both art and literature. Legend has it that Lileth believed herself equal to Adam, and so she would not lie beneath him. When Adam tried to force her she flew off in an enraged frenzy, to reside with demons at the edge of the Red Sea. God told her to return but she refused, preferring the punishment of the loss of her demon children to the confines of a patriarchal marriage. She took her revenge on both God and Adam by injuring male babies – a clear symbol of the fear of the devouring mother and of the dangers she can exact on man.

Gabriel Rossetti's painting *Lady Lileth* stands as a classic example of the artistic representation of this passionate, fearful woman and has been subjected to the scrutiny of scholars since its appearance in the late nineteenth century. It is a painting of a beautiful, almost haughty woman whose hand toys with her luxurious long hair as she gazes unsmiling at her own reflection in a mirror. She is engaged and satisfied with herself, not with any male voyeur. She is sexual, dangerously seductive, and does not give the appearance of an acquiescent femininity which will be easily satisfied. The reaction of a contemporary critic demonstrates the power of this picture:

> As Rossetti painted Lileth she appears in the ardent languor of triumphant luxury and beauty . . . the abundance of pale gold hair falls about her Venus-like throat, bust and shoulders, and with voluptuous self applause . . . she contemplates her features in the mirror . . . The haughty luxuriousness of the beautiful modern witch's face, the tale of cold soul amid its charms, does not belie . . . the fires of a voluptuous physique. She has passion without love, and languor without anxiety – energy without heart, and beauty without tenderness or sympathy for other.
>
> F. G. STEPHENS, the *Porfolio*[51]

Here fear of and desire for 'woman' is incarnated in one painting. She is both sexual and selfish, gazing upon herself with satisfaction, symbolizing her rejection of 'man'. She is described as a witch by Rossetti – 'Adam's first wife . . . the witch he loved before the gift of Eve' – so she is not innocent. She is a witch who is cruel and castrating, because she is powerful and strong. The art historian Griselda Pollock has argued that 'the Lileth figure of painting and poem stands for the debased but highly desirable dangerous figure of female sexuality deformed in this representation by the projection of a complex of inconsistent fantasies and fears.'[52]

Another pictorial representation of the fearful, castrating woman is Judith beheading Holofernes, in an ancient legend in which woman is blatantly the aggressor. Judith has been depicted by scores of artists as a merciless, voluptuous woman, exacting her terrible revenge, through implacably cutting off the head of Holofernes as he sleeps. Or she is shown holding his head as a trophy, calmly triumphant with her prize. An analogous image is that of Salome demanding the head of John the Baptist, which is then delivered to her on a platter. All are symbolic representations of women castrating man – wielding the sword herself, or forcing others to carry out her nefarious desires. Shakespeare gives us Lady Macbeth, a witch-like woman with a desire for power who is represented as being so eternally cruel that she would kill her own children:

> LADY MACBETH:
>   I have given suck, and know
>   How tender 'tis to love the babe that milks me:
>   I would, while it was smiling in my face,
>   Have plucked my nipple from his boneless gums
>   And dashed the brains out, had I so sworn as you
>   Have done to this.

It is, arguably, fear of the vengeful mother which is at the root of 'woman' as witch. As Melanie Klein has argued, this fear originates in early relations with the mother, the first woman, who held absolute power over the child and could give or withhold pleasure at will.[53] In fantasy, the child splits the mother into idealized angel and demon witch as a means of coping with the feelings of vulnerability which infantile dependency brings. Karen Horney has seen this as a fear particular to men:

> In the male we frequently find the following residuals of his early relationship to his mother. First of all there is the recoiling from the forbidding female. Since it is the mother who is usually entrusted with the care of the infant, it is the mother from whom we receive not only our earliest experiences of warmth, care and tenderness, but also our earliest prohibitions. A second trait that betrays an unresolved dependency relation to the mother is the idea of the saintliness of woman, which has reached its most exalted expression in the cult of the Virgin.[54]

This splitting of 'woman' into 'angel' or 'witch' acts as a psychic defence against rage, anxiety and fear. The idealized image of 'woman' is protected from such negative emotions, and thus (in fantasy at least) will never retaliate or withdraw. And as we have already seen, the process of idealization serves to annihilate her threat. At the same time, the witch-like 'woman' deserves to be the object of untrammelled rage and, in fantasy, is destroyed (as in all the best fairy tales). There are a plethora of films conveying this message. Film noir provides many classic examples.

Film Noir: The Danger of the Female Sex

> Film noir is a fantasy, as is most of our art. Thus woman here as elsewhere is defined by her sexuality: the dark lady has access to it and the virgin does not ... Film noir is hardly progressive ... but it does give us one of the few periods of film in which women are active, not static symbols, are intelligent and powerful, if destructively so, and derive power, not weakness, from their sexuality.[55]

> Film noir offers us again and again examples of abnormal or monstrous behaviour, which defy patterns established for human social interaction.[56]

The monster in film noir is always the woman. If Hollywood film has traditionally been most notable for its portrayal of hapless, hopeless women, sexually available or nurturing in the home, film noir goes against the grain. 'Film noir' describes a movement in American film-making current during and immediately after the Second World War.[57] Film noir is characterized by a specific set of visual, narrative and iconographic conventions, one of the most dominant being the portrayal of the active, sexual woman. Women are not peripheral in these films, they are central to the drama. But they are not contained within the family or positioned as passive and in need of protection. For this reason, film noir has been seen by some feminist critics not as condemnatory, but as a movement which opens up a space for women which was hitherto unknown, and a space which acknowledges the contradictions inherent within the feminine masquerade.[58]

In film noir the woman is both desirable and dangerous. Here, as film critic Ann Kaplan argues, 'the woman functions as the obstacle to the male quest.'[59] The male hero must overcome his dangerous desire, the lure of the woman, in order to succeed. His success, marked by the destruction of the woman, restores order. His failure to resist marks his own destruction. This is typified by the death of the hero Walter in the closing sequence of *Double Indemnity*. Having killed the husband of the woman he desires, by his own admission 'for money – and for a woman,' Walter demonstrates his inability to resist her lure and pays the price with his own life. He sums up his own position, 'I didn't get the woman and I didn't get the money.' Yet a more common conclusion within film noir is the return of 'woman' to her rightful place – subjugated to man. For example, in *Mildred Pierce*, the strong, dominant heroine who replaces the man in the family, through having both an independent income and autonomous sexuality, is united with her man at the end. The film closes with a symbolic depiction of the rightful role of woman – a shot of two women literally down on their knees, cleaning the floor.

In film noir, the *femme fatale* is contrasted with her opposite, the nurturing Madonna, or 'woman' as redeemer. Ann Kaplan has said of her:

> she offers the possibility of integration for the alienated, lost man into the stable world of secure values, roles and identities. She gives love, understanding (or at least forgiveness) and is generally passive and static.[60]

This 'good' woman is often associated with rural environments or appears in a dream of the past; it is as if her perfection, or her purity, are too intangible to grasp. The man who rejects the safe woman in favour of seething sexuality is doomed. For, in film noir, man either controls (rejects) the sexual woman, or is destroyed by her.

So the male professor in *Woman in the Window* embarks upon an affair with a woman he cannot resist (her sexuality evidenced by the fact that she is already involved with another man) when his family is away and is implicated in a murder as a result. That it is all a dream does not detract from the central message. In film noir the family is a source of sterility, of boredom, but also of safety. Sex, desire, danger and, ultimately, death lie outside the safe family walls.

The style of film noir is central to its effect. It has been argued that 'visually, film noir is fluid, sensual, extraordinarily expressive, making the sexually expressive woman, which is its dominant image of woman, extremely powerful.'[61] Because of this style, the memorable image is not of the woman's demise or destruction, but that of her strong, powerful sexuality. The woman is dominant in the composition of the imagery, seemingly controlling both the gaze of the hero and the gaze of the camera. She is active not static. She is also narcissistic, gazing at her own reflection, not at the man. This can represent her own self-absorption, and thereby her transgression of the feminine role, and her duplicity – 'visually split, thus not to be trusted'.[62] Reminiscent of the fetishized face in the Pre-Raphaelite painting (Lady Lileth gazing at her own beauty) the *femme fatale* of film noir continues a long-held tradition of imagining the unattainable sexuality of woman.

Film noir has been seen as a movement very much of its time – reflecting fears of loss of identity and security and the instability of the post-war period[63] – yet is it very different from the representations of woman pervading film or other forms of mass media today? The mixture of fascination and fear associated with strong female sexuality continues half a century later in films such as *The Last Seduction* or *Basic Instinct*, in which the strong female heroines are the literal undoing of men, killing them after sex, and not getting caught. Yet not all women get away with it.

Fantasies of Possession and the Glorification of Rape

> It is the avid and ambitious desire to take possession of the object for the benefit of the owner or even of the spectator which seems to me to constitute one of the outstanding original features of the art of Western civilization.[64]
>   LEVI STRAUSS

Whilst representations of 'woman' arguably contain her potential danger, sanitizing and simultaneously sealing her seeping sexuality, they also feed fantasies of possession. This possession can take place literally through ownership of art or film (or ownership of a woman who has turned herself into a fetish object made flesh). Or it can take place through possession being depicted within literary or visual representation. Two of the most popular paintings of the late nineteenth century,[65] depicted women enslaved by men, naked and available, scrutinized and examined prior to the man taking control: Jean-Leon Genome's *Oriental Slave Market* and Edwin Long's *Babylonian Slave Market* present woman as slave, man as her possessor. They depict groups of semi-clad, vulnerable women being inspected by clothed, powerful men. An equally celebrated work, Hiram Powers' sculpture *The Greek Slave*, romanticized the capture of woman and reinforced the attraction of innocent beauty easily violated. Depicting a beautiful young woman standing passively waiting, gazing down, chained to a post, it was one of the most popular exhibits at the Great Exhibition of 1851: 'Woman' at the mercy of 'man', to be used (and abused) as he desires. The message of *Boxing Helena* has clearly pervaded art for over a century.

These slave women are not being bought solely as household helpers – they are destined to service their masters sexually. What is implicit in the image of the woman sold as slave is explicit in the representation of rape – a ubiquitous theme in art and film (as well as pornography). It is a strange form of 'entertainment', at least from the point of view of women.

Representations of rape are invariably presented as seductions (reminiscent of romantic fiction, as well as rape law, as we will see in Chapter Five). The woman raped is invariably ripe and ready, her assailant powerfully taking her as his rightful prize. She is the fruit to be picked, succumbing to his overwhelming strength, ultimately helpless in the face of his masculine power. She is usually depicted as struggling, her attempted escape adding a sense of excitement and mastery to man's possession. This is misogynistic rape-fantasy glorified as 'art', as far from real rape as the seduction fantasies that dominate romantic fiction.

Examples of this genre are depressingly widespread. For centuries mythical symbolism in the world of art protected depictions of sex and sexual violation behind the veil of allegorical disguise. An early example, a sculpture from the Hellenistic period (the third century BC) depicts Hermaphrodite struggling with a satyr. In a pose that was to be repeated over centuries in art and film, the woman is seen struggling and resisting, but man's greater physical strength will ensure that she is eventually overcome.[66] There is evidence of erotic representation in medieval art and sculpture, both in church frescoes and in religious art. However, this often stands as a warning against sexual activity, for example, in the case of the fresco of *The Last Judgement* (1303–10) by Giotto in the Arena chapel at Padua, in which four naked sinners are depicted hanging by the part of the body that led to their sin – the tongue, the hair and the sexual organs.[67] Libidinous satyrs assaulting vulnerable women were a common theme in European art – sixth-century Greek images of man as beast revisited in fourteenth-century Europe. Many images show the actual attack – for example, in a painting by Fantuzzi, *A Satyr Assaulting a Woman Defended by Three Cupids* (1542) in which a struggling woman attempts to escape from the grasp of a mythical beast. Or a sculpture by Géricault, *A Nymph being Raped by a Satyr* (1817–29), which needs no explanation – its title says it all. Allegorical representations of anticipated attack show women being led to their rape, for example, in the print by L.D. after Primaticco, *Woman being Carried to a Libidinous Satyr* (1547), which depicts two women carrying another to a waiting satyr who sits with penis already erect. His animalistic desire is juxtaposed with her vulnerable beauty in a timeless, erotic fantasy. A later example, painted by Raphael's assistant Giulio Romano for the Palazzo del Te in Mantua, depicts Jove, disguised as a dragon, preparing to ravish Olympia.

In the late sixteenth century realism became the norm. This was the time when 'woman' as nude came into its own: woman stripped and waiting, lying voluptuously spread for the visual gratification of man. It was only a short step perhaps to the myriad images portraying women being forcibly taken or raped, which range from the coy, for example, *The Bolt*, an engraving by M. Blot (1784), in which a man is shown reaching to shoot the bolt of the door, symbolically signifying the sexual act that will follow, whilst the woman he holds in his arms struggles to escape, to more candid depictions of rape, such as Van Cowenburgh's 1632 painting *The Rape of the Negress*, which shows three white men laughing as they hold down a struggling black woman. One man is naked, holding the woman on his knee, one is half clothed and stands in front of her, and one is fully clothed, presumably waiting his turn. A fantasy of group rape common in today's pornographic literature and imagery: 'Man' demonstrating phallic mastery in front of his competitors, other men. It also represents one of the dominant images of black women in art (and pornography) – as sexual toy for the pleasure of men.

Some rape imagery shows 'woman' symbolically penetrated, through the use of the image of arrow or sword held erect and unyielding. Perhaps the most well-known representation of this is that of Bernini's *The Ecstasy of St Teresa* (1642–52), a sculpture which depicts the unmistakably orgasmic St Teresa lying with her eyes shut, head back, as she is about to be pierced with the symbolic (phallic) arrow of the angel. The same theme is echoed in Titian's painting *Tarquin and Lucretia* (1571), in which the unwilling Lucretia – vulnerable in her nakedness in comparison to her aggressor's clothed invulnerability – is driven back on to a bed as Tarquin thrusts his knee between her legs, holding aloft the symbolically loaded dagger. The spectator can identify with her possessor or with the 'substitute voyeur' who peers at the pair from the side of the scene.[68] Or, masochistically, he (or she) can identify with the violated woman.

Fantasies of Torture and Heroic Saviours

> The male fear of female aggression is matched, and even overmatched
> . . . by sadistic impulses towards women.[69]   KAREN HORNEY

Artists did not stop at objectification and rape in their treatment of women. More savage sadism, more overt evidence of aggressive impulse is illustrated in the images of women tortured or taking their own lives – often by stabbing. Perhaps a precursor to the sexualized torture beloved of certain of today's pornographers and the torture acted out in material reality by sexual murderers, the world of art is littered with examples of woman bound, captured and driven painfully to death.

In the most innocuous representations the woman is merely bound, her rape and torture implied, and in many cases man as hero comes to her rescue. It is a fantasy of phallic mastery and of possession of the fetishized object, who is captured from the clutches of another man (or beast). Here, the heroic man both gets the woman and beats his male competitor. For example, in Titian's *Perseus and Andromeda* (1554) a chained, naked woman is shown being rescued from a dangerous dragon, whose mouth gapes ominously at the strong hero who cleaves the air with his symbolically raised dagger. Yet this painting is not merely about ravishment or man's power over beast with 'woman as his prize'. It is also about what Karen Horney described so clearly: Man's dread of the vagina, the gaping jaws of the beast representing the horror of the 'vagina dentata'.[70] This is man's fear of losing part of himself when his essence, his penis, disappears inside the woman in the act of penetrative sex; he is literally made impotent at the moment of detumescence – '*le petit mort*'. He is stripped of his phallic power. So he faces, and masters, his fear through art.

This horror of powerlessness can be dispelled through vicious penetration. In the case of allegorical art, this is done with the piercing dagger. One example of this genre is Ingres' painting *Ruggerio and Angelica* (1819), in which a chained, naked maiden is saved from a beast by an armour-clad suitor on a winged stallion. Ingres does not baulk at penetration of the mouth of the beast – his rescuing hero plunges his extended lance into the gaping chasm with ill-concealed rancour. This has as its theme both the symbolic representation of the gaping vagina, the hero demonstrating his phallic mastery in front of the helpless and waiting victim, and, potentially, man homoerotically penetrating his sexual competitor, a message disguised by the sexual aggressor being portrayed as beast.

The depiction of the torture of women saints centres the aggression more directly on the woman. There is no need for symbolism here. Piombo's *Martyrdom of St Agatha* (1520) shows two salacious torturers clamping the nipples of a semi-clad female saint with two immense metal pliers. A knife lies in the foreground, both symbolizing phallic power and warning of the attack which is to come. At the periphery, a number of male voyeurs languidly look on at this scene of sexual violation.

It is interesting how little the paraphernalia of torture and the fantasies its depiction may suggest have changed over the centuries. Phallic sticks, vices, ropes, and a ball and chain surround the body of a naked (dead or waiting?) woman in Cagnacci's *The Young Martyr* (1600–81). Her nakedness, her thrusting young breasts and the open nature of her pose (arms bent, legs slightly parted) serve only to intensify the invitation to the viewer she inadvertently offers. This is the fantasy we see in romantic fiction or fairy tales, in which the unconscious woman is 'taken' by the man. In more intensely misogynistic imagery there are echoes of the diabolic machines to which women are attached in a certain section of hard-core porn today. For example, Lelio Orsi's *St Catherine* (1569) depicts a benignly expressioned female saint, stripped and trussed to an unholy wooden contraption, a cross between a rack and a wheel of fortune, whilst a collection of grimacing men – wielding spears, sticks and clubs – regale themselves at her feet. Her near nakedness, her youth and the familiar sensual depiction of her breasts leaves no doubt as to the pleasure that would be gained from her torture.

Is it a coincidence that the women subjected to the most vile treatment in artistic representations are often women who were strong, independent and rejected the rules of 'man'? The martyrs and the saints were women willing to die for their beliefs; they were also women unwilling to submit themselves to the confines of heterosexuality, preferring worship of God to worship of man. For centuries, such women have been punished. That the representations of the saints are eroticized and often express an almost orgasmic fervour in their reactions to torture and immolation (such as in Bernini's *St Teresa*, *St Catherine* and *St Agatha*) is no doubt a reflection of the familiar misogynistic belief that women enjoy forcible sexual attentions (even if they involve great pain). It may also be a reflection of the myth associated with celibate (or lesbian) women for centuries: Any woman who withholds her sexual favours from man is all the more ready to be sexually awakened – 'All she needs is a good fuck.'

These mythical or religious representations of torture are not all centred on women – men are also represented in positions of torture, being murdered or maimed in a sexualized manner. St Sebastian is a favourite; paintings showing his martyrdom through being pierced by scores of arrows are again strongly reminiscent of imagery in sado-masochistic erotica today. The paintings of Caravaggio are perhaps the most well-known examples of this genre. What is notable is that these erotically tortured saints are often depicted in the archetypal feminine pose – passive, gazing obliquely – and they are often androgynous, or feminine, in appearance.[71] The symbolism in the repeated penetration of vulnerable, sexualized man is clear – attack and sexual mastery of the homoerotic, repression of the feminine aspects of 'man'.

Arguably, similar themes are explored in the depictions of gang-rape which populate literature: Man living out his repressed homoerotic desire through penetrating women still warm with another man's sperm. The same process is at work in the desire to possess the woman owned by another man – a symbolic rape or seduction of the man himself. Take this description of the first rape in *The Story of O*:

> She was then drawn to her feet, and they were probably about to detach her hands so as to tie her to some post or other or to the wall, when someone interrupted, saying that before anything else he wanted her – immediately. She was forced upon her knees again, but this time a hassock was placed as a support under her chest; her hands were still fixed behind her back, her haunches were higher than her torso. One of the men grabbed her buttocks and sank himself into her womb. When he was done, he ceded his place to a second. The third wanted to drive his way into the narrower passage and, pushing hard, violently, wrung a scream from her lips. When at last he let go of her, moaning and tears streaming down under her blindfold, she slipped sideways to the floor only to discover by the pressure of two knees against her face that her mouth was not to be spared either. Finally, finished with her, they moved off, leaving her, a captive in her finery, huddled collapsed on the carpet on the floor.[72]

This is another example of rape as entertainment. 'Woman' degraded and fetishized in every way – by her posture (like an animal, or kneeling like a servant), by the penetration of every orifice, by being left in a heap at the end of the 'game'. But this is as much an act of sex between the men as it is a sexual act or exploitation of the woman, an act which for the heterosexual man is amongst the most taboo, as it would threaten his status as 'man' and undermine his difference and distance from 'woman'.

Filming Rape and Sexual Murder

Before the sixties there were few representations of women being raped or murdered in film. 'Woman' was contained primarily through mechanisms of fetishized objectification or through overvaluation. Post-1960s, there has been a rise in the representation of women in active sexual roles and a concomitant increase in representations of women violated. An early example was a film by Michael Powell, *Peeping Tom*, in which a murderous psychopath lures women to their death by asking them to pose as models, and then, while he and the camera capture the woman in the classic masculine gaze – he watches, the camera films – he strikes the fatal blow. Ann Kaplan has interpreted this film as a literal example of how the camera can be used to seduce women: The women are captured, ravished and finally silenced because they want to be looked at, to be the spectacle, they *want* to take up the position of fetish and are punished as a result. It can also be seen as an example of how cinema can act as a reflection of woman's masochism, encouraging her essentially passive identification with the victim, as the women depicted in the film are forced to witness their own murder through a mirror attached to the murderer's camera. Kaplan argues:

> The woman spectator is thus in the position of witnessing a doubly masochistic identification; first, she identifies with the female figure and *her* construction as masochistic spectator; and second, there is her own position in the cinema as spectator identifying with the female victim.[73]

So women lose on two counts. In contrast, the male spectator of the film is always the phallic master, as long as he identifies with the masculine position. As the 'hero' of the film, he is shown watching and murdering; as film viewer he watches the murder in the position of voyeur.

During the seventies a whole host of films in which sexually active women were brutally treated were produced. In Stanley Kubrick's infamous *A Clockwork Orange* women are repeatedly savaged and raped, both by the penis of the anti-hero (whose actual violence towards women is matched by his violence towards men) and by a huge statue of a penis, which is used to batter and beat a resisting woman. A phallic fantasy made ridiculous, by being so unreal, yet still deadly in its effects. In the film the women themselves are shown to be unsympathetic, colourless, cold characters; their brutalization (and eventual death) is seen not as a result of a violent outburst of misogyny but of what Molly Haskell has termed 'a fashionable and fastidious distaste'[74] about all that is feminine. This stands as a direct parallel to rape and violation in art and with the treatment of raped women in the law. In another classic, *Klute*, the heroine's rejection of the feminine masquerade is symbolized by her choice of the life of a prostitute, which maintains her independence and ensures she avoids the emotional trap of falling for a man. Her complete disdain for men is demonstrated by the act of looking at her watch during sex – the man cannot satisfy. 'Man's' fear of impotence in the face of the voracious, rejecting woman is thus made real – so she is raped and murdered. Her murderer, in his final emotional speech, pronounces that she, like all women, deserves her punishment for taunting and arousing him through her base desire for sex – a desire that he sees in all women.

Other films followed, continuing the theme. *Last Tango in Paris* and *Straw Dogs* depicted sexual women raped and abused but aroused by the abuse, perpetuating the myth that all women want to be raped. In the eighties *Dressed to Kill* portrayed a sexually insatiable (and neurotic) woman violently attacked as a punishment for her open desire. *Fatal Attraction* allied madness and sexuality most closely in its representation of a sexually crazed 'mistress' whose obsession with sex and with the good family man finally leads to her brutal end.[75] As she stalks her errant lover, who has returned to the bosom of his wife (the 'good woman'), regretting his passionate affair, he stabs her. Another allegorical phallic attack in which her danger is penetrated and destroyed. It is a moral tale for all who watch. A warning to both women and men.

The fact that these films first emerged during the late sixties and seventies is no coincidence. This was a time of unprecedented change for women, as feminists challenged many of the taken-for-granted roles and rules that had restricted women's lives for centuries. The 'second wave' of feminism[76] resulted in women entering the workplace and the world of education in numbers previously unimagined and rejecting the archetypal feminine role of house and home as their sole mission in life. This was a time of high visibility for the women's movement and a time when changes to family structures brought about by contraception, abortion and less rigid rules around marriage and divorce were starting to have wide social impact, most notably in women's increased autonomy. Arguably, mainstream cinema reflected the deep ambivalence many men were feeling in response to such changes. Lip-service was frequently paid to female liberation; it certainly appeared to have many advantages for men in the sexual sphere, as sexual freedom came to be seen as a sign of a liberated woman.[77] But 'free love' aside, female emancipation was not greeted with open arms – why should it be? Why should those who held the power – in theory if not in practice – give it up without a struggle?[78]

The increase in depictions of sexual violence on the cinema screen was one of the least subtle reactions to this threat to masculine authority. As the restrictive and misogynistic theories of the early-twentieth-century sexologists, including their denunciation of the independent woman as 'sick lesbian', can be seen partly as a response to first-wave feminism (see Chapter Four), it could also be argued that film-makers attempted to contain the threat of female rebellion, which activated pre-Oedipal fears, through visual representation. Man threatened by woman's sexuality fights back in the arena that is the focus of his dread. He hits her in the place he fears most – her sex.

One of the first films to represent this ambivalence most explicitly was *Looking for Mr Goodbar*. It has been described as a film that bridges the transition between the overtly misogynistic films depicting sexual violence which were current in the sixties and the new genre of 'women's films' which appeared in mainstream cinema in the eighties. Released in 1977, it is a film that clearly reflects a cultural milieu which was reeling from the threat posed by the women's movement but which had not yet integrated the notion of female equality into its social structures. For whilst the cinema of the nineties may portray an independent sexual woman as an integrated (or token) part of society, not simply as a 'whore', in the seventies, she was still an aberration.

The heroine of *Looking for Mr Goodbar*, Teresa, works as a caring teacher by day and lives as a sexual free spirit at night – a classic representation of the archetypal Madonna–whore. Teresa seeks 'liberation' through chasing a life which is the antithesis of the feminine role – taking drugs and drink (the lush), living in squalor (the slut) and engaging in sexual relationships with 'unsuitable' men (the whore). Whilst Teresa's behaviour is shown to arise from a motivation to punish her father, who did not love her, rather than from an enlightened position of female liberation,[79] she does stand as a representation of female autonomy – of the woman who has rejected, in psychoanalytic terms, the law of the father. The film celebrates as righteous the anger of men – whom Teresa uses and abuses. She rejects her father through disobeying his rules; she rejects the 'good men' who want to cosset (ensnare?) her in protective monogamy; she rejects the impotent man who is not sexual enough. All express rage, verbally and physically. One calls Teresa a 'cunt'; one (her father) sends her to hell; another wrecks her apartment – the collective rage of 'man' directed at the perilous 'woman'. The denouement is provided by her last lover, George, who completely annihilates her threat – through rape and murder. By stepping out of her allotted role, Teresa courts death and denigration. Man's fear and disgust, his dread of difference and of impotence in the face of that difference, leads inevitably to her brutal end. This is how film critic Ann Kaplan has interpreted this message:

> The nakedness of Teresa's desire together with her insistence on a certain distance (not letting men stay overnight) prove too much for George. He becomes impotent, and then confesses his weak sense of masculinity . . . As his rage accelerates, he jumps on her and begins to rape her; while his rage makes him potent, he still has to kill her for the threat she offers. Phallus and knife coalesce here, the knife simply adding to the phallus instead of . . . standing in for it. The link between Goodbar and the cycle of films showing violence towards women [*Klute*, *Clockwork Orange*, *Last Tango in Paris* (Kaplan's list)] . . . is clear when George shouts as he rapes and kills: 'That's what you want, bitch, right? That's what you want.'[80]

'Woman' attempting to openly own her sexuality, to be active subject not passive object, eschews the protection of one man and courts violation and degradation from all others.

This theme has continued in mainstream film throughout the eighties and nineties. Sometimes the message is crude and clear; at other times it is disguised with a veneer of celebration of female independence and strength. A crude example is that of Martin Scorceses' *Cape Fear*, a misogynistic remake of an earlier Hollywood classic, in which a crazed psychopath convicted of rape takes his revenge on his defence lawyer, and his wife and daughter. The whole subtext of the film is the threat of sexual violence – as the rapist plans to exact the worst punishment he can imagine on his adversary – the sexual assault of his women. The more transgressive the woman, the more violent the attack. So violent rape and assault (including the biting off of her cheek) are meted out to the lawyer's lover – a career woman who lives independently, has an affair with a married man, drinks in a bar on her own and is willing to have 'sex' with a man she has just met (the rapist). That this 'sex' turns into a savage attack – both on her person and on her lover, the lawyer – is the punishment she courts, for she has transgressed. Her attack is also an act of sexual aggression between the two men: the lawyer, her lover, and the rapist, his adversary.

The other two objects of the rapist's attentions are the lawyer's daughter and his wife. The wife is not an image of perfection, as she drinks and criticizes – the archetypal scold. So punishment is again her due. The daughter is both innocent and ripe for a sexual awakening, a paedophilic fantasy made flesh. She is depicted as being infused with desire for her intended attacker as he builds up to his 'seduction'. A repeated theme in art and film – the spoiling of innocence, the turning of Madonna into whore through the awakening of female desire. In the climax of the film, the husband is humiliated, tied and degraded, so he can be forced to watch the rape of his wife and daughter. Here the vulnerability of woman in the face of man's violent passion is reinforced. That the lawyer husband breaks free and saves his women from this fate worse than death, killing his protagonist in the process, serves only to reinforce the belief that woman needs a (good) man to protect her from the dangers of other (bad) men.

These are not isolated examples nor 'minority' viewing – a number of recent films centring on rape were nominated for Oscars.[81] In *Leaving Las Vegas* (which won the Best Picture Award) we see a prostitute gang-raped by a group of college students; in *Rob Roy* the Scottish heroine is raped at knife point by an English fop; in *Dead Man Walking* we see a protracted and detailed rape of a young woman; in *Showgirls* the heroine's best friend is beaten and gang-raped by a man she idolizes and his bodyguards, and *Eye for an Eye* depicts a woman raped and killed whilst her mother listens helplessly on a car phone. A particularly violent rape and murder is shown in *Strange Days*, directed by one of the few successful female Hollywood directors, Kathryn Bigelow, which centres on a man who films the humiliation and murder of a prostitute. This is in many ways reminiscent of the imagery in *Klute*. However, rather than having the murderer make his victim merely watch herself being raped and killed, in *Strange Days* he uses a futuristic device to relay perverse sensations back into the victim's brain.

These themes of rape and sexual violence are not confined to cinematic representations. Some of the most popular television series and programmes appear to celebrate rape and sexual violence towards women in their gory depiction of gruesome murders and attacks. In Britain popular detective series which attract audiences in the millions, such as *Cracker* or *Prime Suspect*, regularly feature stories of rape and murder for lust. The women raped are frequently prostitutes, 'loose women' or women existing outside of man's protection (or control). For example, in a three-part edition of *Cracker* broadcast in the mid-nineties the crime to be solved was that of three women prostitutes who were sexually attacked with a chisel inserted in the vagina, then left for dead. No details were spared. For whom is this 'entertainment'? The women who fear for their lives and believe that rape and sexual violence is rife on the streets as a result? Or the men who might fantasize about such attacks, living out vengeful fantasies by being a voyeur? We don't see the depiction of sexual attacks on men as a regular part of film and television viewing (Tarantino's *Pulp Fiction* contained a male-rape scene, a notable exception). Perhaps it is less likely to be seen as entertainment. It just isn't funny, is it?

The Challenge to the Masculine Gaze: Feminist Art – Subverting the Discipline

Man as Artist: Woman as Muse

> When a Woman inclines to learning, there is usually something wrong with her sex apparatus.   F. W. NIETZSCHE, 1844–1900

> There are no women composers, never have been, and possibly never
> will be . . . Women ruin music. If the ladies are not well favoured the
> men do not want to play next to them, and if they are well favoured,
> they can't. SIR THOMAS BEECHAM, 1879–1961

> The serious intrusion of women into Art would be an irremediable
> disaster. GUSTAVE MOREAU, 1826–98

> No woman can paint. JOHN RUSKIN, 1819–1900[82]

> Literature is not the business of a woman's life, and it cannot be.
> ROBERT SOUTHEY, writing to Charlotte Brontë, 1837[83]

Twenty years of feminist criticism have demonstrated that in art and
film, framed within the masculine gaze, 'woman' is object and 'man'
is subject. She is sexualized and objectified. Her danger is literally framed
and contained within the canvas or the film screen. She is made perfect,
idealized; or she is denigrated, exposed. Her complexity is concealed
through the illusion of exposure of all her parts. However, as the creative
process has been construed as analogous to the sexual act – an act in
which 'man' is assumed to be active and in control – it isn't surprising that
the masculine gaze, and men as artists or film-makers, have dominated for
so long.

Conflating creation with sexuality arguably maintains woman's
exclusion. As Catharine MacKinnon has represented heterosexual sex
as Man Fucks Woman (subject, verb, object), we might represent 'art'
as Man Paints Woman (subject, verb, object). Neither of these scenarios
is inevitably 'true'. But as fairy tales and romantic fiction position 'man'
as sexually active and 'woman' as sexually receptive, the gatekeepers of
'high culture' have traditionally positioned the artist as *naturally* man,
with woman present in this revered sphere only as the object of his
all-powerful sexualized gaze, as his muse. This idea is crystallized in the
comment of one male writer:

> Poetry, the creative act, the act of life, the archetypal sexual act. Sexuality
> is poetry. The lady of our creation, or Pygmalion's statue. The lady is the
> poem; Petrarch's Laura is, really, poetry.[84]

Artists themselves conflate the creative process with sexuality,
accepting and living out the status of sexual god accorded them in the

popular imagination (the fables associated with the sexual lives of Picasso and Dali being the most blatant examples in the twentieth century). Auguste Renoir, asked how he maintained his artistic output despite being crippled with arthritis, declared that he painted with his 'prick'. Whether he was talking literally or metaphorically, he was certainly not alone. The conflation of the artist's brush, the film-maker's camera, as well as the writer's pen, with the penis, is as old as the creative process itself. As one critic commented:

> If a woman lacks generative literary power, then a man who loses or abuses such power becomes like a eunuch – or like a woman. When the imprisoned Marquis de Sade was denied 'any use of pencil, ink, pen, and paper' declares Roland Barthes, he was figuratively emasculated, for the 'scriptural sperm' could flow no longer, and 'without exercise, without a pen, Sade [became] *bloated*, [became] a eunuch.[85]

As creativity is seen as an essentially masculine enterprise, historically, women who have attempted to enter the hallowed halls of creative endeavour have been treated with disdain. Film theory and art history reinforce this process, discussing the creative process in masculine terms. As Lynda Nead has argued:

> the practice of applying paint to canvas has been charged with sexual connotations. Light caresses form, shapes become voluptuous, colour is sensuous, and the paint itself is luxuriously physical. This representation of artistic production supports the dominant stereotype of the male artist as productive, active, controlling, a man whose sexuality is channelled through his brush.[86]

When talking of the 'great' works of art, the term 'old master' speaks for itself. This is not an arbitrary term[87] – as the creators of the old masters were men. The 'masterpieces' we revere are not those produced by the handful of women who have managed to escape penury and prejudice to exhibit creative work over the centuries – they are all by men. That a woman was incapable of creating great art was for centuries unquestioned. As Sir Thomas More commented in the seventeenth century, 'Howe'er man rules in science and in art/The sphere of woman's glories is the heart.' The fact that women who did paint were traditionally considered mere dabblers is illustrated by the comments of this nineteenth-century art critic, who dismissed women's art as trivial 'taste':

> Male genius has nothing to fear from female taste. Let men of genius conceive of great architectural projects, monumental sculpture, and elevated forms of painting. In a word, let men busy themselves with all that has to do with great art. Let women occupy themselves with those types of art they have always preferred, such as pastels, portraits or miniatures . . . those painstaking arts which correspond so well to the role of abnegation and devotion which the honest woman happily fills here on earth, and which is her religion.[88]

This is a view of 'man' as great genius, and 'woman' as painstaking, petty producer of prettiness – a dismissal of women's art that has been repeated across the centuries. For example, over a century later, in the early 1980s, one art critic praised a woman painter for revealing 'none of the needle-threading eye and taste for detail that is the bug bear of women artists when left to their own devices; a preoccupation that invariably favours presentation at the expense of content'.[89] As women's achievements in every intellectual sphere have been dismissed as the result of hard work, not intelligence; luck or the casting couch, not planning or perseverance, in negating women artists (and as a consequence those who might produce a female gaze), the masculine gaze has been allowed to reign supreme.

Women have also had to 'kill the angel in the house' – the creature whom Virginia Woolf described as appearing at her elbow whenever she took up her pen to write, admonishing her to be true to the feminine masquerade – in order to create:

> Directly . . . I took my pen in my hand to review that novel by a famous man, she (the Angel) slipped behind me and whispered: 'My dear, you are a young Woman. You are writing about a book that has been written by a man. Be sympathetic; be tender; flatter; deceive; use all the arts and wiles of your sex. Never let anybody guess you have a mind of your own. Above all be pure.' And she made as if to guide my pen . . . I turned upon her and caught her by the throat. I did my best to kill her.[90]

So it isn't surprising that the gender of the artist is remarked upon when 'greatness' is achieved by (or ascribed to) a woman: They have had to transgress the script of femininity. As the celebrated artist (and teacher) Hans Hofman commented on the work of women artists he admired, 'this painting is so good you'd never know it was done by a woman.'[91] Faint praise, indeed. But it is not the case that 'no woman can paint,' as John Ruskin confidently proclaimed over a century ago, rather that, historically, art which is produced by women has been systematically ignored. Arguably, 'great' women artists *have* existed for centuries[92] – it is just that their work has not always been recognized within the closed, élite, world of 'high art'.[93]

In the early, heady days of second-wave feminism, certain hopeful critics believed that all we had to do was widen the opportunities open to women and they too would produce works of artistic genius, and thus masculine hegemony and the dominance of the masculine gaze would be challenged. For example, in 1973, Linda Nochlin published a controversial article asking the question 'Where are all the great women artists?' She demanded an opening-up of male-dominated institutions in 'the arts' so that women could be given a chance to compete for the label of 'greatness' alongside men.[94] Nochlin – like many other liberal feminists – believed that equal opportunities were the answer to women's invisibility and the absence of positive images of 'woman' in the creative world.

Yet this presupposes that there is something essentially different about the art that is produced by a woman – something that has been bitterly contested by many women artists.[95] For example, the celebrated American artist Georgia O'Keefe, whose paintings of flowers have been interpreted (and celebrated by feminists) as symbolic representations of female genitalia and sexuality, protested that the biological fact of her being female was being seen as more important than her talent or skill as an artist. She remonstrated that two of her male contemporaries who produced flower paintings, Marsden Hartley and Charles Demuth, did not find their work interpreted as erotic or associated with their gender. In contrast, O'Keefe's work was seen as inseparable from her self. As one critic, Paul Rosenfield, commented in 1924, 'in these curves and spots and prismatic colour there is the woman referring the universe to her own frame, her own balance; and rendering in her picture of things her body's subconscious knowledge of itself.'[96]

In many ways O'Keefe was right: Why should she be assumed to produce a 'female gaze' because of her biological sex? But the issue here is not simply about *who* creates representations of 'woman' or 'man', it is about the conscious and unconscious *meaning* of the images that are produced – the perspective and intentions of the artist or film-maker[97] and the interpretations which are made by the spectator. Art and film which is constructed within an explicitly female gaze, or within a feminist frame, arguably conveys different meanings and allows different interpretations about what it means to be 'woman'.

'Feminist' art or film is not one stylistic type or entity; it does not follow one recognizable form or adopt one medium. To talk of feminist art is to talk of subversion, to talk of a challenge to the existing order, the dominant *Zeitgeist* which produces a certain set of fictions about 'woman'. Feminist art is necessarily deconstructive in that it works to question the basis of existing aesthetic norms and values, whilst also extending the possibilities of these codes and offering alternative and progressive representations of what it means to be 'woman'.[98] What feminist artists and film-makers (as well as writers) invariably struggle to do is to create representations of women as active, questioning subjects, not as passive objects or simple projections of 'man's' unconscious fears and fantasies. There is also an attempt to produce a 'female gaze', to represent the world from the perspective of 'woman'. In this way, feminist art stands as a disruption and deconstruction of the 'dominative pleasures of the patriarchal visual field',[99] yet also as a space within which new meanings and new pleasures can be formed. It is an implicit social critique and as such cannot be seen as separate from the social and cultural context in which the meanings it expresses are created. These new meanings take many different forms.

Woman Constructing the Sexual Other: Imagining the Male Nude

Skilled in his art and sexually dominant, the artist . . . is the maker, the female figure both the object of his gaze and the result of his contemplation.[100]

Women artists no longer have either to ape their male colleagues or produce pretty little 'feminine' things. They are free to assert their independent voices – to be quiet or loud, aggressive or introspective, feminist or apolitical – to explore the full range of personal expression or political commitment without being considered insipid weaklings or hysterical harridans.[101]

It is an interesting question: If women dominated the word of art, film or literature, would we see so much emphasis on the female nude, on glorified sexual violence, on male action-heroes? Would we see so much celebration of masculine power, or so much deification of phallocentric heterosexuality? What would be the focus of a 'female gaze'? The most simple answer is 'man'. If the female nude has been viewed as the embodiment of masculine fantasies about 'woman', what better way to subvert this genre than to depict the male nude?

It is only in the last thirty years – a brief moment in time in relation to the long history of art – that women have been producing images of the male nude (two exceptions being Alice Neal and Suzanne Valadon, who painted male nudes in the first half of this century). Yet the women who have painted the male nude have not been simply celebrating or idealizing the sexuality of man – many examples of this genre contain elements of subversion or open parody. Sylvia Sleigh parodied traditional depictions of the female nude in two paintings, *Philip Golun Reclining* (1971) and *The Turkish Bath* (1973). In the former, a woman artist is portrayed sitting upright and in control, contemplating the male nude who lies before her, gazing at his own reflection in a manner which is reminiscent of the female nudes produced for centuries. In *The Turkish Bath* six men lounge in languid, naked splendour in the manner of Manet's naked women or Ingres' harem. In less sympathetic parody, Linda Nochlin mocked the use of women's bodies, and particularly their breasts, as metaphors for fruit or flowers (for example, in Gauguin's painting of *Tahitian Women with Mango Blossoms* (1889), which shows a bare-breasted woman holding a tray of rounded fruit), by photographing a naked man gazing vacantly into the distance whilst holding a tray of bananas. His penis dangles above the bananas in the way that women's breasts seductively brush trays of apples or pears. In a similar vein of parody, the film *Planet Earth* (Marc Daniels, 1974), depicted a post-apocalyptic world in which a tribe of women warriors – the Confederacy of Ruth – have turned men into their servants and sex slaves. It is a play on the most crude form of chauvinism – women are shown leering, treating men as sex objects (an early version of *The Girlie Show*?) and dismissing the very idea of men having views or rights. The Stepford Wives in role reversal – but in this case with each woman having a harem of men.

Yet these images are *not* simple role reversals. Nochlin's *Buy Some*

Bananas shows 'man' as ridiculous and asexual. Sleigh's male nudes are not mere mounds of sexualized flesh, laid out for our pleasure or delectation. They are confident, relaxed, clearly individuals in their own right; not objects, but subjects. Griselda Pollock and Rozsita Parker have argued that 'these contemporary naked men indicate relaxation, athleticism, familiarity, but not sexuality. They belong to a Dionysian or Apollonian tradition.'[102] An image of a man without clothes takes on a different symbolic meaning to a woman without clothes. A passive man rarely serves as an erotic object for women in the same way that a passive, sexually available woman can for men — at least not within the boundaries of traditional heterosexuality. Women's response to 'cheesecake' pictures of passive, naked men in erotica aimed at women (such as *Playgirl*, or *For Women*) says it all:

> 'They're just not sexy, not erotic at all. I can't imagine getting turned on by looking at pictures of a man lying down waiting for a woman to come along. They look a bit ridiculous. Nice bodies, though.'

> 'They just look stupid — with vacuous grins, and a soft penis. I wouldn't mind if they were shown erect and aroused, but they don't look as if they're up to much, do they?'

I have yet to meet a woman who uses such material for masturbation, in stark contrast to men, for whom the passive, splayed woman in soft- or hard-core porn, seems to be the standard masturbatory stimulus (see Chapter Three).

The fact that the passive, splayed *male* nude is not found sexy by heterosexual women, but similar representations of the female nude stand as powerful erotic images for heterosexual men, draws attention to the power difference implicitly deployed in representations of 'woman' and 'man'. Male passivity just isn't sexy for most women; heterosexual women want men to be able to perform. The flaccid penis of the pin-up or the acquiescent obedience of the simple role reversal leads to boredom in bed — 'In full working order, getting a hard-on whenever I want him to, but never challenging my independence or autonomy out of bed,' is how one woman I interviewed described her ideal man. The only arena where we can see a reversal in roles is in the depiction of men as sex objects in the ubiquitous 'sex-and-shopping' novels, where woman is not sexual object but active, striving conqueror, and man is her prey. Yet as with the conquering of the hero in romantic fiction, these are fantasies of women overpowering the strong, phallic man. No fun (or erotic interest) if he's waiting (or wilting) and weak.

It is only in gay male art and photography that this passive positioning of 'man' is explored to the full – such as in the work of Caravaggio, Robert Mapplethorpe, David Hockney, or Gilbert and George – the closest to the male 'nude' (where nakedness signifies sexuality) that we have yet arrived at. That these images disturb the gaze and often invoke strong emotions in heterosexual men[103] is not surprising – they expose, in the field of vision, homosexual sexuality and desire, making heterosexual men face homoerotic desire in themselves. It's not surprising such work is frequently categorized as 'obscene' and banned. Men are not supposed to look at men with a sexualized gaze. But then neither are women.

The outrage expressed by many male critics at the very notion of women taking up 'the sexual gaze' was brought into focus by an art exhibition, 'Women's Images of Men', which toured Britain in the 1980s.[104] It was highly successful as a public exhibition – record attendances were registered. Yet the audacity of women at taking up the role which men had adopted for so long – chronicler of the naked body of the sexual other – appeared to strike deeply at the heart of those sent to pass their expert judgement. One art critic, Waldemar Januszczak, writing for the *Guardian*,[105] dismissed the exhibition for having 'an aura of sensationalism, of penises for penises' sake [which] undermines the savagery with which some of the exhibitors have entered the arena.' Women's depiction of the penis was clearly viewed as an enterprise that could only be motivated by the desire to shock or attack, and thus seen as trivial and unthinking, certainly outside the world of 'art'. Other critics were so incensed they could not hold back their bile, variously describing the exhibition as consisting of 'hysterical overkill', a 'shrill scream of pain and frustration', 'full frontal assaults' and 'nothing but the male organs'.[106] In point of fact, there were only twenty nudes amongst ninety-eight works, with only two focusing on the genitals.

The outrage provoked by these reversals of traditional roles acts to draw attention to the fact that the positions of 'woman' and 'man' in the field of vision are taken for granted. This exhibition cut across the assumption that 'men act and women appear.'[107] If 'men look at women,' and 'women watch themselves being looked at,' as John Berger has claimed, the act of women imagining men as objects of desire is more

than merely subversive, it is catastrophic to those intent on preserving
the status quo, in both the world of art and the material world which
it both reflects and constructs. For as Sarah Kent and Jaqueline Morreau,
two women artists associated with the exhibition, commented, female
depictions of 'man' act to undermine 'carefully protected masculine
myths'. No wonder men were outraged, for 'nobody wants an informer
in the kitchen or bedroom, and as wives, mothers and lovers, women
know far too much about men to be allowed to speak freely.'[108]

Yet the reaction of many women to this plethora of images of men
was very different. Here was a chance to see 'man' as women see him
– a far cry from the phallic action-hero who populates much of art
constructed within a masculine gaze. For here, 'as well as being loved
and respected companions, men were portrayed as dependent and
frightened babies, as persecutors and thugs, as foolish poseurs or objects
of sexual desire.'[109] The very act of revealing 'man' in a different –
often less flattering – light was intended to expose the relationship
between women and men for what it is[110] – a complex balance of power
and powerlessness, desire and nurturing, fear and loathing, admiration
and disgust. A far cry from the romantic myths 'art' traditionally
reinforces.

Women Viewing Woman: Exploring Femininity and Celebrating the Female Form

> If the tradition of the female nude emphasizes the exterior of the body
> and the completion of its surfaces, then women's body art reveals the
> interior, the terrifying secret that is hidden inside this idealized exterior.[111]

The female gaze is not confined to imagining men. Women can also
frame 'woman' within a female gaze, thereby exposing the asymmetry
of power and the restraints within the codes of art which act to regulate
what is produced. In the early seventies feminist artists focused on
those aspects of female experience that had historically been hidden or
ignored in mainstream 'art'. One of the notable examples of this was
'Womanhouse', an avant-garde art installation in an actual house in
Hollywood, opened in 1972, under the direction of Judy Chicago and
Miriam Shapiro, which explored the everyday life of an ordinary
housewife.[112] Chicago described 'Womanhouse' as 'an environment

that housed the work of women artists working out of their own experiences and the "house" of female reality into which one entered to experience the real facts of women's lives, feelings and concerns'.[113] So Camille Grey produced *Lipstick Bathroom*, a mixed-media site painted in bright red, depicting a sink, a mirror and an array of cosmetics and hair rollers; Beth Bachenheimer produced *Shoe Closet*, a mixed-media site which was literally a closet containing rows and rows of shoes (mostly high-heeled); Kathy Huberland produced *Bridal Staircase*, a bride fully bedecked in white veil and dress, who moved down a garlanded staircase:

> The bride is portrayed as an offering – encased in lace, flowers, and dreamy sky blue. As she descends the stairs the blue slowly changes to grey. The bride's failure to look clearly where she is going leaves her up against the wall.[114]

Sandy Orgel produced *Linen Closet*, a model of a naked woman half in and half out of a closet filled with folded sheets. Orgel explains, 'As one woman visitor to my room commented "This is exactly where women have always been – in between the sheets and on the shelf." It is time now to come out of the closet.'[115] *Nurturant Kitchen*, by Susan Frazier, Vicki Hodgetts and Robin Weltch showed a typical fifties kitchen, with models of breasts lining the walls; Judy Chicago's *Menstruation Bathroom* was a bathroom containing a bin overflowing with used sanitary towels. The artist described the room as 'very, very white and clean and deodorized – except for the blood, the only thing that cannot be covered up. However we feel about our menstruation is how we feel about seeing its image in front of us.'[116] *Leah's Room* by Karen LeCoq and Nancy Youdelman showed a performance of a woman continually applying layers of make-up as she sits in front of a mirror. The artists described this as:

> the pain of aging, of losing beauty, the pain of competition with other women. We want to deal with the way women are intimidated by the culture to constantly maintain their beauty and the feeling of desperation and helplessness once this beauty is lost.[117]

This representation of the 'unspoken' aspect of women's lives (minus lesbianism, which was still omitted) and the exposure of hypocrisy behind the feminine masquerade through art produced by women, from an explicitly female perspective, has had an inordinate influence on both artists and the art audience. It provided an inspiration for succeeding generations and directly challenged the view of 'woman' and women's lives that has traditionally been depicted within so called 'high art'. In the late eighties, a similar project was conducted in England, in the Nicolas Treadwell Gallery in Womenswold, Kent,[118] a converted mansion with a series of rooms depicting women's representations of their lives. On both sides of the Atlantic, legions of individual women artists have continued to explore the meaning of being 'woman' through art and performance work. As Arlene Raven has commented, reflecting on 'Womanhouse' over twenty years later, ' "Womanhouse" held the raw, explicit expression of an incipient feminist sensibility that has, to this day, provided a source and reference for a tradition of innovative and socially concerned contemporary art made by women.'[119]

It was also in the early seventies that a number of notable feminist artists started to subvert the positioning of the female as a central unquestioned motif in 'art', by portraying vivid, explicit images of the internal secret side of female sexuality, in particular the female genitals. To expose or celebrate the hidden aspects of female sexuality was seen by many as an act of reclamation of the body. For example, Judy Chicago's *Red Flag* depicted the removal of a bloody tampon – pushing the boundaries of the acceptable to what many would claim was the limit. Here, the interior of the woman was revealed, in all its gory glory; thus, the function of art as containment of 'woman' and her seeping boundaries is subverted. Other work which Chicago produced was more symbolic, including *Female Rejection Drawing*, an abstract image which metaphorically suggested the vagina, a theme repeated many times over in her celebrated monument to women and their achievements *The Dinner Party*. Completed in 1978 and exhibited to thousands of people in both Europe and North America, it was the result of the efforts of over a hundred women and consisted of an equilateral triangle, each side forty-eight feet long, symbolizing a dinner party, where places were set for thirty-nine influential women past and present (including such luminaries as Virginia Woolf). Each place setting contained a ceramic plate decorated specifically for the particular woman who was being honoured – a cup, and a brightly coloured needlework runner, decorated individually. Many of the decorations on the plates were unmistakably symbolic representations of female genitalia. For this reason, this work is at risk of entering the realm of the 'obscene'.

One example of this was the treatment of the work of Susanne Santoro, who had embarked on a critique of the idealization of the female nude in classical art and sculpture, which she saw as a symbol of the colonization of women's bodies and the annulment of their sex. In *Towards New Expressions* (Rome: Rivolta Feminine, 1974) she entreated women to take control of their own sexuality. Santoro juxtaposed images of vulvic flowers, shells and the female clitoris with those of Ancient Greek figures as a means of exploring and demystifying the reality of women's sexuality and thereby exposing the way 'woman' has been misrepresented in traditional art.[120] In 1976 Santoro's book was banned by the British Arts Council from an exhibition in which it was supposed to take part on the grounds that it was 'obscene', therefore not 'art'. The point of departure from the hallowed boundaries of art was the self-avowed claim of the artist that the work act as a 'plea for sexual self-expression' – grounds for censorship in the eyes of the gatekeepers of artistic merit. 'Art' has served this same purpose for male artists for centuries, without any question (Picasso and Dali being two obvious examples) and without the artist being cast to the outside, 'beyond the boundaries of art'. As Lynda Nead notes, 'the problem it seems is not so much sexual self-expression but *female* sexual self-expression.'[121] It is more than ironic that in the same exhibition from which Santoro's work was banned, exhibits by Allen Jones showing women in degrading poses were displayed: as furniture (*á la Clockwork Orange*, with 'woman' on hands and knees as a table); as fetishized fantasy, dressed in leather, with whips, stocks and phallic stilettos, genitals *naturally* all concealed. 'Woman' as fetish or sexualized object is obviously not 'obscene'; woman's self-expression of sexuality is. No ambiguity about whose values are at work here. The same process operates in the nineties, where sexually explicit work by the lesbian photographer Della Grace has been banned from bookshops as 'obscene', as was the lesbian erotic magazine *Quim* before its premature demise.

Women's body art is a further example of the reclaiming of the sexual body of 'woman' by feminist artists. Body art literally centres on the use of the female body *as* art – invariably the artist's own body. It has been claimed that body art acts to subvert the masculine gaze, allowing women to becoming speaking subjects as opposed to mere objects of the gaze. It also prevents the fetishization of the female body, for the woman artist is herself in control. Lynda Nead has argued that:

> whereas with painting or sculpture the viewer is able to relish the object at his chosen speed, to carry out repeated examinations and to select viewing positions, the mobility of the performance artist prevents this colonization of the female body. She . . . determines the way she is experienced by her audience and, in this way, takes control of her own image.[122]

Body art has taken the form of photographic, mixed-media or painted representations of the female body, as well as the form of performance art. It was seen very much as fringe, but has recently become mainstream. In 1995 one of the four shortlisted candidates for the art world's prestigious Turner Prize in Britain was the artist Mona Hatoum, whose work consisted of a camera travelling inside her body, exploring the forbidden insides of 'woman', as we see her cervix, vagina and the inside of her arteries. In the same month, Annie Sprinkle, an ex-porn-star turned performance artist, could be seen at the ICA, a mainstream London art venue. Her previous performances had included audience viewing of her cervix through a speculum. In this show she demonstrated a self-induced orgasm onstage.

Women's body art can act to subvert expectations by presenting images of women who are not perfect commodities, women who do not enact the traditional feminine masquerade. For example, the British artist Jo Spence photographed her own naked body both before and after her diagnosis of breast cancer, going on to create a photomontage history of her invasive lumpectomy treatment. Graphic images of her disfigured breasts parodied the traditional treatment of the feminine sexual body in a series of images that were both moving and satirical. Her explicit aim was to 'make visible in public the taboo subject – the unhealthy and aging female body'.[123] In a similar vein Mary Duffy, a performance artist with no arms, used her naked body to 'confront issues of gender, representation, disability'. By provoking reaction to their difference, these women violently confront us with the knowledge that the female body that is represented in art is the perfect, whole, young body – an image that is rarely representative of the bodies of 'real' women.

Yet this celebration of the female body is not without its detractors.

It could be seen to reify the connection between 'woman' and biology, the age-old association between woman and nature – the connection that artists such as Georgia O'Keefe have eschewed. Feminist art historians and critics Rozsita Parker and Griselda Pollock have argued that vaginal iconography is dangerous, as it 'merely perpetuate[s] the exclusively sexual identity of women, not only as body but explicitly as cunt'.[124] In this view, the conflation of 'woman' and sexuality inherent in more traditional art forms is not broken but reinforced by feminist body art, allowing easy co-option of the imagery and the possibility of its being read as supportive of the long-standing view of woman as sexual object to be conquered and owned. As nothing but a body.

It is true that in other contexts vaginal iconography has a very different meaning. The splayed genitals in a pornographic magazine, the detailed depiction of the Japanese courtesan – face and cunt – in the Vaginal albums of the Ukiyo-e tradition (a guide to the woman, her price, her attributes and her location for the desiring man), are strongly reminiscent of the sexual imagery adopted by many feminist artists. The artist may be a woman, the intention subversion rather than titillation, but is this intention enough to prevent sexualized objectification? Does it not depend on the reading of the imagery by the spectator? Those taking a masculine subject position may not distinguish between the 'gynaecological' porn festooning the pages of *Hustler* magazine and subversive feminist art. Both may be dubbed 'obscene', providing titillation rather than subversion. The context in which they are displayed signifies their different meaning – a privately viewed porn magazine and an art gallery are very different spheres of representation. But the distinction is not always made.

The same critique has been levied at the exposure of the transformation of 'woman' through the feminine masquerade which is at the centre of the work of photographer Cindy Sherman. She has produced an extensive series of untitled self-portraits showing 'woman' in various guises – Madonna, whore, angel, slut. The style is reminiscent of Hollywood film stills – 'woman' frozen, part object, perfect and manicured – as well as presenting us with apparent realism, catching women unawares. That all these photo-narratives are of the same person is startling – Sherman remoulds herself in every guise woman can adopt, dramatically illustrating the falseness in the masquerade of beauty celebrated in traditional 'art', film and photography (and the mass media):

It is rarely 'natural' or uncontrived. Jo Spence has conducted a similar critique of both femininity and social class with her photographic self-portraits of 'woman' as mother, daughter, bride and victim.[125] As both subject and object of their own art, like many other feminist artists and photographers, Sherman and Spence undermine the notion that women cannot be active in the creation of modes of representation. Yet to the unknowing viewer are Sherman's photographs anything other than 'sexy'? As the critic Jeff Perrone commented:

> Sherman poses herself in Playboy-like centerfolds, albeit clothed in little school-girl outfits that make her appear both withdrawn and New Wave, seductive and scared – a punk virgin waiting to get laid. I think some people (men) like it so much because some critics and collectors (men) like a little blonde served up in juicy colour. That her photographs are ostensibly about female representation in popular culture seems beside the point, not to mention evasive. Her work is, from the consumer's point of view, having your cheesecake and eating it too.[126]

Yet as critics Norma Broude and Mary D. Gerrard counter in their excellent anthology *The Power of Feminist Art*:

> Perhaps as a result of post-modernism's denunciation of essentialism, the only acceptable way remaining for post-70s women to represent themselves appears to be in slightly ironized versions of the old familiar images of femininity – i.e. as sex objects and victims – that have been traditionally devised by and for men.[127]

Sherman is thus reframing the archetypal image of 'woman' within a knowing female gaze. However, whilst these images might be meant as ironic critique, as Jeff Perrone points out, it is not inevitable that they will be interpreted so. In the same way that a woman who knowingly dresses herself in the fetishistic garb of stilettos, stockings and suspenders may claim she is making a post-feminist statement about her ability to *choose* to masquerade as sex object, but a man may see her *as* sex object, we cannot predict or proscribe the reading of a particular vision of 'woman'. It depends on whether we take up a masculine or feminine position as spectators or viewers, whether we position ourselves as 'woman' or 'man'.

Cindy Sherman's work translates women's knowing manipulation of the feminine masquerade into 'art'. That some will interpret it differently from the way in which Sherman intends should not surprise us – is this not the very point that is being made? For as is the case with the practice of femininity itself, those who take up the positions of 'woman' and 'man' often make very different readings of the performance: Women see themselves as '*doing* girl'; men appear to believe that women *are* girl (which is exactly what the careful masquerade sets out to achieve). Neither is more 'true' – it is simply that the world is viewed through a different, gendered gaze.

Post-modernism and Feminist Representation

Post-modernism has also inspired a more abstract form of feminist art, which requires some understanding of feminist theory, and of psychoanalysis, in order to interpret its meaning.[128] For example, Mary Kelly exhibited a mixed-media work, *Post-Partum Document*, in London in 1979, which addressed the position of women in male-dominated culture and the oppressive nature of dominant social constructions of female sexuality. Drawing on psychoanalytic conceptualizations of the mother–child relationship,[129] Kelly produced a six-section, 165-part work, which chronicled the early relationship between herself and her son. She challenged the concept of 'art' through documenting this mother–child relationship not through visual representation, but through fragments of text, diaries, objects (such as nappies/diapers), feeding charts and faecal stains – each mounted individually. Kelly's work directly challenged myths about motherhood, documenting the way in which women are expected to *know* instinctively about children and the difficult process of child-rearing. It was a direct challenge to archetypal images of Madonna and child.

For example, in one section, *Weaning from the Breast*, she charted the anxieties and tensions inherent in the process of weaning through the traces of faeces on nappy liners accompanied by clinical feeding charts. Kelly argued that 'the normal faeces is not only an index of the infant's health but also within the patriarchy it is appropriated as proof of the female's natural capacity for maternity and childcare.'[130] Kelly intended to expose the judgement made upon woman as mother, through the juxtaposition of the hard, excreted evidence and the medical charts which express the difficulty of the weaning process. Other sections dealt with the relationship between the mother, child and father, the mother's fears, fantasies and fetishization of the child (her focusing on part of the child or on objects as means of gaining gratification), and the feelings of loss which underlie our knowledge of sexual difference. The importance of language in the development of her son's sense of himself as 'I' and his consequent adoption of a masculine identity was indicated by fragments of text depicting her son's first words, his adoption of language and her diary reactions at this time. Through these, the invisible work and worries of mothering were made visible, legitimated as works of 'art', and the complex relationship between mother and child was explored. Kelly thus set out to undermine the notions of naturalness and instinct implicit within dominant ideologies of motherhood.[131]

Another example of women's art influenced by psychoanalysis and post-modernism is that of Barbara Kruger, who used photographic images juxtaposed with fragments of text to deconstruct mass media and advertising imagery. In representations which subvert the power of art and the gaze, Kruger draws attention to the notion of masculine control of language and representation. One example is that of a woman's head, in profile, juxtaposed with the text, 'Your gaze hits the side of my face.'[132] Other work in this vein includes the photo-histories of Annette Kuhn documenting her childhood and her relationship with her mother;[133] the video and photographic work of Valerie Walkerdine, where themes of class and femininity are explored;[134] and the photo and text installations of Laura Simpson, where issues of race and gender are explored. These and the legions of other feminist artists explore what it means to *be* 'woman' from the perspective of those who are attempting to negotiate the feminine masquerade. It is a rich and varied field, as Broude and Gerrard indicate in their citation of recent feminist work in the US, which I will quote at length, as it illustrates the breadth and range of what could be characterized as a 'female gaze':

> Lynne Yamamoto's autobiographical sculptures, Polly Apfelbaum's fabric constructions, Nicole Eisenman's wall drawings, Liz Larner's soft knots and wax forms, Deborah Kass's appropriations of Andy Warhol, Erika Rothenberg's politicized greeting cards, Lorraine O'Grady's race conscious performances and portraits, Sue Williams's visceral renderings of female victimization, Janine Antoni's body works, Karen Finley's subjectively-female performances, Beverly Semme's clothing sculptures,

Catherine Opie's cross dressing portraits, Andrea Fraser's museum interventions, Susan Silas's conceptual works, Zoe Leonard's photographic explorations in museography, Marlene McCarty's text-based canvases, Holly Hughes's lesbian-explicit performances, Rona Pondick's psychologically-suggestive body sculptures, Ilona Granet's billboards for abortion rights, Cheryl Donegan's video send-ups of Abstract Expressionism, Patty Matori's domestics of violence, Lauren Szold's floor spills, Ann Hamilton's feminization of the Protestant work ethic, Ashley King's female confessions, Marilyn Minter's portraits of sex and food, Mary Weatherford's floral paintings, Carrie Mae Weems's photographic documents of identity, Ava Gerber's feminized, sculpturized assemblages, Catherine Howe's interrogations of painterly styles and imagery, Rachel Lachowitz's works in lipstick, Julian Scher's surveillance monitors, Jessica Diamond's wall paintings, Annette Kapon's bathroom-scale comment on assemblages, Kay Rosen's word plays, Millie Wilson's *Museum of Lesbian Dreams*, Chysanne Stathacos's hair paintings, Kiki Smith's bodily forms, Sadie Benning's youthful videos of lesbian love, Cady Noland's Patty Hearst, Robin Kahn's embroidered fabric pieces, and Kathe Burkhardt's 'bad' paintings.

As Broude and Gerrard conclude, 'All of these artists incorporate an understanding of women's experience – and of women's historic devaluation and cultural exclusion – in their works': Evidence enough (if we still need it) that women *can* create; and that there can be an alternative to the masculine gaze.

In a different vein, in an attempt to challenge ownership of the gaze, a number of feminist artists and photographers have deliberately refused the notions of authorship and originality in their work. Sherrie Levine has repainted and rephotographed major works of modernist art – the paintings of Kasmir Malevich, Egon Shiele and Vladimir Tatlin and the photographs of Walker Evans and Edward Weston – and has exhibited them as her own, deliberately undermining the concept of a work of 'art' as the original output or property of one man. Levine does not pretend that she has produced an 'original' image. She deliberately sets out to draw attention to the emphasis placed on original self-expression in art appreciation and valuation, highlighting the fact that this process is a reflection of patriarchal values, as 'originality' and 'subjective expression' are almost inevitably seen to be the property of men. As many of the 'original' photographic prints (which Levine was sued for 'copying') would not have been actually produced by the named artist himself anyway – in the same way that many paintings attributed to the great masters may have been produced by their pupils – it could be argued that Levine's prints are in reality no different from those which have existed for centuries.[135] What she *is* doing differently is making clear the process of creation, and deliberately drawing attention to the question of ownership of artistic genius. Levine's work has been embraced by many critics as the emblem of an era of post-modernist deconstruction and radical critique,[136] which undermines the notion of art as commodity.

However, this process can work against the female artist, who would otherwise benefit from the post-modernist disempowerment of the 'great master'.[137] For if fame, canonization and public celebration of the artist and her work and positioning of art as commodity becomes politically incorrect in the post-modernist era, women's work runs the risk of remaining anonymous and invisible. So rather than celebrating the 'death of the artist', feminist critics such as Luce Irigaray have deemed post–modernism 'the last ruse of patriarchy'; or, as Craig Owens suggests, merely 'another masculine invention to exclude women'.[138] This is perhaps why Sherrie Levine has latterly claimed that her own work *can* be seen as commodity, and why she has criticized the way her (male) critics have praised her work only as emblem of deconstruction: It means they can overlook her artistic talents.[139]

Feminist Film as Counter-Culture: Avant-Garde Feminist Film

Semiotic and psychoanalytic theory has also been used in a series of avant-garde films[140] which both examine the position of 'woman' within the phallocentric sphere and, through drawing attention to their own cinematic process (preventing complete suspension of disbelief), make the spectator aware of the role of cinema itself in perpetuating woman's positioning as 'other'. For example, Laura Mulvey and Peter Wollen's *Riddles of the Sphinx* (1976) broke new ground in dealing with mother–daughter relationships. Taking the mother's position as the starting point of analysis, the film used Jacques Lacan's notions of the imaginary and the symbolic to explore the ways in which the voice of the mother is traditionally silenced, and then looked at the way in which a mother attempts to find a voice in a symbolic order that has no place for her. It was a film which involved a direct exploration of the 'law of the father'.

Sigmund Freud's Dora (Tyndall, McCall, Pajaczkowska & Weinskock, 1979) further developed the exploration of both the position of woman within the symbolic order (outside) and the role of psychoanalysis in maintaining this position. Through an examination of the case of Dora, the young woman accused of hysteria after a series of events, including an attempted seduction by her father's friend, the film depicts the way in which 'man' speaks and 'woman' is spoken about. In a dramatization of his case notes, Freud speaks about Dora, placing her sexuality and her distress within a phallocentric framework where Dora has no voice of her own, even when she speaks herself – illustrated by the device of her adding 'she said', or 'she confirmed' to each of her responses. The place of 'woman' as site of multiple and contradictory meanings within the sphere of representation is examined through the juxtaposition of images of 'good' and 'bad' women as seen in advertisements and pornography – each positioned in relation to the male gaze. The absence or repression of the mother within traditional psychoanalytic analyses of Dora's case is highlighted through Dora's writing a series of letters to her mother. Avoiding what many have seen as a masculine obsession for closure and answers, Dora poses a series of questions, but does not attempt to answer them.

Sally Potter's *Thriller* worked within a similar theoretical vein, examining how classic narratives construct and represent 'woman' and how a male model of creativity works to exclude the female voice. Her more recent film, *Orlando*, took Virginia Woolf's novel of the heroine who changed sex from man to woman to man and back again as a means of examining the relationship between gender, creativity and desire. *Amy!* (Laura Mulvey & Peter Wollen, 1980) also explored the theme of women's exclusion from masculine culture and language, but focused on 'woman's' position in the mass media, through the story of Amy Johnson, the first woman to fly the world solo. The film explored how her enormous achievement, and as a consequence her threat, was contained and dismissed – through her representation as 'cute' in popular music, and the psychoanalytic notions of substitution of career for love which pervaded stories of her in the popular press.

This may all seem potentially heavy going for those outside the élite world of post-structuralist theory. Yet what these films illustrate are the ways in which critics steeped in feminist film theory have moved beyond deconstruction, beyond the apparent doom-ridden analysis presented by Lacan, Barthes and the like, to produce films which both reflect their critical theories and attempt to move into a new territory, beyond the traditional spheres of representation they so vociferously condemn. Whilst Ann Kaplan may be being too optimistic in her conclusion that such films will become more accessible as the theories on which they are based reach a wider audience, these avant-garde films stand as an important milestone in the sphere of feminist resistance.

The Response of the Mainstream: Films for Women

One of the most evident consequences of two decades of feminist critique is the apparent change in the representations of 'woman' available in the mainstream. I say 'apparent' because the traditional objectification and blatant misogyny have not disappeared. But there has been a notable development of films *for* women which differ from the romantic, chocolate-box fantasies deemed suitable for female viewing in the unenlightened pre-feminist era of cinema. No longer is a 'woman's film' inevitably expected to be a tear-jerker or a happy romance (although such films continue to exert influence and maintain a loyal following). Women can be shown outside of the narrow confines of the role of Madonna or whore and can take up the traditionally masculine subject position without being destroyed (as was the case in film noir).

One way in which this genre evolved was through the use of documentary films, which were deliberately polemical and addressed the concerns of the second wave of feminism head-on. In many, the values inherent in traditional film were exposed through a revaluing and viewing of previously ignored aspects of women's lives: women sewing (*The Song of the Shirt*), women's ambivalence in their relationships with each other (*Daughter Rite*), women carrying out vaginal examin-ations (*Self Health*), women talking about their own lives (*The Women's Film: Three Lives*).[141] These films attempted to 'reconquer' spaces pre-viously colonized – through, for example, allowing women to see in detail the cervix, the vagina and the details of a vaginal examination, providing information about the body previously unknown to many women (many were surprised at the size and shape of the cervix in *Self Health*). Other documentary films contain a wider political message. *Not a Love Story* deals with the controversy surrounding pornography; *Taking Our Bodies Back* with the health-care system. All took on the same role as the conscious-raising groups of the seventies – exposing women's oppression and moving towards enlightenment.

This detailed depiction and revaluing of women's lives is a theme repeated in a number of feature films made subsequently – for example, women cooking and following an exacting domestic routine (as well as engaging in prostitution) in *Jeanne Dielman* (Chantal Akerman), or the family relationships of a young woman living in Northern Ireland in the seventies in *Maeve* (Pat Murphy). The relationship between sisters is explored in *Marianne and Julianne* (Margarethe von Trotta). Hollywood followed suit, cashing in on the newly recognized audience, the 'modern' woman. The spate of films aimed at women in the seventies and eighties includes *Alice Doesn't Live Here Any More* (1974), *Girlfriends* (1978), *Gloria* (1980), *Nine to Five* (1980), *Lianna* (1982) and *Fried Green Tomatoes at the Whistle Stop Café* (1991). There have also been a number of films which centre on the mother as a strong woman, such as *Distant Voices Still Lives*, directed by Terence Davies, or *The Piano*, directed by Jane Campion. Other mainstream films which grossed large profits at the box office contained female heroines who in many ways broke the previously restrictive mould: Carrie Fisher as Princess Leila in the *Star Wars* series, Sigourney Weaver in the *Alien* series and Linda Hamilton in *Terminator II*, being some of the most well-known examples.

There have also been a number of examples of explicit subversion of traditional representations of a narrow feminine role. In *Thelma and Louise, the* women's road movie of the late eighties, female friendship and solidarity between two strong, rebellious women form the core of the film. Thelma and Louise are two women fighting back – literally – as they leave their previous existence, which centred on men, and travelled across North America together. They have more fun together than they did with any man.

The fairy-tale theme which predominates in Hollywood films was deliberately parodied in *Muriel's Wedding*, an Australian film which tells the tale of an unhappy young woman, Muriel who is desperately looking for a man (as all girls are). She is cast out by the other girls, in the manner of Cinderella and her ugly sisters – except that these girls are beautiful; they have no trouble getting a man (or at least sex with a man – the form 'getting' takes today). Muriel does everything she can to achieve her aims (changing her appearance, behaving in the way 'nice' girls do), but is only able to get a man to marry her by agreeing to a marriage of convenience – her handsome 'prince' is a South African swimming star who needs her nationality to compete internationally. He falls in love with Muriel. She leaves him in order to live with her best friend. The film ends with the two women singing as they drive off in a taxi together. The moral of the modern fairy tale: It's better to have a good time with the girls?

In another recent parody, *Clueless*, where 'doing girl' is both celebrated and ridiculed – the heroine, Cher, is a rich and beautiful high-school girl, an expert player in the game of feminine wiles and attraction, who transforms her ugly-duckling classmate through a skilfully executed 'make-over' – there is a more traditional 'girl gets boy' ending. The twist is that the boy that is 'got' is the 'boy next door' (in this case, the son of one of Cher's father's other marriages), who has seen the 'real girl' under her mask of beauty and carefully executed sexual ploys. This film is perhaps the cinematic equivalent of teenage girls' magazines – openly acknowledging the way in which young women believe they have to '*do*' girl' in order to attract a man and the disdainful attitude towards young men who are fooled by this masquerade. However, at the same time, there is a frustration that boys do not bother; in one scene, Cher comments on the unattractive appearance of the majority of the high-school boys, who wear sloppy clothes, have greasy hair and still expect to get the girl. The only boy she fancies turns out to be gay. That Cher ends up with a boy who is both 'nice', attractive, and who knows her for who she really is (as she wasn't trying to impress him with her beauty or charms) is a subversive message indeed: It suggests that whilst girls might *enjoy* shopping, clothes, being beautiful or playing out the feminine masquerade, they should acknowledge it for the game it actually is, and that 'true love' comes with a man who loves her for herself. We could read this as merely an updated version of the traditional fairy-tale story (or an update of Jane Austen's *Emma*), but there is a power and a pleasure in the deliberate 'doing' of femininity in this film, which puts the masochism and self-sacrifice of the likes of Cinderella to shame.

Lesbian Desire in Film: Exploring Forbidden Fruit

> Whatever is unnamed, undepicted in images, whatever is omitted from biography, censored in collections of letters, whatever is misnamed as something else, made difficult-to-come-by, whatever is buried in memory by the collapse of meaning under an inadequate or lying language – this will become, not merely unspoken, but unspeakable.[142]

Another interesting challenge to the notion of 'woman' as inevitably frozen in the gaze of 'man' is the representation of lesbian sexuality and desire in mainstream film. Prior to the twentieth century, few of the images of 'woman' produced *by* women have had explicit erotic intentions, due to the suppression of the lesbian voice or view. Notable exceptions – such as the poetic work of Sappho – stand out as rarities in a symbolic sphere which is almost exclusively heterosexual. Until the seventies, lesbianism was entirely invisible in film – it was deemed a 'perversion' by Hollywood between the thirties and sixties. So when Lillian Hellman's play *The Children's Hour* was filmed in 1936 as *These Three*, the 'lesbian secret' which formed the centre of the play's narrative was transformed into heterosexual adultery.[143] The cross-dressing of Marlene Dietrich in *Morocco* or of Greta Garbo in *Queen Christina* was the nearest to transgression of heterosexual femininity that film-makers dared to show.

In the seventies, this was all to change. On the one hand, a number of 'coming-out movies' portrayed lesbian existence from the perspective of lesbians – for example, *Getting Ready* and *Greta's Girls* (1978). When mainstream film took up the lesbian motif, a very different picture emerged. One example was the film *Black Widow*, which tracked the relationship between a female detective, Alex, and a *femme fatale*, Catherine, who marries men for their money and then murders them – the proverbial black widow. Catherine transforms herself into the ideal woman that each of her husbands desires – alternately playing girlie, cute, challenging or intellectual, depending on each man's weak spot – an obvious exposure of the shallow nature of the feminine masquerade, used very blatantly to trap and ensnare 'man'. Yet the *real* desire and tension in the film runs between the two women. And whilst lesbian sexual activity is not explicitly acted out, merely hinted at, overt themes of female identification and shifting notions of gender and power are played out within the story. Both women have sex with the same man – as close to an erotic connection with each other as they can get without crossing the forbidden divide.

Explicit desire and sex between women featured in *Basic Instinct*, the film that had gay lobbyists out in force in protest at the representation of a lesbian as murderer. Catherine Trammell (notoriously played by Sharon Stone), the anti-heroine of the film, was a strong, affluent, intelligent woman, who flaunts her sexuality and her desire for both women and men, yet always stays in control. She implicitly challenges the feminine script: She does not respect any boundaries, she is power incarnate – yet she also epitomizes female desirability, a desirability which does not result in her being contained or condemned. Lesbian sex is represented as glamorous and exciting – certainly not sickness or second-best – coinciding with the ubiquitous media image of the lipstick lesbian in the early nineties. In both *Black Widow* and *Basic Instinct* the 'Catherine' character is reminiscent of 'woman' as witch, the modern-day Lileth, who poses only danger for 'man'. What elevates both women above the status of whore and consequent derogation by man is their social class – they are rich, stylish women whose attractiveness is increased by this fact.[144] Money can't buy you love, but it can buy you out of whoredom. In these incarnations of 'woman' as witch, their desirability and danger is doubled by their sexuality being outside of the control of man. This eroticized representation of the dangerous lesbian has been more explicitly played out in vampire films, where the lesbian vampire both pleasures and murders her lovers: In *The Vampire Lovers* the lesbian seductress Carmilla brings her female victims to orgasm before she pierces their throats; in *Vampyres* we see female vampires murdered by enraged men because they are lesbians; in *The Hunger* the female vampire (played by Catherine Deneuve) is impossibly attractive and seductive, to both women and men.

Whilst *Black Widow*, *Basic Instinct* and *The Hunger* showed the 'lesbian' character also sexually engaged with men, a number of mainstream films have been released which directly challenge the assumed presence of heterosexual desire. In *Desert Hearts* two women are shown gradually falling in love and lust with each other, their desire as real and powerful as that traditionally shown between women and men. It was a film which used many of the traditional narratives of a Hollywood love story; it was only the fact that the sex and love were between two women that set it apart from the established norms for romantic narrative. For this it has received some criticism,[145] and it is certainly not as challenging as many of the films in the avant-garde tradition. But are lesbian women to be denied the pleasure and suspension of disbelief heterosexual women take for granted in their viewing of film? This pleasure has been explored in a series of smaller budget and less widely seen 'lesbian films', such as *I've Heard the Mermaids Sing*, *Lianna*, *Clare of the Moon* and *Go Fish*: Women desiring women being celebrated, not condemned. And by the very fact of showing 'woman' as sexual and desirable outside the boundaries of phallocentric sex and romance, acting to challenge the unquestioned normality of the heterosexual 'original' and the position of 'woman' in relation to 'man'.

Black Women: A Different Voice?

Whilst we might now see the odd appearance of lesbianism, in Anglo-American film and art, 'woman' is still predominantly white. Black women have been absent from art and film confined within an archetypal masculine gaze, and have also arguably been left out of many 'feminist' analyses or critiques. Traditionally, in both art and film, the black woman has been represented as sexualized, as slave, or as 'Black Momma' in the home: In *Gone with the Wind*, we saw the Momma; in *Hallelujah*, *Porgy and Bess* and *Carmen Jones*, we saw the seductress; in recent years we see black women engaging in exotic, almost circus-like acts – Tina Turner in *Mad Max: Beyond Thunderdome* and Grace Jones in *A View to a Kill*. Spike Lee's *She's Gotta Have It*, whose central character is a sexually empowered black woman is one exception, but has been criticized for depicting a black woman as promiscuous and as learning to enjoy a sexual attack. (However, the choice of camera angles and position holds all three men in *her* gaze, placing her in the dominant position.)[146] *The Color Purple* portrayed strong black women as central characters, showing violence, sexual assault and victimization alongside female solidarity, as did a more recent film, *Boys on the Side*, a female 'road movie', where one of the three central characters is black. Yet these films could be criticized for presenting us with stereotypes: *The Color Purple* and *Boys on the Side* show lesbianism, 'black mommas' and violence. Hollywood's female stars still remain almost solely white women.[147]

There are a growing number of black women artists, who are challenging the dominance and superiority of white culture and its representations of 'woman' in their production of Black Art. In the introduction to the catalogue of 'The Essential Black Art' exhibition, which took place in London in 1988, Rasheed Araeen argued:

> Black Art, if this term must be used, is in fact a specific historical development within contemporary art practices and has emerged from the joint struggle of Asian, African and Caribbean people against racism, and the art work itself . . . it specifically deals with and expresses a human condition of Afro-Asian people resulting from . . . a racist society or, in global terms, from Western cultural imperialism.[148]

There have been a number of exhibitions featuring the work of black women. In London in 1981 there was an exhibition, 'Four Indian Women Artists', and in 1982 'Between Two Cultures' and 'Five Black Women' focusing on the work of black and Afro-Caribbean women. In the United States, the work of native American women was exhibited in a 1985 exhibition 'Women of Sweetgrass, Cedar and Sage', and in a 1988 exhibition 'Autobiography: Her Own Image'. Many individual women artists continue in this vein. So the viewing of 'woman' within a western imperialist frame is also beginning to be challenged.

The Death of the Masculine Gaze?

Anyone who is aware of the dominant representation of women in mainstream film and literature must welcome these new gazes, as women are represented as central and are often strong and heroic. Yet it isn't time for us to stop being critical. When Hollywood adopts feminist imagery, any serious ideological critique is inevitably watered down, as commercial success is the aim. It is also arguable that as the women represented in many supposedly enlightened Hollywood films are not ordinary in any way, their success can be attributed to their superhuman powers. Charlotte Brunson has argued that the problems women face in the new Hollywood version of the 'women's film' are individualized, thereby distracting attention away from the overall oppression of women as a group.[149] A cynical view might be that it is only the existence of a receptive, paying audience that motivates Hollywood film directors and promoters to accede to feminist critics – it is the mighty dollar that speaks, not the conscience. For every *Thelma and Louise* with women living independent lives, there is a *Cape Fear* with woman terrorized and assaulted, sex object and victim. For every *The Piano*, depicting a strong resilient woman, there are films such as *Misery*, *The Hand that Rocks the Cradle* or *Single White Female*, portraying woman as monster incarnate, destroying both children and men. In Hollywood 'woman' is still portrayed as sex object, either as idealized, fought-over 'girl' (for example, in *The Mask*, or *Batman Returns*) or as voracious 'post-feminist' seducer – most notably in *Fatal Attraction* or *Disclosure*, where it is man who is positioned as victim of female sexual harassment.

The archetypal masculine gaze isn't a thing of the past, and it isn't only present in art and film – we see it in literature, in the mass media, in every form of representation produced and consumed by men. Sometimes it is positioned as humour or irony, and criticism can be warded off. When asked to justify his representations of sexually humiliated women, the artist David Salle stated tersely that they were 'irony'.[150] Art critics supported this view. Of one of his pieces of work, *Autopsy* (1981), which showed a naked woman sitting on the side of a bed, wearing a dunce's cap on her head and on both her breasts, the critic Donald Kuspit wrote, '[this] is to stimulate, not critically provoke – to muse, not reveal.'[151] Feminist critic Mira Schor expounds a more cynical view: 'Salle's work was an act of gender revenge, conscious or unconscious, perhaps against the loss of total centrality which by all rights a talented young male artist might feel entitled to and would have enjoyed in any art school.'[152]

After twenty years of feminist critiques of art these images cannot be 'unknowing'. Deeming them 'ironic' merely legitimates a sexualized masculine gaze, which is arguably being celebrated as part of the backlash against feminism and as an assertion of phallocentric hegemony in a world where masculine power is increasingly being questioned. Is this why a crude masculine gaze still proliferates in mass media imagery aimed at men? For example, in the British comic *Viz* we see representations of two overweight, voraciously sexual women in *The Fat Slags*, who lurch through life frightening and sexually devouring men. This is sold (and bought) as 'humour'. Or the advertising images of a buxom model in a Wonderbra, with the inscriptions 'Hello Boys,' 'Are you just pleased to see me?' or 'Don't worry, they're with me.' This is not supposed to be 'sexist' but 'cute and funny' (so says the photographer, Ellen von

Unwerth) – images of a powerful sexual woman with a knowing 'post-feminist' gaze.[153] But do men read it as such? As one critic, Carter Ratcliff, has said of the sexualized depictions of nude women by the artist David Salle, 'to see his paintings is to empathize with his intentions, which is to deploy images in configurations that permit them to be possessed.'[154] Is this very different from the traditional image of the female nude, who permits a fantasy of possession on the part of the spectator? The only difference today appears to be that 'woman' is more likely to be portrayed as being humiliated as part of this possession, apparently legitimating the ascription of ironic intent by creator and critic alike.

Representations of supposedly strong women within the mainstream may not be particularly emancipatory, but may merely serve the function of inoculation. For example, when we see the strong intelligent heroine – the paleobotanist researcher in Spielberg's film *Jurassic Park* – we might falsely assume that this reflects a world in which men and women are judged equal in intelligence and strength, a factor influencing many women and men in their (erroneous) belief that we are now in a 'post-feminist' era, and therefore that the aims and claims of feminism are now redundant. These 'strong women' may also serve the same purpose as the acting out of anger against men in romance – providing a safety valve for women's frustration,[155] thus providing inoculation against any *real* resistance. For whilst it is clear that women *are* active in resisting the narrow restrictions of the feminine masquerade, we are still a long way from the position where we can say that we have freedom to decide what being 'woman' means to us. For centuries, women have been severely sanctioned for stepping out of line, for daring to challenge phallocentricism at all, those who stand up and declare themselves 'feminist' more so than any others.

This is not just since the so-called 'feminist backlash' of which Susan Faludi has written began. Take the 'Rokeby Venus' incident: On 10 March 1914 Mary Richardson, a suffragette, concealed an axe upon her person, walked into the National Portrait Gallery in London and in front of horrified observers repeatedly slashed the painting *The Rokeby Venus* by Velazquez.[156] Her action was ostensibly carried out in protest at the government's treatment of Emmeline Pankhurst, who was being force-fed as a result of her hunger-strike protest at the fact that women did not have the right to vote. Yet this incident came to be seen in the minds of art critics and public alike as the epitome of monstrous feminist rejection of the hallowed world of art[157] – a desecration of what is most venerated. It was certainly not coincidental that this act of vandalism was directed at a female nude. Richardson was protesting at the objectification of 'woman' in more ways than one. The 'Rokeby Venus' incident and the attendant anti-suffragette propaganda that it served to polarize stand as early examples of the strong reactions provoked when women dare to resist.

The reaction to Richardson's protest was arguably out of all proportion to the scale of her actions (the painting was not destroyed and stands in the gallery to this day). There was a public outcry. The gallery was closed, and Richardson was vilified as an example of all that was evil and unruly about women – in particular, feminist women. She was described as a 'wildwoman', who was captured whilst hacking at the painting in a 'wild frenzy'.[158] Her actions proved an ideal target for those whose intention was to warn *all* women – the ugly caricature of 'feminism' serving the same purpose as the caricature of 'lesbian' propagated in legal and sexological dictates to this day – ensuring women remained in their 'proper' feminine role. The depiction of Richardson as animalistic harks back to Darwinian theories of woman as closer to nature, and consequently as both more bestial and uncontrolled than man. It was a view reinforced by the pictorial depiction of the suffragettes as ugly, coarse, harridans.[159] These images have much in common with the physiognomic diagrams popularized by Conrad Lorenz, who claimed to be able to distinguish criminals by their facial features. This anti-suffragette imagery with the 'flushed expressions, wild gestures, and cognate lapses from womanly decorum'[160] exposed a deviant femininity, all propriety lost, the woman fallen as far as woman could fall. Lisa Tickner has argued that what this imagery serves to do is 'give feminism a sexual pathology which makes it a 'law and order problem', not only for the interests of the Empire and the state, but at the deepest levels of sexual identity.[161] The feminist was not really 'woman'. She could therefore be dismissed, and her dismissal act as a warning to all women. This is not dissimilar to many of the negative stereotypes of 'feminism' perpetuated by 'backlash' propaganda today,[162] which ensure that few women adopt this label to describe themselves, despite their avowal of 'feminist' principles.

Similar vilification of overt feminist critiques has continued across the century. Take the case of Kate Millett, who with her ground-breaking book *Sexual Politics*, published in 1970, pursued the connection between man's representations of 'woman' and women's place in a patriarchal world. Millett documented the explicit sexual representation of 'woman' in male writing, focusing on D. H. Lawrence, Henry Miller, Norman Mailer and Jean Genet, ensuring that we could no longer read explicit descriptions of heterosexual sex without being aware of its ideological intent – the intention to position 'woman' as cunt, as hole, as object to be fucked. Whilst her book was an international bestseller, it provoked outrage on the part of many of the accused. Norman Mailer published a vitriolic attack in his own defence, in his book *The Prisoner of Sex*. He described Millett's style as 'suggestive of a night-school lawyer who sips Metrecal to keep his figure, and therefore is so full of isolated proteins, factory vitamins, reconstituted cyclamates, and artificial flavours that one has to pore over the passages like a business contract. What explosives are buried in those droning clauses . . .'[163] Emotive reactions to the worm who has turned. Masculine hegemony is not given up easily.

Equally, the work of feminist artists continues to be marginalized in the mainstream art institutions. As Mira Schor has documented, in the eighties 'major national and international exhibitions routinely excluded almost all women.'[164] Paranoia? This is her case:

> The *Zeitgeist* exhibition in Berlin in 1982 included only one woman, Susan Rotenberg. 'Documenta 7' in 1982 included 28 women to 144 men, 'Documenta 8' in 1987, 47 women out of 409 artists! The 1985 'Carnegie International' included 4 women to 42 men, the 1988 exhibition included 10 women to 42 men. In June 1984 the Museum of Modern Art reopened its enlarged facilities with an exhibition 'An international survey of painting and sculpture'. Of the 164 artists chosen, only 13 were women.[165]

In response to this continued marginalization of a female voice, a campaign was launched in 1985 by the self-styled 'Guerrilla Girls – Conscience of the Art World', consisting of a series of posters that were plastered all over New York's Soho, which drew attention to the sexism still inherent in the art world. Two 1986 posters declared 'ONLY 4 OF THE 42 ARTISTS IN THE CARNEGIE INTERNATIONAL ARE WOMEN' and 'THE GUGGENHEIM TRANSFORMED 4 DECADES OF

SCULPTURE BY EXCLUDING WOMEN ARTISTS.' A 1987 poster
headed 'THE ADVANTAGES OF BEING A WOMAN ARTIST' listed the
following:

WORKING WITHOUT THE PRESSURE OF SUCCESS

NOT HAVING TO BE IN SHOWS WITH MEN

HAVING AN ESCAPE FROM THE ART WORLD IN YOUR FOUR FREE-
LANCE JOBS

KNOWING YOUR CAREER MIGHT PICK UP AFTER YOU'RE EIGHTY

BEING REASSURED THAT WHATEVER KIND OF ART YOU MAKE, IT
WILL BE LABELLED FEMININE

NOT BEING STUCK IN A TENURED TEACHING POSITION

SEEING YOUR IDEAS LIVE ON IN THE WORK OF OTHERS

HAVING THE OPPORTUNITY TO CHOOSE BETWEEN CAREER AND
MOTHERHOOD

NOT HAVING TO CHOKE ON THOSE BIG CIGARS OR PAINT IN
ITALIAN SUITS

HAVING MORE TIME TO WORK AFTER YOUR MATE DUMPS YOU
FOR SOMEONE YOUNGER

BEING INCLUDED IN REVISED VERSIONS OF ART HISTORY

NOT HAVING TO UNDERGO THE EMBARRASSMENT OF BEING
CALLED A GENIUS

GETTING YOUR PICTURE IN THE ART MAGAZINES WEARING A
GORILLA SUIT

The response of the art world? The Leo Castelli Gallery declared,
'There is absolutely no discrimination against good women artists.
There are just fewer women artists.'[166] In a similar vein, in 1990, the
critic Paul Schjeldahl commented, 'What there are now, after feminism's
long march through the art culture, are more and more top women
sculptors, photographic artists, and artists of installation and performance
. . . But no truly great painters. Is it biology? The very suggestion seems
sexist, but what if it happens to be true?'[167]

So over a hundred years later, we still seem to be harking back to the sentiments of Ruskin. However, perhaps it is more true to say that 'No woman who challenges the masculine gaze is easily allowed entry into the world of "high art".' In a phallocentric sphere, we should not be surprised to find that what threatens to unthrone or subvert the archetypal masculine gaze is denigrated or dismissed. The very fact of its being unsettling because it exposes the fantasies and fears at the heart of dominant representations of 'woman' will lead to it being excluded or marginalized within what is still a masculine domain. 'Woman' being depicted from the perspective of those who are expected to act out the feminine masquerade is perhaps too much of a challenge to heterosexual masculine hegemony. It exposes as artificial and constructed what is supposed to be 'natural' and unquestioned – the power of 'man' and the passivity and sexual vulnerability of 'woman'.

NOTES

1. Berger, John, *Ways of Seeing*, London: Penguin, 1972, p. 47.
2. Mulvey, Laura, 'Visual Pleasure and Narrative Cinema', *Screen*, 16 (3) pp. 1–16.
3. I cannot examine *all* art and film framed within the masculine gaze. I am taking a selective journey through the dominant representations of 'woman' and female sexuality in work which mostly has Anglo-American origins (touching on similar themes in European art). See Mellencamp, Patricia, *A Fine Romance: Five Ages of Film Feminism*, Philadelphia: Temple University Press, 1995, for an analysis of feminist critiques of film over the last few decades.
4. Literature and poetry are also considered 'high culture' and have also been subjected to feminist critiques. In this context I am focusing on art and film because they are pervasive media open to a wide public gaze (not confined to the literate or 'chattering' classes); because women have been historically excluded from the creation of art or film, whilst for centuries women have been able to write; and because, arguably, in recent years at least, women are one of the major audiences for literary representations of 'woman', particularly with the rise of the 'woman author'. For feminist critiques of literature see: Humm, Maggie, *Feminist Criticism*, Brighton: Harvester, 1986.
Warhol, Robyn R. & Herndl, Diane P., *Feminisms: An Anthology of*

Literary Theory and Criticism, New Brunswick, NJ: Rutgers University Press, 1995.

K. K. Ruthven-Canto (ed.), *Feminist Literary Studies: An Introduction*, Cambridge: Cambridge University Press, 1996.

5. Seiter, E., Borchers, H., Kreutzner, G. & Warth, E. M., *Remote Control: Television, Audiences and Cultural Power*, London and New York: Routledge, 1991.

6. Mulvey, 1975.

7. Men literally dominate the film industry, even in the late nineties.

8. Mulvey, 1975, p. 11.

9. The 'gaze' of the artist is essentially masculine – traditionally it is men who paint. Within the artist's frame, the woman is always looked at, rarely looking. And dominant representations of women in art are those which are pleasing or satisfying to men.

10. Quoted by Pam Morris, *Literature and Feminism*, Oxford: Blackwell, 1993, p. 13.

11. This is not to say that all men see women in this way, or that there is only one gaze. However, there are a number of dominant themes which can be identified and tied to conscious and unconscious fears and fantasies of man.

12. In western art at least.

13. The same process was taking place in North America. See Banta, M., *Imagining American Women: Ideas and Ideals in Cultural History*, New York: Columbia University Press, 1987.

14. Nead, Lynda, 'The Magdalen in Modern Times: The Mythology of the Fallen Woman in Pre-Raphaelite Painting', in Betterton, R., *Looking on: Images of Femininity in the Visual Arts and Media*, London: Pandora, 1987.

15. See Pollock, G., *Vision and Difference: Femininity, Feminism and Histories of Art*, London: Routledge, 1988, Ch. 6, for a detailed analysis of the significance of Rossetti's paintings.

16. See Berger, 1972.

17. Milton, quoted by Gilbert, S. & Gubar, S., *The Madwoman in the Attic: The Woman Writer and the Nineteenth-Century Literary Imagination*, New Haven: Yale University Press, 1979, p. 21.

18. The feminist critics Sandra Gilbert and Susan Gubar have seen this novel as a good summary of the 'philosophical background of the angel in the house'.

19. Eichner, Hans, 'The Eternal Feminine: An Aspect of Goethe's Ethics', in van Goethe, J. W., *Faust*, Norton Critical Edition, Walter Arndt (trans.), Cyrus Hamlin (ed.), New York: Norton, 1976, p. 620. Quoted by Gilbert & Gubar, 1979, p. 22.

20. Haskell, Molly, *From Reverence to Rape: The Treatment of Women in the Movies*, New York: Penguin Books, 1974.

21. Homosexuality was officially deemed a 'perversion' in Hollywood between the 1930s and 1960s.

22. Horney, Karen, 'The Dread of Woman', in Horney, K., *Feminine Psychology*, H. Kelman (ed.), London: Norton (first published in 1932), 1967, p. 136.

23. Ibid., p. 142.

24. Ibid., p. 143.

25. Persons, Ethel S., *Dreams of Love and Fateful Encounters: The Power of Romantic Passion*, New York: Norton, 1988, p. 265.

26. I am talking here about desire in the context of heterosexual relationships. In gay male relationships the object of desire would be a man and, arguably, fears of merger would be directed towards men.

27. Pribam, Deirdre (ed.), *Female Spectators. Looking at Film and Television*, London: Verso, 1988, p. 1.

28. Horney, 1967, p. 60.

29. See Martin, Emily, *The Woman in the Body: A Cultural Analysis of Reproduction*, Milton Keynes: Open University Press, 1989; and Ussher, Jane M., *The Psychology of the Female Body*, London: Routledge, 1989.

30. Benjamin, Jessica, *Bonds of Love: Psychoanalysis, Feminism and the Problem of Domination*, New York: Pantheon, 1988, p. 106.

31. See Chodorow, Nancy J., *Femininities, Masculinities, Sensualities. Freud and Beyond*, London: Free Association Books, 1994, p. 59.

32. Mayhew, Henry, 'London Labour and the London Poor', p. xxxix. Quoted in Nead, L., *The Female Nude: Art, Obscenity and Sexuality*, 1992, p. 82.

33. Letter from Dante Gabriel Rossetti, 30 January 1885, to Holman Hunt, cited in Nochlin L., *Women, Art and Power and Other Essays*, London: Thames & Hudson, 1988, p. 58.

34. Nochlin, 1988, p. 67.

35. Pacteau, Françette, *The Symptom of Beauty*, London: Reaktion Books, 1994, p. 62.

36. Nead, L. 1992, p. 1.

37. Kuhn, A., *The Power of the Image: Essays on Representation and Sexuality*, London: Routledge, 1985, p. 11.

38. Nead, L. 1992, p. 2.

39. Ibid., p. 7.

40. See ibid., p. 11, and Berger and others.

41. Schor, Mira, 'Backlash and Appropriation', in *The Power of Feminist Art: Emergence, Impact and Triumph of the American Feminist Movement*, Norma Broude and Mary D. Gerrard (eds.), New York: Harry N. Abrams, 1994, pp. 248–63, p. 251.

42. Pollock, 1988, p. 148.

43. Classically, fetish objects have been women's shoes, legs, underclothes, or silk and fur. It isn't surprising. These are the objects which become eroticized because they are associated with the early infantile phase of discovery of woman's difference. Because of this, these objects elicit anxiety; yet through mastery of them, through their use in a sexual scenario, man can disavow the knowledge of his own dread and fear. So reaching arousal and climax with a woman's shoe gives a temporary illusion of control and wards off anxiety about separation, merger and loss of identity. See Kaplan, Louise J., *Female Perversions*, London: Penguin, 1991.

44. Many have argued that if the early carer were not a woman, these fantasies would not be directed solely at the female sex and would not be manifested in misogyny. Shared parenting between women and men has been advocated as a result. Yet this has not (yet) come about. Even if it did, generations of men now in adulthood have experienced this relationship with woman as mother and continue to project their fears and fantasies on to women (and 'woman') in adult life.

45. Kaplan, Ann, *Women and Film. Both Sides of the Camera*, London: Methuen, 1983.

46. Even the anodyne Madonna is depicted with infant at breast, her role as mother legitimating this bodily exposure. In film the tradition continues, with greater exposure of the breast gradually taking place over the century, from the titillating fantasy produced by 'stars' such as Marilyn Monroe or Jane Russell in the fifties and sixties, where the gaze of the camera focused on the cleavage, to the almost mandatory exposure of full-frontal naked breasts by the modern female star.

47. The other sexual fetishization is the focus on the genitals in the realm of the obscene – porn.

48. This could also be seen as an example of infantile rage directed at the mother, acted out in the fantasy of dismemberment of this woman.

49. Gilbert & Gubar, 1979, p. 79.

50. Holbrooke, David, *Images of Women in Literature*, New York: New York University Press, 1989, p. 160.

51. *Portfolio*, May 1984, pp. 68–9. Quoted by Pollock, 1988, p. 141.

52. Ibid., p. 144.

53. See the work of Melanie Klein or Donald Winnicott for descriptions of this.

54. Horney, 1967, p. 126.

55. Place, Janey, 'Women in Film Noir', in *Women in Film Noir*, Ann Kaplan (ed.), London: BFI, 1980, pp. 35–68, p. 35.

56. Harvey, Sylvia, 'Woman's Place: The Absent Family of Film Noir', in Kaplan, 1980, pp. 22–34.

57. It has been suggested that the film-noir period was short, running between *The Maltese Falcon* in 1941 and *Touch of Evil* in 1958. See ibid.

58. Kaplan, 1980.

59. Ibid., Introduction, pp. 1–5, p. 3.

60. Ibid., p. 50.

61. Place, in Kaplan, 1980, p. 36.

62. Ibid., p. 47.

63. Ibid., p. 37.

64. Quoted by Berger, 1972, p. 84.

65. Powers' sculpture *The Greek Slave* was a huge success at the Great Exhibition of 1851, and Long's *Babylonian Slave Market* fetched what was then a record price for a work of art. Genome's painting *Oriental Slave Market* is an example of a popular genre. See Lucie-Smith, Edward, *Sexuality in Western Art*, London: Thames & Hudson, 1991.

66. The 'seduction' of woman was certainly not the only sexual fantasy represented in art of this period. Proud, powerful phalluses, active sexual congress between man, woman and beast (in all possible combinations) and vivid depictions of the naked female form were commonplace during this time, as the Victorians found to their chagrin and horror when excavating the remains of Pompeii, where the volcanic tomb had preserved what had elsewhere been destroyed during centuries of puritanical religious fervour. See Kendrick, Walter, *The Secret Museum*, London: Viking, 1987.

67. See Lucie-Smith, 1991, p. 34.

68. Ibid., p. 192.

69. Ibid., p. 239.

70. Ibid., p. 212.

71. Ibid., p. 216, for a discussion of this.

72. Réage, Pauline, *The Story of O*, London: Corgi, 1980, pp. 10–11.

73. Kaplan, 1983, p. 74.

74. Haskell, 1974, p. 362.

75. The original director's cut of *Fatal Attraction*, re-released in 1993, had a different ending, in which it is the husband who pays the price for his adulterous sexuality, as the family is split up and the mistress survives. The version presented to the cinema audience in the 1980s was a much more moral tale.

76. The first wave in Europe and North America occurred at the beginning of the nineteenth century. See Humm, M., *Feminisms: A Reader*, Hemel Hempstead: Harvester Wheatsheaf, 1989, for accounts of women at these different stages.

77. In retrospect, many feminists have challenged this 'freedom', seeing it as yet another means of objectifying women, turning them into sexual objects to be used and abused, this time under the guise of 'free love'. See Segal, Lynn, *Straight Sex: The Politics of Pleasure*, London: Virago, 1994.

78. This is not to suggest that all men are in power over all women – the situation is clearly more complicated than that. However, in a patriarchal society, the structures are set up to support male interests and maintain certain groups of men in positions of power.

79. See Kaplan, 1983, p. 79, for a psychoanalytic reading of this film, which accounts for Teresa's behaviour in terms of rejections and rivalries.

80. Ibid., p. 81–2.

81. In 1996.

82. Morgan, Fidelis, *A Misogynist's Source Book*, London: Jonathan Cape, 1989, p. 165.

83. Quoted in Gérin, Winifred, *Charlotte Brontë: The Evolution of Genius*, Oxford: Oxford University Press, 1967, p. 110.

84. Quoted by Gilbert & Gubar, 1979, p. 13.

85. Gilbert & Gubar, 1979, p. 10.

86. Nead, 1991, p. 56.

87. In the way that those incensed by 'political correctness' would cry that the use of the generic term 'man' (as in 'history of man', 'chairman') to

refer to the human species is a linguistic device, not an example of sexism or the systematic exclusion of women (a point with which I would naturally disagree).

88. Sir Thomas More, 'Du rang des femmes dans l'art', *Gazette des beaux arts*, 1860. Quoted in Parker, R. & Pollock, G., *Old Mistresses: Women, Art and Ideology*, London: Pandora, 1981, p. 13.

89. McEwan, John, 'Beleaguered', *Spectator*, 9 September 1978. Quoted by Parker & Pollock, 1981, p. 7.

90. Virginia Woolf, in a lecture to the National Society for Women's Service, 21 January 1931. Published posthumously in *The Death of the Moth*, London: Hogarth Press, 1946.

91. Chadwick, Whitney, *Women, Art and Society*, London: Thames & Hudson, 1990, p. 302.

92. For example, in an extensive anthology entitled *Women Artists: Recognition and Reappraisal from the Early Middle Ages to the Twentieth Century* (New York: Women's Press, 1996), Peterson and Wilson criticized the tendency of art history to focus on the 'greats' to the expense of the rest. Their volume, along with others, such as the book *Women Artists 1550–1950* written by Linda Nochlin and Ann Sutherland Harris (Los Angeles County Museum of Art, 1976), firmly placed women within the mainstream of art history.

93. For example, Whitney Chadwick has argued that ' "Greatness" remains tied to specific forms of artistic lineage', Chadwick, 1990, p. 10.

94. Nochlin (Nochlin, Linda, *Women, Art and Power, and Other Essays*, New York: Harper & Row, 1988) also argues that only a change in women's roles will allow us to recognize that women are equal to and able to achieve as much as men.

95. As so many other factors influence creativity – class, age and ethnicity arguably being as important as gender – the emphasis on the artist being a woman may seem inappropriate and essentialist. If the gender of male artists or film-makers is not remarked upon, why should we focus on gender if the artist is a woman? It reinforces the notion that women are somehow more tied to their biological sex than men, and therefore that their work can only be judged in relation to their sex. This is a perennial argument, a double-edged sword for women.

96. Quoted in Chadwick, 1990, p. 285.

97. These intentions or interpretations are not always conscious; it is not always possible for a woman (or man) to leave behind gender, and the

perspective which our gender gives us of the world, or the unconscious fantasies and desires which are tied to our development as 'woman' or as 'man'.

98. Nead, 1992, p. 62.

99. Pollock, 1988, p. 15.

100. Parker & Pollock, 1981, p. 124.

101. Kent, Sarah, 'Scratching and Biting Savagery', in *Women's Images of Men*, Sarah Kent and Jaqueline Morreau (eds.), London: Writers and Readers Publishing, 1985, p. 10.

102. Parker & Pollock, 1981, p. 126.

103. Such work is frequently banned, or seen as obscene, whereas similar images of nude women are commonplace. For example, Robert Mapplethorpe's work was banned for many years.

104. The tour started in 1980, following a successful showing at the prestigious London Institute of Contemporary Arts.

105. *Guardian*, 3 October 1980.

106. See Kent, Sarah, 'Looking Back', in Kent & Morreau, 1985, pp. 55–74, p. 58 op. cit.

107. Berger, 1972, p. 47.

108. Kent & Morreau, Preface, in Kent & Morreau, 1985, pp. 1–2, p. 1.

109. Ibid., p. 1.

110. The organizers of the exhibition state their first aim to be 'to show the comments of a diverse group of women on men and patriarchy'. Morreau, J. & Elwes, C., *Lighting a Candle*, in Kent & Morreau, 1985, pp. 13–26, p. 15.

111. Nead, 1992, p. 66.

112. Raven, Arlene, 'Womanhouse', in *The Power of Feminist Art*, Norma Broude and Mary D. Gerrard (eds.), New York: H. N. Abrams, 1994, pp. 48–65.

113. Chicago, Judy, *Through the Flower: My Struggle as a Woman Artist*, New York: Penguin, 1993, p. 114.

114. Raven, 1994, p. 52, quoting Hubbard.

115. Ibid., p. 55, quoting Orgel.

116. Ibid., p. 57.

117. Ibid., p. 60.

118. The Nicolas Treadwell Gallery was subsequently moved to Bradford and has now closed down. It held art by men as well as women, but many of the pieces by women artists were reminiscent of 'Womanhouse'. See

Treadwell, Nicolas, *Sex Female: Occupation Artist. The Art of Contemporary Women*, Womenswold, Kent: Nicolas Treadwell Publications, 1984.

119. Raven, 1994, p. 61.
120. See Parker & Pollock, 1981, p. 127.
121. Nead, 1992, p. 66.
122. Ibid., p. 68.
123. Quoted in ibid., p. 80.
124. Parker & Pollock, 1981, p. 127.
125. Spence, Jo, *Cultural Sniping. The Art of Transgression*, London: Routledge, 1995.
126. Quoted in Broude, Norma and Gerrard, Mary D., 'Introduction: Feminism and Art in the Twentieth Century', in Broude & Gerrard, 1994, pp. 10–29, p. 28.
127. Ibid., p. 28.
128. Cottingham, Laura, 'The Feminist Continuum: Art after 1970', in Broude & Gerrard, 1994, pp. 276–87, p. 279.
129. In particular, Lacan's emphasis on language and Foucault's views of sexuality as the result of both institutional and discursive practices.
130. Quoted by Parker & Pollock, 1981, p. 164.
131. Ibid., pp. 162–8, for a more detailed discussion of this work.
132. This emphasis on re-reading the female body and the celebration of female sexuality has also been an underlying theme in the writing of an influential group of French psychoanalytic feminists, most notably Luce Irigaray, Julia Kristeva and Hélène Cixous. Whilst there are many differences between these four women, they share a belief in the need to move away from the invisibility of 'woman' within phallocentric language. They all advocate a dethroning of the phallus, a move away from 'man' (as phallic subject) as 'I' within language, from 'woman', in contrast, being 'not-I, or 'other'.
133. Kuhn, Annette, *Family Secrets: Acts of Memory and Imagination*, London: Verso, 1995.
134. Walkerdine, Valerie, *Schoolgirl Fictions*, London: Verso, 1990.
135. The critic Abigail Godeau has argued this. See Chadwick, 1990, p. 359.
136. See Abigail Soloman-Godeau, 'Living with Contradictions, Critical Practices in the Age of Supply-Side Aesthetics', in Squiers, S., *The Critical Image*, New York: Bag Press, 1990, for a critical analysis of Leine and her work.
137. See Broude & Gerrard, 1994, p. 17.

138. Owens, Craig, 'The Discourse of Others: Feminists and Postmodernism', in *The Anti-Aesthetic: Essays on Postmodern Culture*, Hal Foster (ed.), Post Townsend Walsh: Bag Press, 1983, pp. 60–79.

139. Interview with Gerald Marzorati, 'Art in the (Re)Making', *Artnews*, May 1986.

140. See Kaplan, 1983, chs. 11 & 12, for a detailed discussion of the following films.

141. See Lesage, Julia, 'Political Aesthetics of the Feminist Documentary Film', in Brunson, Charlotte, *Films for Women*, London: BFI, 1986, pp. 14–23.

142. Rich, Adrienne, *Sinister Wisdom*, no. 6. Quoted in Raven, 1994, in Broude & Gerrard, 1994, p. 63.

143. Russo, Vito, *The Celluloid Closet: Homosexuality in the Movies*, New York: Harper & Row, 1981.

144. On similar lines *Four Weddings and a Funeral* sees the beautiful (heterosexual) female heroine run through her (endless) list of ex-lovers, scoring them for interest, to the amazement of her would-be suitor. This seems to enhance rather than detract from her desirability, and she *does* get her man in the end.

145. See Teresa De Lauretis, *Alice Doesn't: Feminism, Semiotics, Cinema*, London: Macmillan, 1990, pp. 24–5.

146. Simmonds, '*She's Gotta Have It*', in Bonner, F., *Imagining Women: Cultural Representations and Gender*, Cambridge: Polity Press & Open University, 1992.

147. Whoopi Goldberg and Whitney Houston being two notable exceptions in the mainstream.

148. Quoted by Chadwick, 1990, p. 365.

149. See Brunston, 1986, pp. 14–23, p. 19.

150. Schor, 1994, p. 248.

151. Ibid., p. 249.

152. Ibid., p. 249.

153. It is the fact that these images are produced by a woman which apparently gives them a different reading. Ellen von Unwerth comments: 'they *would* be different if they had been taken by a man.' As interviewed by Gaby Wood, *Observer*, 24 March 1996, p. 8.

154. Cited by Schor, 1994, p. 249.

155. See Kaplan, Ann, 'Is the Gaze Male?', in A. Snitow, C. Stansell & S. Thompson (eds.), *Desire: The Politics of Sexuality*, London: Virago, p. 331.

156. See Nead, 1992, pp. 34–8, for a discussion of this event and its implications.

157. As art historian Linda Nead has argued, 1992, 'the incident has come to symbolize a particular perception of feminist attitudes towards the female nude; in a sense, it has come to represent a specific stereotypical image of feminism,' p. 34.

158. Nead, 1992, p. 38.

159. See Banta, 1987.

160. Tickner, L., *The Spectacle of Woman: Imagery of the Suffrage Campaign 1907– 14*, London: Chatto & Windus, 1987, pp. 204–5.

161. Ibid., p. 204.

162. See Faludi, Susan, *Backlash: The Undeclared War against Women*, London: Vintage, 1992.

163. Mailer, N., *A Prisoner of Sex*, London: Sphere Books, 1971, pp. 57–8.

164. Schor, 1994, p. 253.

165. Ibid., p. 253.

166. Quoted in Schor, ibid., p. 253.

167. Quoted in Schor, ibid., p. 257.

CHAPTER THREE

Pornography: Denigration of 'Woman' or Exploration of Fantasy and Transgression?

defining difference . . .

Pornography as a genre wants to be about sex. On close inspection, however, it always proves to be more about gender. The raw materials of sexual difference are dramatically at play in pornography.

LINDA WILLIAMS[1]

dread . . .

Man strives to rid himself of his dread of woman by objectifying it. 'It is not,' he says, 'that I dread her; it is that she herself is malignant, capable of any crime, a beast of prey, a vampire, a witch, insatiable in her desires. She is the very personification of what is sinister.' KAREN HORNEY[2]

flesh . . .

The secret message in the pornographic revelation of beauty . . . is to rob the female body of both its natural power and its spiritual presence. So in the striptease, culture realizes its revenge against nature. The mystery of the female body is revealed to be nothing more than flesh, and flesh under culture's control.

SUSAN GRIFFIN[3]

power . . .

In the sphere of sexuality, pornography is a significant source of ideas and narratives. It transmits to those who use it – primarily men but also women – notions of transcendence and mastery as intrinsic to sexual pleasure. These ideas . . . pervade our everyday, unremarkable sexual encounters as surely as they do the grotesque acts of Ted Bundy and his ilk.

DEBORAH CAMERON AND LIZ FRAZER[4]

pleasure ...

What is pornography?

In my mind's eye I imagine how we look, my long-limbed naked body in the tub of water, legs slightly spread, hands clutched at my chest, flushed face giving away my excitement. Her leaning over me, fully dressed, breasts spilling from her low-cut shirt, baby browns peeking out behind long black dreads, touching me. My mind snaps photographs of us, her hand on my cunt, my body tense, her eyes intent on mine, my face a state of controlled lust ...   *Quim*[5]

desire ...

'Pornography turns me on. I use it on my own, when I masturbate. But I also watch it before having sex sometimes. It acts to increase my desire, and because it feels as if I shouldn't be watching it, I enjoy it all the more. It makes me feel powerful.'   *Woman reader of porn*[6]

Pornography:[7] The ultimate denigration of woman or an expression of erotic possibility within the realm of fantasy? The most explicit exposure of man's dread of what is female or a celebration of the rich tapestry of his desire? There is no simple answer. The question of the power and permissibility of pornography has incited more debate and dissent, both public and private, than any other subject in the representational sphere. The arguments rage on: How do we define pornography? How do we measure its impact? Should it be banned? Whatever standpoint we decide to take, it is in pornographic representation that female sexuality is most explicitly examined and laid bare; it is experimented with and exposed in the most detailed manner imaginable. No shroud of respectability is necessary, no pretence of artistic integrity, unlike in the more rarefied worlds of art or film. No lip-service to the god of romance or to supposed female sensitivities, unlike mass media imagery aimed at women.

If art represents the idealization and glorification of 'woman', pornography celebrates her denigration. If film presents her as a foil or a trophy, pornography depicts what it really means to 'have' her. If in romantic fiction woman is seduced, in porn she is fucked. In pornography sex defines 'woman's' meaning, her usefulness and her relationship to 'man'. She is body and she is flesh. She is splayed for the world to see. Yet it is not just the body of woman that is exposed in pornography, but also the myths and misogynies within the script of heterosexual desire.

Despite the absence of subtlety, pornography cannot be separated from every other representation of 'woman' frozen in the masculine gaze, in the manner that many of its critics would insist. For the image of 'woman' purveyed in pornography is not unique, it is the extreme end of a continuum. It is perhaps the last bastion of the unfettered masculine gaze, where the influence of 'woman' as spectator is absent from the scene and the power of 'man' as phallic hero is unthreatened or untamed. In pornography, the process of fetishization and objectification of 'woman' we have seen in art and film is merely more obviously played out. It is perhaps the last politically incorrect playground for those who believe in (or fantasize about) the *natural* power of 'man' over 'woman'. Pornography provides us with a script of how to *do* 'sex', of how to *do* femininity and masculinity that is crudely heterosexist, phallocentric and sympathetic to the fantasies of 'man'. The only way in which it is different from the many other scripts that circulate in the masculine gaze is that the narrow configurations of 'woman' and 'sex' are in no way concealed or disguised.

The necessary exposure to pornography – both 'soft' and 'hard' – that I carried out as part of the research for this book left little doubt that pornography elicits a direct and visceral response. Its impact is incomparable to any other medium in the sexual sphere. It is designed to provoke emotion, if not action, and undoubtedly succeeds. Never before have I found the boundaries between personal and professional life so strained. I could not simply split off what I was reading or seeing at the end of the day or pretend that I was not moved by the pornography I saw. Looking back, I almost lost sense of myself. The constant exposure was nearly too much. Its impact certainly seeped into my personal life and I began to see the boundaries of acceptability in the sphere of sexuality very differently than I had before. Only by stopping for some time and coming back to complete this writing could I rise above my own unavoidable reactions to pornography in an attempt to understand what it means and to unravel the competing arguments about its influence and effects.

Try it. Spend a day absorbed in heterosexual pornography aimed at men. What you will find is a representation of 'man' always in control. In soft-core porn the sexualized masculine gaze is unchallenged, incontestable. In hard-core, 'man' pumps and pounds and penetrates, possessing the body of 'woman' and thereby possessing her. There seems scant need for a subtle reading of the pornographic text, little controversy in the analysis of the significance of nuances of representation, of gaze, of posture. Pornography is crude: Man wants woman and he has her, in as many different postures and guises as his imagination can allow; he always comes out as the winner, even when his masochistic fantasies are being played out and she feigns domination, because it is clear that in giving up power he is merely playing a game.

Critics of pornography have seen this as a reflection of reality, of men's power over women, of women's subjugation through heterosexual sex, at the very least as what men would *like* to do to women, given the chance. In these anti-porn critiques, as in pornography itself, the meaning of what it is to be 'woman' is narrowly – and negatively – defined. 'Woman' is object, victim, her body subjugated and exposed; in contrast, 'man' is a misogynist, his heart's desire being to violate and control.

However, others have argued that pornography does not simply reflect or reinforce men's power and women's powerlessness – it reflects man's fantasies, fears and anxieties about 'woman', his fantasies, fears and anxieties about 'sex'. In this view, pornography is the ultimate foil for the flaccid, fearful, phallocentric man. In pornography he is always hard. He is unquestionably 'man'; 'woman' is always *imagined* as object, rarely resisting or, if so, always overcome. At all levels of the pornographic gaze, man is able to maintain the illusion that the penis *is* the phallus – that possession of that particular biological organ *naturally* leads to power, authority and control – and thus free himself from his fear that it is nothing but a piece of flesh. It is an impossible dream – the ultimate phallic illusion. So in this view, the representation of 'woman' in porn is not a reflection of what women are or even what men would *really* like them to be, but a transgressive fantasy in the realm of the forbidden.

It was in order to untangle these opposing positions, and to examine how 'woman' is positioned in the pornographic gaze, that I turned to pornography itself. In collecting pornographic material I have never been so aware of myself as 'woman'. In my local newsagent I bought a copy of every 'pornographic' magazine available on the top shelf. The man serving in the shop was incredulous, and was driven to ask what I wanted them for. Would a man have been asked? I told him they were for research. I now wish I'd said I was going to have an orgy: What could he have said? I also spent time visiting hard-core porn shops in London's Soho, and in Amsterdam, where illegal material is freely available on the shelves. Women are obviously an unusual sight in such an arena – in a number of shops the male customers seemed to disappear as soon as their closed territory was invaded. The assistants were all engaged in hard sell: What do you like?; Try this one; Are you into . . . ? were common rejoinders to greet my entrance. That I was in a sex shop accompanied by a man perhaps legitimated the intensely probing questions into my own sexual preferences (invariably assumed to be our joint preferences). Perhaps the sight of a woman scouring shelves of material showing women being penetrated from every con-ceivable angle, in every possible orifice (often all at once), persuaded the purveyors of porn that they were being visited by a connoisseur. Was this why nearly all of them tried to show us various videos as we browsed through their wares? Or was it the slightly voyeuristic titillation of demonstrating pain and perversion to a relatively naïve-looking pair, who clearly didn't know what they wanted to buy? I was left with more questions than answers: Why is this material so arousing? (I defy anyone to watch a broad range of pornography and not find *some* of it erotic); Why is it so repetitive?; What does the content of pornography say about the viewer?; What is its relation to other forms of represen-tation? Perhaps the most important question is: What is the significance of the particular vision of 'woman' we see produced in the pornographic imagination?

About Porn

The Secret Museum and the Birth of Modern 'Pornography'

'Pornography' is inherently difficult to define. Many people would agree with Justice Potter Stewart, who commented, 'I don't know what it is, but I know it when I see it.'[8] The very essence of pornography is that it is 'obscene'; it is an explicit representation of sex, intended to incite lewd behaviour or thoughts, and as a result is subject to censorship in various degrees. 'Pornography' itself is not a late-twentieth-century phenomenon. Historians have traced explicit sexual representation back to the ancient Greeks.[9] Yet it is only in recent centuries that defining the boundaries of the 'pornographic' has become an issue of such public concern and that the influence of pornography has been deemed so detrimental. As Michel Foucault has argued, prior to the mid seventeenth century sexuality was freely spoken about and the taboos and secrecy which came to characterize the Victorian era of sexual silence from which we are still smarting[10] were as yet unknown:

> At the beginning of the seventeenth century a sexual frankness was still common . . . Sexual practices had little need of secrecy; words were said without undue reticence, and things were done without too much concealment; one had a tolerant familiarity with the illicit. Codes regulating the coarse, the obscene, and the indecent were quite lax compared to those of the nineteenth century. It was a time of direct gestures, shameless discourse, and open transgressions, when anatomies were shown and intermingled with will . . . a period when bodies 'made a display of themselves'.[11]

The mid seventeenth century heralded both a prohibition and a proliferation of discourse on sexuality. What Foucault has referred to as the 'beginning of an age of repression'[12] was characterized by both an institutionalized restraint on the public acknowledgement of sex – be it in the form of speech, writing or visual representation – and the simultaneous 'steady proliferation of discourses concerned with sex,'[13] as rules and regulations for the control of sexuality systematically evolved. So an increase in censorship was paradoxically accompanied by a preoccupation with the sexual – particularly with the 'obscene'. As Foucault argues, 'What is peculiar to modern societies . . . is not that they consigned sex to a shadow existence, but that they dedicated themselves to speaking of it *ad infinitum*, while exploiting it as *the* secret.'[14]

In the mid nineteenth century the regulation of sexuality 'moved into the home' and protection from its influence was extended far beyond those who were attempting to achieve spiritual heights by avoiding the supposed corrupting influence of female lasciviousness through celibacy. Whilst science and medicine superseded religion as the controllers of the boundaries of 'normal' and 'abnormal' sexuality (see Chapter Four), the tentacles of Victorian censorship reached into the sphere of representation to control and condemn. The increasing interest in the supervision of 'suitable' sexuality coincided with the proliferation of printing presses that widened access to what was deemed lewd and obscene and with what was arguably the archaeological find of the century – the discovery of the perfectly preserved relics at Pompeii, which included much explicitly sexual material. Walter Kendrick has argued that this led to the first use of the term 'pornography' in the English language, as well as to the first 'official' collections of what was held to be obscene.

The archaeologists who uncovered Pompeii from its volcanic blanket found myriad buried, and thus perfectly preserved, erotic artefacts – amongst the few to survive the purging of explicit sexual imagery by centuries of repressive Christianity.[15] These learned men exposing the time-frozen world of Pompeii were disconcerted by the ubiquitous nature of the overt sexual iconography. Not confined to the brothels and bathhouses, it was displayed in homes and public places to such an extent it meant that it could be neither denied nor ignored. Yet the status of this material as ancient relic prevented its destruction.

As Walter Kendrick describes in *The Secret Museum*, what was required was a new taxonomy. If Pompeii's priceless obscenities were to be properly managed, they would have to be systematically named and placed. The etymological root of the term chosen for the priceless, priapic treasures – 'pornography' – was the Greek term *'porno graphos'*, meaning 'writing about prostitutes'. They were housed in the 'secret museum' in Naples in order to confine viewing to the select few deemed immune from their supposed untoward influence. Other museums followed the Italian example. Both the Louvre in Paris and the British Museum in London house extensive collections of pornography (the British Museum's Private Case was founded in 1860) – with access initially strictly limited to the bourgeois gentleman. All others were excluded for their own protection.

Yet much of what the Victorians deemed obscene is now accessible to public scrutiny. The artefacts of Pompeii can be viewed by all and sundry. The women, children and working-classes who were previously the main focus of censorship are no longer considered open to corruption from images of satyrs coupling with goats or from paintings of an erect penis.[16] Today, tourists from Greek islands carry home ornaments depicting the erect member of the previously 'pornographic' icons. What was previously deemed obscene or lewd is now often categorized as erotic 'art' or literature; its status as 'high culture' presumably protecting the viewer from being inclined to licentious thought or deed. Books banned in the early twentieth century – such as *Lady Chatterley's Lover* or *Fanny Hill* – are now set texts in schools. Explicit sexual imagery is everywhere; public access is almost impossible to prevent. 'Pornographic' magazines and videos are freely available; in Britain tabloid newspapers sail as close to the wind as they possibly can. We might believe that the media explosion has led to the notion of the 'obscene' or the 'pornographic' being outmoded. But this is not so. It is merely that our boundaries have changed.

'Pornography' in the Late Twentieth Century: The Violation of Woman

> I define pornography as material that combines sex and/or the exposure of genitals with abuse or degradation in a manner that appears to endorse, condone, or encourage such behaviour. RUSSELL[17]

> Sexual explicitness *per se* is not a problem: the sexualised and sexually explicit dominance, subordination and violence of pornography are the problem. ITZEN[18]

Defining pornography has today become an emotive political activity. To both radical feminist critics and conservative campaigners concerned with censorship, 'pornography' appears to have come to mean explicit depictions[19] of sexual violence or degradation. This is now considered the dividing line between acceptable 'erotica' and unacceptable 'pornography'.

In most feminist and right-wing conservative critiques the very term 'pornography' has come to be synonymous with the oppression or objectification of *women*. In order to leave no hostages to fortune, exact descriptions of what should be deemed 'pornographic' – and as a consequence banned – have been produced. For example, Catharine MacKinnon and Andrea Dworkin, in their Minneapolis law ordinance, which was an attempt to ban pornography on the grounds of its assault on civil rights, defined it thus:

> the graphic sexually explicit subordination of women through pictures and/or words that also includes one or more of the following: (i) women are presented as dehumanized sexual objects, things or commodities; (ii)

women are presented as sexual objects who enjoy pain or humiliation; or (iii) women are presented as sexual objects who experience sexual pleasure in being raped; or (iv) women are presented as sexual objects tied up or cut up or mutilated or bruised or physically hurt; or (v) women are presented in positions or postures of sexual submission, servility or display; or (vi) women's body parts – including but not limited to vaginas, breasts or buttocks – are exhibited such that women are reduced to those parts; or (vii) women are presented as whores by nature; or (viii) women are presented being penetrated by animals; or (ix) women are presented in scenarios of degradation, injury, torture, shown as filthy or inferior, bleeding, bruised, or hurt in a context that makes these conditions sexual.[20]

Given this broad definition, much of art, film and other mass media imagery could be banned, as it frequently presents women 'as de-humanized sexual objects, things or commodities', 'in positions or postures of sexual submission, servility or display', or as 'sexual objects who experience sexual pleasure in being raped'. This demonstrates how difficult it is to define 'pornography' operationally, at least at the 'soft' end. Equally, much lesbian 'erotica' would be censored by this definition, as it is not distinguished from heterosexual pornography. Interestingly, gay male pornography – which shows men in such sexualized positions – would lie outside of this definition.[21] Is this because the objectification and denigration of *men* does not sit easily within a radical feminist argument?

There are definitions of pornography which are not gender specific and which do attempt to distinguish between erotica and porn. For example, the Canadian psychologist Charlene Senn, in her research on sexual violence, has distinguished between three different categories of sexual material:

Erotica – Nonexistent and Nonviolent
These images have as their focus the depiction of 'mutually pleasurable, sexual expression between people who have enough power to be [involved] by positive choice . . . They have no sexist or violent conno-tations, are hinged on equal power dynamics as well as between the model(s) and the camera/photographer . . .

Nonviolent Pornography – Sexist and Dehumanizing

These images have no explicitly violent content but may imply acts of submission or violence by the positioning of the models (e.g., guns, whips, chains in the background). They may also imply unequal power by different dress (e.g., male fully dressed, female naked), costuming (e.g., dressing adult models to look like children, models dressed in clothing that implies violence), positioning (e.g., behind bars, in positions of vulnerability) . . . or by setting up the viewer as voyeur (the model is engaged in some solitary activity such as bathing and seems totally unaware or very surprised to find someone looking at her . . .

Violent Pornography – Sexist and Dehumanizing

These images portray explicit violence of varying degrees perpetrated by one individual against another (e.g., hair pulling, slapping, whipping, etc.). This category also includes images that portray self-abuse or self-mutilation . . . Also included are images in which no actual violence is occurring, however the model appears to be suffering from the aftermath of abuse (bruises, black eyes, welts, etc.).[22]

These lengthy descriptions of the 'harder' end of pornography, which are held up to be dissected, make many of the anti-porn arguments strangely synonymous with the very pornographic texts which are condemned. They leave little to the imagination.[23] Paradoxically, the defenders of this particular brand of faith – the anti-censorship lobby – are more circumspect in their descriptions. Equally, there are few detailed analyses of the text of pornography in the reports of experimental studies. Can this be because any foray into the world of porn incites desires and erotic sensibilities otherwise repressed?

These definitions make explicit the vast change in what is deemed a pornographic gaze since the days of the secret museum. Violence, degradation and bondage *appear* to be common features of modern-day pornography. So for those who conjure up air-brushed images of small-waisted, large-breasted women lying on silken cushions (à la *Playboy*) when they are asked to describe 'pornography', the message would seem to be: We've travelled a long way since then.

Yet the MacKinnon–Dworkin definition may be most apposite when applied to what many would call 'hard-core' or 'specialist' porn – Charlene Senn's 'violent porn' – the material which is most likely to be illegal.[24] So there is a danger in taking perhaps the most extreme end of the continuum and seeing it as representative of all pornography. Certainly, there have been criticisms that the US Senate hearings which debated the issue of censorship of pornography focused on 'atypical' violent material, or examined sado-masochistic pornography out of context, with no attention to the meaning behind such representation, and the focus on consensual ritual and role play.[25] So we need to be quite clear what we are talking about when we refer to 'pornography' and its meaning or effects. The problem is that, because of the very fact that it is illicit, there is no common agreement about the contents of pornography currently in distribution. Those who are pro-porn, and those who are anti-porn, present us with a very different picture of what is 'typical' and, as a consequence, a very different picture of how the pornographic gaze positions 'woman'.

A Journey through Pornography

Surveys of the content of recent pornography conducted by anti-pornography campaigners make for sobering and emotive reading. For example, in one study of over 5,000 books, magazines and videos carried out in the USA in 1986,[26] where the authors limited their analysis to the covers of one in five of the myriad titles found in 'adult bookstores' (thereby concluding that they underestimated the extremity of the representations, as more violent images are contained *inside* the covers), it was claimed that 25 per cent of the material depicted violence. Representations of individuals (usually women) either gagged, blind-folded, hooded, handcuffed, in leg or neck restraints, or in some other form of bodily restraint numbered 16 per cent. More violent imagery such as whipping or knifing, rape, forced piercing, spanking, hoisting or stretching on a rack, or other sado-masochistic imagery was present in nearly 15 per cent of the material. Ano-rectal eroticism – including depictions of anal intercourse, fisting, enemas, faeces and defecation – was present in over 12 per cent; fellatio in 21 per cent (cunnilingus was represented in less than 7 per cent of the material) and masturbation or penetration with an inanimate object in 7 per cent. There was also a fair smattering of bestiality (1.1 per cent), leather (4.8 per cent), rubber (1.4 per cent), kinky boots or shoes (2.4 per cent), child-like props or clothing (3.7 per cent), shaved pubic hair (1.6 per cent), extremely large breasts (5.4 per cent), or breasts engorged with milk (1.1 per cent). This is all presented as if it is a fair representation of the current fantasies of the all-American male. It may well be – who knows? As vaginal intercourse was present in only 7 per cent of the material, outstripped by sex between three people (11 per cent), between two women (6 per cent) or two men (8 per cent), one might be forgiven for concluding that the days of 'normal' heterosexual sex in the missionary position are dead – at least in the realm of fantasy.

In a similar vein, a group named Organizing Against Pornography carried out a content analysis of every issue of the mainstream magazines *Playboy*, *Penthouse* and *Hustler*, with the intention of compiling an educational slide show portraying the reality of porn. Themes of violence, denigration and exploitation were presented as common. Below are listed a number of examples extracted from the text that accompanied the resulting slide show:

> *Penthouse*, December 1984, p. 126: A woman is bound into a harness and hangs suspended from a tree, seemingly unconscious.

> *Playboy*, January 1985, p. 104: Model dressed in bondage clothing, with legs open inviting penetration, and superimposed by a shadow of a chain fence, suggesting imprisonment.

> *Best of Hustler*, 1979: In a story, 'The Naked and the Dead', a nude woman is led from a cell by fully dressed guards. Her head and pubic hair is shaved. She is handcuffed, and raped by the male guard. The final scenario shows the woman with gaping mouth and vagina, eyes closed, suggesting unconsciousness or death.

> *Hustler*, 1983: A scantily dressed waitress is shown being gang raped by three men on a pool table. She initially resists the assault, but finally has an orgasm.

> *Hustler Kinky Sex*, 1984: A bear is licking a woman's genitals – her genitalia are completely exposed both to bear and to camera.

> *Playboy*, 1976: A cartoon showing a girl leaving an older man's house after a sexual encounter. She says 'You call *that* being molested,' implying that she seduced him and didn't get enough.[27]

After examining the above, Catherine Itzen has concluded that 'woman hatred underlies all pornography.'[28] If we see this material as representative, then it's hard not to disagree: 'Woman' as dead, defiled and captive. Abuse and violation – of both women and girls – as legitimate action or object of amusement, the violation seen to be desired by the woman. But is this 'typical' pornography? And if it isn't, can we claim that it is simply 'woman hatred' that underlies all pornography? Are there not many other reasons why pornography holds such a lure for many men?

It is understandable why those who take a strongly pro-censorship position argue that violent, hard-core material *is* 'typical' pornography. This material depicts acts which are not only degrading but often illegal. Brutal rape and physical assault are difficult to condone in any context. Only a hardened misogynist[29] will publicly admit to enjoying such representations, so the majority of the pro-porn lobby is effectively silenced. Yet these extremes of degradation are not the only images available in pornography. There is a spectrum of objectification ranging from the cheesecake poses of naked 'girls' to the woman begging to be fucked by a dog or a dildo. The association of sex with violence ranges from the clasping tightly of a straining woman by a dominant (and handsome) man to the full exposure of genitals of a bleeding, bound woman being subjected to rape and physical violence. The snuff movies, where women are dismembered, disembowelled and then die for the camera are clearly the most extreme end of the scale. They are also the most rare (many anti-censorship critics contest the fact of their existing at all). Indeed, in contrast to the arguments of the anti-porn lobby, Lynne Segal has argued that only 3 to 4 per cent of pornography is violent.[30] In my own research, I found that the most common theme was of a woman on her own – no man in the scene at all – strongly reminiscent of the archetypal nude we see in 'art'. Hard-core or violent porn may be the most emotive and the most difficult to defend. But soft-core is certainly more ubiquitous, and if we examine the vision of 'woman' in this context, it is not as easy to say that it can be explained away solely as 'woman hatred'. It appears to be as much about fantasies of untrammelled desire, or about warding off fear, as it is about desecration or dread.

Soft-Core Porn: 'Woman' as Sign of Sexual Desire

Soft-core porn is legal, focusing on woman in various (limited) sexual postures, with man rarely appearing in the sexual scene – except by implication, as spectator. At one end of the soft-core market stands the self-avowedly 'tasteful' – such as *Playboy* – which, in the nineties at least, holds on to pretensions of being a 'men's magazine'. *Playboy* contains features on music, fashion, sport, politics, health, motoring, work and lifestyle. Juxtaposed with stories, features and a problem page are photographs of naked, beautiful women, with pubic hair exposed. These form only a small proportion of the magazine: In one recent edition which contained 162 pages, only 15 were taken up with pictures of naked women. Many of the photographs would not have looked out of place on an advertising hoarding or in a women's magazine – photographs of a naked woman on a beach, or a back shot of a woman lying on the floor. It is only the full-frontal shots of large breasts, the come-hither facial expressions and the exposure of pubic hair that differentiate this material from 'acceptable' mainstream advertising, such as the naked pictures of the model Kate Moss advertising products for Calvin Klein. In many ways, flicking through *Playboy* is a more startling experience than looking at the more explicit magazines that have a naked, splayed woman on every page. The up-market presentation, the presence of mainstream advertising and the lifestyle features serve to position the photographs of naked women as respectable – no pretence at transgression here. It is analogous to the British tabloid newspapers or to men's magazines, such as *Loaded*, which feature semi-clad or naked, sexualized images of women as *normal* pleasure for men.

The majority of the soft-core, 'top-shelf' magazine market does, however, contain a more gynaecological view of 'woman', women lying, typically, in the classic 'beaver' shot, with legs splayed and labia fully exposed (in some cases held open to show the vagina). The women are all of very similar appearance: long hair, heavily made-up eyes and lips, long painted fingernails. They appear to be adopting the normal script of femininity – all wearing the proper mask of 'beauty'. Yet where they differ from representations of 'woman' in non-pornographic contexts, is in the crudeness of their make-up (this is for men, not women, so glossy pink lipstick, dark eye-liner, fake beauty spots and dark arched eyebrows are the norm), their tousled 'bedroom' hair and, again, in their expressions. Mouths are nearly always open – pouting, sighing orgasmically, or, sometimes, smiling vacuously; the representations are of women who aren't threatening (or intelligent). They look as if being 'had' is the only thought in their heads. These pictures are very similar for a reason: They convey the message that this could be *any* woman. This is the fantasy that underneath her cool cosmetic façade, *every* woman is waiting to be fucked; the surface mask of 'beauty' conceals a rampant whore. This is a very different message from the one women and girls are given in their encouragement to adopt the latest beauty tips.

The woman in the pornography gaze is rarely completely naked. Many of the photo-'stories' show women in various stages of undress – the classic striptease – ending with the woman wearing fetishistically inspired underwear – stockings, suspenders or a pulled-down bra. Other common themes are extremely large breasts, schoolgirl clothing, high boots, shaved pubic hair, teacher, housemaid, fur, wedding dress, wet clothes or smeared food. Soft-focus pseudo-lesbian scenes are ubiquitous – two (or three) women touching or kissing each other, invariably dressed in the fetishistic garb of stockings, suspenders and silky underwear. Their long fingernails (no penetration possible here), archetypal 'feminine' demeanour (*both* women passive and coy) and appearance ('big' hair, heavy make-up) are as far from the representations of 'woman' in erotica produced by and for lesbians as one could possibly imagine. This is lesbianism in masculine fantasy with man as voyeur, as the sales blurb for a video advertised in the magazine *For Men* illustrates:

> ### Things Change (Vivid Imagination, certificate 18)
>
> This vid [sic] features two of the loveliest ladies we've ever seen. Lisa has lived with Denise all of her adult life – it is the only heated sexual relationship she has known. Denise has always satisfied Lisa's every burning desire, but now things are changing because Lisa's curiosity is leading her down an erotic path she must experience. Once she feels a man's touch, she knows she can never live without it again. There again, as the title suggests, things can always change. Tastefully shot.[31]

In heterosexual pornography lesbian sex is positioned as entertainment for men and always seen as a prelude to the 'real thing' – phallic penetration or fucking. Legal strictures ensure that this can only be present by implication in the visual imagery in soft-core porn. But it is the focus of every 'story' that accompanies the photographs, often written from the point of view of a woman, implying that 'a good fuck' is what every woman wants. As the narrator of a story in *Lipstick* tells us:

> Sucking Darren's cock in the searing afternoon sun was an absolute joy. This time, however, there was no way he was conning me out of a fuck. Sure, he grumbled a bit, when I withdrew my 'lip service', but he soon cheered up again when I spread my legs. It's such fun fucking outdoors in the summer sun.[32]

What happens in the 'stories' in soft-core porn is, by implication, about to happen in the photographs – 'sex'. This is a vision of 'woman' as both sexually adventurous and appreciative – a match for the sexual skills of the most athletic man. As the heroine in a story in *Fiesta* illustrates:

> He plunged straight in and gave me the best seeing to I've ever had. He wheelbarrowed me for a couple of minutes, shafting me so hard I could feel my buttocks shaking like jellies as he slammed against them. Then we went through a range of positions until I was sitting on his lap, arms around his neck and legs wrapped around his back, with that glorious prick right up me . . . Finally I was practically standing on the bed ramming myself down onto this astonishing piece of Spanish meat and, Sarah later told me, screaming about what he was doing to my cunt.[33]

Yet this explicit representation of woman as desperate for man's 'glorious prick' is not confined to the top-shelf magazines from which children (and women?) are protected. In the British tabloid newspaper the *Sunday Sport* (21 August 1994) there is a similar tale – this time presented as 'news'. Here is an 'exclusive' story by reporter Nicki Lewis on her visit to a local soccer team, reporting that 'They looked really p★★★ed off in the changing rooms but seemed to cheer up when I whipped off my jeans and joined them in the shower.' Things soon progressed:

> As I knelt down in front of him I gave him a mixture of heaven and hell with my mouth, teeth, and nails. At the same time I arched my back and wiggled my bum provocatively to the others, but they didn't move.

> Reluctantly, I left my throbbing comforter and moved in on them. They
> stood like statues as I unzipped them and gave them head to arouse them.
> Once I had them rock hard I went back to the couch but this time I
> didn't need to wiggle anything because as soon as I slid my lips on his
> penis one of them plunged himself into my sopping wet depths from
> behind. It was wonderful as the guy on the couch slid in and out of my
> mouth as the other thrust into my pussy.

The roving reporter goes on to have sex with each man, ending with
the comment 'It took me a while to recover, and I'm just sorry that I
couldn't find a way to get them all up me at the same time!' Readers
are informed that if they want Nicki to 'spice up [their] stag night' or
'if [they'd] like to have her', to write to the *Sunday Sport*. This is literally
an advertisement for sex, and a representation of 'woman' as voracious,
insatiable and wanting nothing more than a 'gang-bang' – in a freely
available 'newspaper'. The only thing that distinguishes it from the
soft-core magazines (allowing it to defy censorship laws and be categorized as 'news'), is that the woman's genitals are not exposed.

Hard-core porn goes a step further – it visually depicts what is merely
left to the imagination (or the story-writers) in the soft-core magazines
– actual sex.

Hard Core Porn: 'Real Sex'?

In 'hard-core' porn phallic penetration and the penis are at the centre
of every scene. The typical scene involves a man having repeated and
vigorous penetrative sex with a woman – vaginally, anally or orally.
There are various combinations: a man and a woman; a lesbian couple
watched by a male voyeur, who then 'joins in'; one woman and two,
three or four men; two or three women and one man; or a series of
couples. Magazines photograph such scenes; films purport to show
them in 'real time'. The more lavish productions will involve some
semblance of a story-line and a brief interlude of foreplay before the
'real' action begins. In the down-market films (the majority of the
market) the opening shot will be of a penis entering a female orifice.
This will continue in every imaginable permutation (and many which
defy the imagination) for hours. There are never any problems with
the man's performance, and the woman is presented as being ecstatically

satisfied by this repeated pounding (which looks excruciatingly uncomfortable, if not painful, to me). It is presented as if it is all she ever wanted. The ultimate phallic illusion of the active controlling man and the passive yet responsive woman – the penis as symbol of his potency and power, literally agent of his mastery and control over woman.

Much of the hard-core pornography I viewed contained the classic scenario, which conflates rape with seduction – the woman taken against her will, who quickly learns that she enjoys being forcibly fucked. It is in many ways an extension of the central theme of romantic fiction – the tall dark hero forcing himself on the ultimately compliant victim. The difference in pornography is that the sexual act is itself the focus of interest, not the supposed seduction or the aftermath of guilt, tears and tremulous desire. The act of penetration and the effects on the woman's sexual arousal are all captured in the goriest detail by the camera: his powerful phallic thrusting; her facial and bodily contortions; and her ultimate experience of pleasure, despite herself. It is all seen from the position of the man – here, *he* is in control.

The very attraction of hard-core pornography is that the sex is 'real', not simulated. The camera focuses closely on the penis as it thrusts into the woman. The 'come' (or money) shots, where the man ejaculates visibly over the woman (often over her face or into her mouth), are common. Most men in 'real life' don't withdraw the penis before ejaculation (unless practising an archaic form of birth control), but in porn it indicates that the sex is *actually* happening, that the man's arousal and pleasure are authentic. The major task of the woman posing in porn (in addition to flexible limbs that allow the contorted sexual positions) would appear to be the ability to simulate orgasm – loudly. Most films are dubbed, so the actress merely has to provide the appropriate facial expressions, her moans, groans and gasps being added at a later date (often with comical consequences, as groans are emitted from a closed mouth, or moans of 'Yes, baby' or some such similar appear from a woman who is grimacing with apparent discomfort, or engaging in fellatio).

Yet this is not simply 'real sex', it is an illusion. The feats performed in hard-core porn are impossible for all but the most unusual man. To maintain an erection whilst carrying out vigorous sexual manoeuvres for a protracted period, in front of a camera crew, with all the stops and starts that are normal in filming, takes a particular (one might say peculiar) type of man. Robert Stoller, in his analysis of hard-core porn, has described how the 'stars' of this genre are a rare breed who show both exhibitionist tendencies and an apparent defiance of normal rules of physiology, both in terms of size (most men in porn have abnormally large penises) and their ability to perform penetrative sex for hours without losing their erection, as well as being able to resume action with a minimal refractory period after ejaculation.[34] One male porn star was described as having a 'leather dick', with hide the thickness of a rhinoceros's, which could take any amount of abuse and still remain erect.

The failure of a few unfortunates who attempt this public display of sexual virility and cannot maintain it is demonstrated in two behind-the-scenes hard-core films: *Exhibition* and *Behind the Scenes of a Blue Movie*. Anthony Crabbe has commented:

> In [*Behind the Scenes*] there is an excruciating scene where a novice actor comes to his first intercourse scene and is completely unable to perform despite the patience of the camera crew and the manual and oral minis-trations of his veteran partner. In *Exhibition* we see French actresses routinely coping with this problem, showing amusing Gallic *ennui*. In an issue of the magazine *Cinema Blue* there is a photograph showing even the seasoned team of Bent Weed and Dawn Cumming arousing a tired actor for the next take.[35]

This is an interesting variation on the effort women exert to overcome sexual problems in the privacy of the bedroom – except that in filming porn the resuscitation is presumably carried out without any of the emotional baggage (at least on the part of the woman), which normally makes it far more significant than a problem with hydraulics.

So whilst undoubtedly violent pornography exists – and the *suggestion* of violence and the demonstration of man's power over woman is central to much of heterosexual pornography – there are many other stories of 'woman' and 'man' being told within the pornographic images and texts. The question that has bedevilled pro- and anti-porn critics alike is what do these images mean and whether pornography has specific effects.

Unravelling Pornography

A Mirror of Masculine Fantasy and Fear ...

> When the pornographer models a figure of a woman, when he fashions her portrait, or captures her in his camera, he is possessing her. And now, by this possession, he controls the one who has captured him, who has ensnared and enchanted him, who causes his death and ensnares him. He has made himself safe from her power.   GRIFFIN[36]

The image of 'woman' framed in the pornographic gaze[37] – and the function of this creature for spectator and creator alike – should be by now a familiar concept. Like other forms of representation constructed within a masculine gaze, pornography acts to deny or alleviate temporarily men's sexual anxiety through identification with phallic mastery. It counters man's underlying fear of woman – his fear of not being good enough, or hard enough, both literally and metaphorically. A fear of the devouring, consuming 'woman', with her apparently insatiable sexuality; of being rejected, laughed at. In heterosexual pornography, where 'man' is positioned as active subject and 'woman' as responsive object, she becomes not a person, but a hole to be penetrated. The symbolic representation of 'woman' in porn acts to denigrate her, to dismiss her and to annihilate her power. She is fetishized in the most obvious manner – split into part object (breast, vagina, mouth) rather than whole object – and the fears she provokes in man (of castration, of not being big enough, of not being 'man') are contained. In pornography the apparent mystery of 'woman' is thoroughly exposed. There is no question of 'What does woman want?' here. No ambiguity about what is inside: As she pulls open her vagina, we can see. Nothing – only flesh. No danger, or horror – nothing to fear. He can even deny any fears of castration – for in the face of *this vagina denta* he is able to look; he can pretend he is not afraid.

The men who read porn are not strong, macho heroes. If women read pornography and believe that this is how men actually are, they are conned. The many men I interviewed were first exposed to pornography as adolescents. They presented a view of it which was not simply one of inculcation into misogyny and violence, but into a world where the images represented were frightening; one man admitted he was 'scared shitless'. For pre-adolescent boys, images of perfect phallic performance or the sight of a waiting, sexual woman can fill the heart with dread. This isn't surprising. Men who have prior experience of their own sexual competence are often filled with dread at the thought of future failure – the fear of not being able to 'get it up' being one of the most common (often unspoken) fears of men. Identifying with the phallic hero in pornography briefly allays that fear. But as the anxiety will return as soon as the pornographic text or picture is put down, the same images must be revisited again and again. That is why pornography is so repetitive. It is not novelty that is being sought, but the desire to master the most repressed desires and fears.

We have already seen evidence of this process in art and film. Here it is more obviously tied to sexual performance. For within dominant constructions of heterosexuality, men have a need to prove their manhood again and again. Feminist psychoanalyst Karen Horney has described 'one of the exigencies of the biological difference between the sexes' as the fact that 'the man is obliged to go on proving his manhood to woman' in sex.[38] He has to prove continually his ability to achieve and maintain an erection, to perform, whereas, in contrast, from a biological and reproductive perspective, she has only to 'be' not to 'do'; to receive, not to act.[39] Within heterosexual sex as it is almost universally constructed, the focus is on the performance of the penis[40]: Heterosexual 'sex' is almost universally defined as penetration of the vagina by the penis. If the penis doesn't work, 'sex' cannot occur, and so the pressure is on man to perform. As one man I interviewed commented:

> 'There's a lot of pressure to be good – to make the woman come. If the woman makes the first move then the pressure is worse. You know, give her five orgasms or something. Thank God for oral sex, that's all I can say.'

Within the traditional script of heterosexual sex, it is the man who gives pleasure to the woman: Sex is something he does *to* her; her pleasure is a reaction to him, a confirmation of his skills as a lover. As another man told me:

> 'Every time a man goes with a woman he wants it to be like the, sort of, the first time . . . the best lover that she's ever had and all that sort of

business . . . women just don't think of men in those terms, of, like, scoring points.'

So his status as 'man' is confirmed by *her* sexual pleasure, as 'sex' comes to be seen as 'good' only if the woman responds:

'[Sex is about] the fact you know you've got this person excited. While you're in the act I don't think you can start to get off until she starts to get off on it, when she starts getting off on it then maybe, yeah.'

Yet, paradoxically, women who show an interest in sex (as increasing numbers of women do) are not the ideal fantasy that readings of pornography might lead us to believe. They simply put more pressure on the man. As one man said:

'If things stay in my control, then I can go at my pace, and do what I want to do, assuming that the woman was compliant. But then the paradox being that it puts the responsibility on me . . . I mean I might be thinking that she wants to be screwed five times in five diverse positions, and feel obliged to produce that, and feel a failure if I didn't make it past the third . . . but then if the woman made it quite clear, "let's go off and make love somewhere," that would make me very scared. It's catch-22 – you're scared because you can't deliver, and then you can't.'

So, women who are open about their sexuality may inspire greater dread.

It's not a coincidence that we find a proliferation of pornography in social contexts in which women are taking up positions of greater independence and power, where women are openly embracing the notion of autonomous female sexuality. As one man I interviewed on the subject of women who make passes at men commented:

'In some ways I think it's great . . . for guys that are too shy to ask women, or for women that want to consume one or two guys each week . . . but the idea of a woman making a pass at me I find quite scary. The prospect of sex with someone new is quite scary anyway. It's to do with feeling whether or not I'd be good enough, whether it would work. There's a fear of rejection, a fear of failure . . . I have anxiety about whether or not I'd get an erection. It's happened sometimes, on the first time, especially if the woman's obviously keen.'

Pornography allows men to avoid facing this fear. As Lynne Segal has written, 'through pornography real women can be avoided, male anxiety soothed, and delusions of phallic prowess indulged, by intimations of the rock-hard, larger than life male organ.'[41] It's no wonder 'real' women pretend to have orgasms during sex with men; the effect on men is potentially catastrophic if they don't. Inordinate pressure is put upon men by this positioning of the penis as a symbol of phallic power. The penis is not positioned simply as a small piece of cylindrical flesh, which in some contexts can become erect and give pleasure to a woman (or man), and in others remain flaccid, leading to exploration of other parts of the sexual repertoire; it is supposed to be all-powerful, always functioning, as it signifies the power and mastery of man. If the penis fails, it is a failure of the very essence of what it is to be 'man'. Given the fragile nature of the organ that the penis really is, it isn't surprising that fears of failure and anxiety underlie the apparent sexual bravado of man, or that women are the primary sites of projected anger, anxiety and despair.[42]

Escaping into pornography allays fears of being unable to produce the performance that signifies phallic power and displaces fears of inadequacy – the perennial masculine obsession with penis size and performance. Freud referred to this as a remnant of the phallic phase of children's development, where the boy 'behaves as if he had a dim idea that [his] member might be and should be larger'.[43] As Horney has argued, this obsession, which is 'displayed naïvely throughout boyhood and persists later as a deeply hidden anxiety about the size of the subject's penis or his potency, or else as a less concealed pride about them'[44] continues throughout life. It is often displaced on to other achievements which symbolically compensate for (or demonstrate) his phallic potency: building bigger, being greater, fighting harder – 'Look at the size of my bank balance, the power of my car, my muscles, my gun . . .'; 'Look at how many contracts I can win, how many achievements I can notch up'; or, most obviously, 'Look how many women I have had' – fighting off the demon of woman's disdain with the symbol of the source of his dread.

The process of proving phallic power, and warding off this anxiety, can assume obsessive proportions in the behaviour of the classic Don Juan, the man who appears driven to possess and conquer woman, after woman, after woman – he who is implicitly celebrated in pornography.

His narcissistic desires are fulfilled through the seduction and possession of desirable women. *His* desirability, *his* power, is demonstrated through his possession of 'woman'. This is necessarily a public demonstration, man's conquest of 'woman' acting as a narcissistic mirror to prove to others that he is 'man'. Repeated sexual conquests prove his phallic mastery; the compulsive repetition is necessary because he is only as good as his last conquest. His security does not come from within, but from his sexual prowess and his ownership of a beautiful woman (beauty being the most important currency, as women well know). Pity the man who attempts to prove his manhood by repetitively conquering women and then boasting about his possession of them. What he reveals is not mastery, but a terrible insecurity within. As his conquests are often only for one night, he is proving to himself that he can always do it 'the first time'.

In pornography, men can act out this fantasy by proxy, in the safety provided by its being within the representational sphere. They can attain the illusion of possession of the women who are photographed and exposed therein; by masturbating over her image they are 'having' her. It is Don Juanism once removed. The fact that these women cannot resist, that they continue to smile vacantly at the man as he comes, adds to his pleasure and sense of power. As he masturbates over his pornography, there is never any question of who is in control. Man can immediately gratify himself without any of the difficulties of arousing or satisfying female desire. As Elizabeth Cowie has argued:

> The image of the woman's genitalia . . . offers a fantasy scenario in time
> – of the woman *already* excited and desiring, a scene into which the
> spectator can step . . . The scene narrates a situation of lack – the sexual
> climax – which will be supplied by the man in fantasy as he completes
> the scene with his penis and even quite literally, in his own masturbation.[45]

Pornography is also a representation of need. As Anne McClintock commented after investigating the world of male pornography, 'Have women been forbidden the world of commercial sex because man's need for woman is there so nakedly on display?'[46] She describes her visit to a men's sex emporium in Manhattan thus:

> Where were the brutish howls, the heady odour of male power, the whiff
> of abuse? I could as well have been looking at the nursery of a maternity

ward during breastfeeding: the men were slumped low in their chairs, slack-jawed and still, mouths wet with longing, a spectacle of glazed infantile enthralment. The vaguely mocking dancer, on the other hand, moved powerfully through her routine.[47]

The representation of 'woman' as weak victim and 'man' as oppressor does not easily fit into this analysis. Yet this doesn't mean that the critics of porn have got it all wrong. As McClintock continues:

> A couple of years later I sat in a porn palace, the only woman amid scores of masturbating men . . . Without warning, the male lead began, in manly rebuke, to club his partner across her face with his penis, and at once the porn palace broke into a roar of glad baritone cries. I was jolted into trauma, any arousal doused by this barrage of male hostility, and I left in disarray.[48]

This is, arguably, the combination of need and rage projected on to 'woman' in the flesh that we have already seen in representations of woman as witch, as whore, or as *femme fatale* in art and film. The only difference in pornography is that the sadistic urges are not disguised as allegory. At root this is still a reflection of the fantasies and rages of the early infantile phase of development, with the overwhelming need and anger towards our first love, our mother. As Jessica Benjamin has argued,[49] much of our early fantasy life is sado-masochistic and so it shouldn't surprise us to find that themes of domination and submission are played out in porn.

Elizabeth Cowie[50] has argued that pornography represents the 'desire to desire'; that it represents most blatantly the fantasies of transcendence and mastery which underpin our sexuality. These are fantasies related to our earliest infantile experiences, where power and desire are irrevocably linked and eroticized. Arguably, sex is not simply about fulfilment of sensual erotic desire for anyone. Through the act of sex, the most intimate action most of us ever engage in, we attempt to re-create the fantasy of completeness, the illusion of unity that was present at the earliest phase of infancy in the relationship with the mother. Sex *does* provide enormous physical pleasure and emotional release – but it is not simply a question of lustful drives. The Don Juan, or his more modern equivalent, may convince himself that he is simply seeking sexual fulfilment, but the desire to re-create the early infantile illusion of unity, of being 'one', in order to compensate for deep feelings of incompleteness and lack is what is being sublimated in 'sex'. This desire is impossible to fulfil, for the unity with the mother in infancy is as illusory as the possibility of achieving complete psychic fulfilment in adult sexual or emotional bonds. Those who hold it in highest esteem, through attempting to achieve complete unity within a relationship, or desperately seeking the perfect woman (or man) are most likely to be disappointed. The repetition, the continual searching for the ideal, drives many men from woman to woman. Chasing a fantasy and, paradoxically, desperately driving away a fear. A fear of the omnipotent mother and of man's sense of lack in the face of her power. Pornography is the archetypal representation of this repetitive fantasy – an illusion of mastery and power which must be returned to again and again as it only temporarily provides satisfaction.

Multiple Readings of the Pornographic Image and Text: The Case of the Money Shot

What the above discussion suggests is that there are many different levels at which we can read or identify with pornography, and that the viewer of pornography is not a passive, unthinking subject. We should not simply assume that all men identify with the phallic 'man' in the pornographic image (or that all women identify with the position of 'woman' as victim). Take the classic 'come shot' (or 'money shot') in hard-core porn, where the man ejaculates on the face or body of the woman. There are a number of readings of this particular image that can be made, and the one that we make may well depend on the meaning pornography (and sexuality) has for us. At one level, it simply shows that the sex is 'real', as is argued above. A more malevolent interpretation is that it epitomizes man's disgust and disdain for the sexuality of women. As this pornographer, Bill, interviewed by Robert Stoller, explains:

> I like to bring more violence into my creations. I'd like to bring what I call erotic terror . . . I'd like to show what I believe men want to see: violence against women. I firmly believe that we serve a purpose by showing that. The most violent we can get is the cum shot in the face. Men get off on that, because they get even with the women they can't have.[51]

So by identifying with the man who ejaculates, men can vent their hatred of women, which Karen Horney so clearly spelt out (see Chapter Two). A very different interpretation is made by critic Gary Day, who argues:

> If pornography in part involves a realization of the incestuous phantasy, then the come shot takes on a very different meaning. For what the man does in ejaculating over the woman is in a sense to replicate the role of the mother in giving milk to the infant.[52]

Here the male spectator is seen as taking up the position of the mother, and revealing both an incestuous wish and his desire for complete merger with her – he can *be* her. A different view again is expressed by Anthony Crabbe, who argues that 'the *raison d'être* of the come shot is to provide evidence of the actor's real pleasure, while the actress's manipulation of the semen is witness to her endorsement of masculine fulfilment'[53] – a more seedy version of the script of romantic fiction. According to Anne McClintock, it stands for the forbidden desire for another man: 'the cum shot is potentially homoerotic: men who time their orgasms to the cum shot identify vicariously with the spectacle of another man's pleasure.'[54] In contrast, Linda Williams has argued that it could be interpreted as standing for women's desire: 'the money shot . . . attempt[s] to substitute for what the film could not show: the visible, involuntary convulsions that would be proof of the woman's pleasure . . . the invisible female orgasm.'[55] It signifies the 'success' of the sexual act (as defined by phallocenticism): Woman is pleasured by man.

There is no 'correct' interpretation. Different men may make different identifications at different points in time, always influenced by their current and past psychological anxieties and fears. They may switch between identification with the active phallic subject and with the denigrated object during one session of pornographic viewing. As the cultural theorist Jonathon Dollimore has commented, 'I find if I look at a video of a man and a woman having sex, I very much identify with both positions.'[56] For many men, it is the masochistic position – the traditional position of 'woman' – which is more erotic. This is why one of the common representations in porn is of men being subjugated by women (something which is ignored in many of the radical feminist critiques), and why many men who visit sex workers seek to be beaten or dominated, not to dominate themselves. But men can also identify with the objectified woman in pornography in order to explore these fantasies – as women identify with the phallic hero in romantic fiction. As Dollimore continues, in describing his viewing of pornographic videos, 'I want to be fucked by that man as a woman – my experience is very strongly with the woman – my desire is going very strongly through the woman. To put it quite simply, there are times when I want the vagina. I'm not just wanting to position myself in the position of the woman as a man.'[57] So porn may be seen to be as much a representation of man's desire to be subjugated as it is of his desire to subjugate women. If the script of heterosexual sex and desire were not so rigid in defining 'man' as having to be strong and in control, perhaps we would see more open playing-out of the masochistic side of masculine desire. We certainly see it in porn for gay males, where subjugation, femininity or 'doing girl' is not so feared. Heterosexual men mostly have to make do with projecting their desires on to 'woman'. This allows them to take up the masochistic position in fantasy, with no threat to their position as a 'real man'.

Yet whilst we might explore the *meaning* of the representations in pornography, the debates clearly do not end here. The question is, do readers of pornography confine their acting-out of the role of phallic hero (or subjugated slave) to fantasy, or does this have an impact on their treatment of women or their enactment of 'sex' in material reality? Is pornography, as many of its critics would claim, an education in sadistic sex?

Pornography: An Education in Sex?

Certainly pornography is not simply seen and used by a relatively small number of men with 'special' problems. Men usually see pornography when they are quite young: it is clandestinely circulated on the way home from school, or, increasingly, watched on parents' video-cassette players. Many young men see pornography belonging to their fathers or other, older male relatives and friends. One childhood friend of mine found a box of pornography in a tree in his local park; he then kept it hidden in a locked suitcase in the back of his wardrobe.[58]

As Peter Baker demonstrates, pornography is not the preserve of a select few 'perverts', but is widely read by men and boys. In one American study[59] the men interviewed reported that they saw their first issue of *Playboy* or similar magazine at eleven years of age. All the high-school-age males had experience of soft-core porn, and 84 per cent had experience of hard-core porn. So it appears to be a statistically normal part of masculine existence, as ubiquitous as television, cinema and other mass media images which define the boundaries of 'woman' and 'man'.

One of the ways in which pornography does differ from other forms of representation is that by definition it is forbidden and therefore imbued with secrecy and excitement. The taboos surrounding its viewing add to the transgressive nature of the sexual thrill it sets out to provoke. This doesn't mean that viewing porn is a solitary, shameful activity. The sharing of pornography in childhood described by Peter Baker continues into adult life, particularly in all-male environments, where magazines are passed around at work and 'girlie' calendars bedeck the walls. Yet the public display and consumption of porn is not solely about group denigration or objectification of women, the main reason why many women (and men) object to the open display of such material in the workplace. It can also be seen as an act of male bonding, a shared secret – a game for the 'boys' to be kept private from the girls – in the same way that shared reading of teenage magazines or talking about pop stars is an act of solidarity between girls. It can be seen as a means of publicly signifying masculinity (as well signifying masculine power and male territory). It signifies 'I'm in control (and therefore not afraid) of women.' Peter Baker has described pornography as a 'rite of passage into manhood'.[60] For many, it is certainly an important part of the establishment of a masculine sexual identity, providing essential cues for the establishment of 'normal' heterosexuality. Publicly displaying or talking about porn demonstrates that young men are unquestioningly 'man', with unquestioned heterosexual desires and appropriate masculine feelings towards women.[61] It signifies 'I *know* about women, I fancy them, and I can "do" sex.' The sexual bravado or bragging associated with the group sharing of pornography alleviates the dread that any of these points may be untrue (which they so often are) and serves, as do the other visions of 'woman' framed in a masculine gaze, as a defence against psychic anxiety and dread.

Interestingly, whilst many of the men I interviewed were happy to talk about when they first saw porn or about public sharing, I initially had great difficulty in finding men who would admit to *regularly* reading or owning pornography, particularly hard-core. Yet in later discussions about the imagery pervading these magazines and videos all these men were unsurprised at what I had found and were invariably able to provide me with more extreme examples of every 'specialism' I described. An interesting contradiction. A shame at owning, but not at viewing? In response to my question why no man would admit to being a regular reader of pornography, a colleague commented, 'It's like masturbation and voting Tory: Everyone does it but no one admits to it.'[62] When viewed *privately*, pornography is invariably associated with masturbation. Arguably, it is its main purpose. As these men commented:

> 'They're like a tool – they make it easier to come. Just getting them out and looking at them turns me on. As soon as I've come I'm not in the slightest bit interested. They suddenly seem boring.'

> 'It's just a picture. And it's just the fact that there's a naked woman as an aid to your fantasy. I mean an aid for your fantasy when you're having a wank . . .'

Pornography provides a ready-made sexual fantasy which aids arousal. It works – as any man (or woman) who has ever used it in such a way will testify. Sex researchers testing arousal or orgasm in the laboratory give pornography to their experimental participants – both men and women. Sex therapists use it for the same purpose, as do those collecting male semen for artificial insemination – one semen donor talked of the incongruity of being given a bottle and a soft-core-porn magazine and then being sent to the toilets in his local clinic to produce the 'goods'.

We could view this use of porn in a purely functional way: It allows men to reach orgasm quickly and provides them with private release of sexual tension. However, many critics have argued that this use of pornography as a masturbatory tool provides men with sexually explicit material that has a direct effect on their views of women. As Catherine Itzen argues:

> Pornography . . . plays a part, together with other forms of sex-objectified, sex-stereotyped presentations, in the social and psychological conditioning of all men – constructing *normal* masculinity . . . and maintaining the whole system of male power. Pornography presents to men how it is

permissible to look at and see women . . . in terms of their sexuality and sexual inequality as presented by pornography.[63]

Pornography is undoubtedly shared amongst boys as a means of gaining knowledge about the mysteries of women, promising the 'truth' – finally – of what woman is really like, as these young men interviewed by Ben Gurney Smith commented:

> 'I first found a pornographic magazine, my brother's porn mag, that was the first time I had seen . . . er . . . muff and all that. And that was very interesting!'

> 'It's the first opportunity to see a woman, unless you've been in bed with her, a grown woman.'

> 'You see things, like, it does, like, give you a better understanding, not all the stories and stuff, but just looking at the female body.'

If pornography *is* educational, it is clearly providing a very skewed education about both sex and about 'woman.' Susan Griffin has argued that 'the pornographer reduces a woman to a mere thing, to an entirely material object without a soul, who can only be loved physically.'[64] Pornography undoubtedly emphasizes man's difference and distance from woman and the requirement for man to be in control, to be conqueror. So it could be seen as an education in power, in being the phallic hero. As these two men interviewed by Corrine Sweet commented:

> 'Pornography gives you a sense of sex divorced from any relationship, it also treats sex as something geared towards performance – it's like football, you've got to train for it, you've got to learn to "do the business".'

> 'Pornography confused me about what women are really like. It communicated two main things: One is that women are merely sexual objects to satisfy my lust, and two that women are insatiably sexual. So it made me contemptuous of women and it also made me feel inadequate.'[65]

Heterosexual pornography aimed at men *does* depict sex without emotion, without commitment – arguably, without humanity. It is sex without conversation or intimacy, something men do *to* women. Love is anathema to the pornographer. But it would be wrong to say that pornography *causes* these fantasies of man as active and woman as object to be used, for as we have seen, they are based in deep-rooted phantasy and fears and are not unique to porn. Yet men who claim to have been influenced by porn are not the only ones to have taken up this position.

Pornography and Violence: A Cause-and-Effect Relationship?

Pornography is the theory, and rape is the practice.

ROBIN MORGAN[66]

Pornography predisposes some men to want to rape women or intensifies that predisposition in other men already so predisposed; it undermines some men's internal inhibitions against acting out their desire to rape; and it undermines some men's social inhibitions against acting out their desire to rape.

DIANA RUSSELL[67]

Analyses of the denigration of 'woman' in pornography by feminist critics such as Robin Morgan, Andrea Dworkin, Catharine MacKinnon and Susan Kappeler have led to the view that it should be condemned and then banned. Put simply, the argument is that men see, and then believe; that they follow the pornographic script and enact violence against the bodies of women. The contention that 'pornography is the theory, and rape is the practice' is not merely feminist rhetoric. It was the premise underpinning a number of legal commissions in the USA, Canada, Britain and Australia which were set up to assess the effects of pornography on the general population. Yet, perhaps unsurprisingly, there is as much disagreement about the impact of pornography as there is about its definition.[68] For example, a congress commission set up in 1967 in the USA, which reported to President Nixon in 1970, concluded unequivocally that 'empirical research designed to clarify the question has found no evidence to date that exposure to explicit sexual material plays a significant role in the causation of delinquent or criminal behaviour among young youth or adults.'[69] Contrary to expectations, the commission recommended the repeal of legislation prohibiting the 'sale, exhibition, or distribution of sexual materials to consenting adults'[70] – the complete abolition of censorship. The more conservative United States Senate rejected the report – by a majority of sixty votes (only five senators voted in favour). The president supported the senate vote and, in an emotional speech, linked pornography with not only sexual licentiousness, but with a general threat to social order:

'So long as I am in the White House there will be no relaxation of the
national effort to control and eliminate smut from our national life . . .
Pornography is to freedom of expression what anarchy is to liberty; as
free men willingly restrain a measure of their freedom to prevent anarchy,
so must we draw the line against pornography to protect freedom of
expression . . . If an attitude of permissiveness were to be adopted regarding
pornography, this would contribute to an atmosphere condoning anarchy
in every other field – and would increase the threat to our social order
as well as to our moral principles.'[71]

So pornography was seen to stand for not only unbridled sexuality,
but an unleashing of anarchy – which meant it must be controlled. But
this was the public view, the official line, espoused by one with his eye
on opinion polls. And pornography continued to proliferate.

The US Attorney-General's Commission on Pornography, which
reported in 1986 to the conservative, 'family-values' president Ronald
Reagan, came to the conclusion that there *was* a causal link between
both violent and non-violent pornography and harm to women.[72]
However, similar commissions in Britain in 1979, Canada in 1985 and
Australia in 1988 came to the conclusion that the evidence available
could not support such a contention – there was no consensus in
the existing research on the effects of pornography. Yet censorship
campaigns continued defiantly. In 1983 the Minneapolis City Council
in Indianapolis held hearings, spurred by anti-pornography campaigners
Andrea Dworkin and Catharine MacKinnon, which passed legislation
against pornography on the grounds that it contravened women's civil
rights, inciting men to misogyny and violence. The legislation was
never enacted, being outvoted at later appeals. However, at a Federal
Court appeal hearing in 1985, which decided to maintain the legality
of pornography on the grounds of free speech, it was officially acknowledged that pornography can be harmful *to women*. The Court of Appeals
concluded:

Indianapolis justifies the ordinance on the ground that pornography affects
thoughts. Men who see women depicted as subordinate are more likely
to treat them so. Pornography is an aspect of dominance. It does not
persuade people as much as change them. It works by socializing, by
establishing the expected and the permissible. In this view pornography
is not an idea: pornography is the injury . . . Depictions of subordination

tend to perpetuate subordination. The subordinate status of women in turn leads to affront and lower pay at work, insult and injury at home, battery and rape on the streets. In the language of the legislation, 'pornography is central in creating and maintaining sex as a basis of discrimination. Pornography is a systematic practice of exploitation and subordination based on sex which differentially harms women. The bigotry and contempt it produces, with the acts of aggression it fosters, harm women's opportunities for equality and rights.'[73]

Similar conclusions were drawn by the Canadian Fraser Committee on Pornography and Prostitution in 1985 and the Canadian Supreme Court in 1992: Feminist rhetoric (for perhaps the only time) was harnessed by the machinery of the law in an attempt to enact legislation. Yet again because of attention to free speech, the majority of what is defined as 'pornography' remains available – merely being limited (officially) to adult viewing.

In Britain, where an exact definition of pornography has *not* been established within the law – the vague notions of 'obscenity' (that which threatens to deprave or corrupt) or 'indecency' (that which an ordinary decent man or woman would find to be shocking, disgusting or revolting) being the basis of censorship[74] – the laws are acknowledged to be amongst the strictest in existence. Yet a public acknowledgement of the purported harmful effects of pornography on women, in the manner of recent American pronouncements, has not been forthcoming. Perhaps the prurient British attitude to sexuality maintains tight controls on any public depiction of the sexual without there having to be any appeals to the rights of women. Or perhaps the feminist lobby is merely less powerful. In contrast to the respectful treatment of feminist campaigners Catharine MacKinnon and Andrea Dworkin by various US Senate hearings, the Labour MP Clare Short was vilified both by parliamentary colleagues and the press when she attempted in 1989 to introduce censorship of the topless page three girls in tabloid newspapers, such as the *Sun*.[75] Her (mostly male) critics were reduced to mirth at the notion that such 'harmless fun' could be taken seriously. She was positioned as a sexless, humourless harridan, in the way that feminists have been vilified for over a century.

But feminist backlash (or British parliamentary misogyny) aside, is there a case to be made? It is undoubtedly the case that the majority of heterosexual porn – be it hard or soft – positions man as dominant, woman as sexual object. But do men see the images of 'woman' writhing in the hands of a group of thrusting men, every orifice filled with a penis, and believe that this is what women actually want? That it is legitimate to truss a woman up and ejaculate all over her, having repeatedly anally penetrated her against her will? That women enjoy sex with horses, dogs and pigs? For even if we argue that the sexual fantasies that are contained in pornography have a complex aetiological root, is it possible that pornography provides permission (and a detailed script) for sexual subjugation and violence, as many critics would declare? To demonstrate its widespread effects, attention has turned to the effects of pornography on 'normal' men (those who have not been convicted of sexually violent crimes) – and in particular to the results of experimental-psychology research.

Pornography and the 'Normal' Man

It would be ethically impossible to carry out research involving exposure to pornography and *actual* sexual violence in order to measure its effects. But in a laboratory situation men *have* been exposed to pornography and their reactions measured, in terms of both their fantasies and desires and their subsequent attitudes and behaviour towards women. Much of this work has been conducted in psychology laboratories in North America, predominantly using college students as research participants.

For example, experiments carried out by the psychologist Neil Malamuth[76] have demonstrated that male college students exposed to violent pornography were more likely to create violent images in their subsequent sexual fantasies. Diana Russell has used this research to support her argument that pornography influences men's sexuality through associative learning. She has also described research in which men have become conditioned to be sexually aroused by a woman's boot through repeatedly being shown slides of boots juxtaposed with slides of nude women[77] – the evolution of a foot fetishist – as evidence for the power of association.

The experimental research appears to suggest that men are more likely to find sexual violence erotic when the violence is presented as exciting for the woman. For example, in one study where men and women were presented with both violent and non-violent pornography (a rape scene: one with pain, one without) the men were found to be more aroused by the violent scene, but only the rape victim is shown experiencing an orgasm as well as pain. Women were most likely to be aroused by the scenario of orgasm without pain.[78]

It has also been argued that exposure to sexually violent material results in greater acceptance of rape myths and that if the woman is shown enjoying the violence, men are more likely to report the possibility of engaging in similar behaviour.[79] Evidence cited in support of this view is that men watching aggressive pornography are more aggressive towards women in a laboratory situation: Men shown a film depicting a rape subsequently behaved more aggressively towards women (but not men), their aggression being measured by (pseudo)shock intensity given in an experiment. Men shown explicit sexual but non-violent material, or a neutral film, were not affected in the same manner.[80]

Researchers have tended to focus on the effects of *violent* sexual material. But non-violent porn has not been immune from such scrutiny. For example, in one study that examined exposure to non-violent pornography, it was reported that rape was likely to be trivialized and viewed as having less serious effects on the victim; callousness towards women increased; the acceptability of male dominance in intimate relationships increased; and the acceptability of female equality in relationships or everyday life decreased.[81]

It is perhaps ironic – given the supposed effects of pornography on women's lives – that when compared to the vast body of work examining men's reactions to and use of pornography, there is very little research that has examined women's experiences of pornography. It is as if the answers are taken for granted. The research that has been conducted has tended to introduce women as a comparison group to men in the experimental studies carried out in the laboratory – with mixed results being reported. Some women respond much more negatively to pornography than men, others show a similar response – or no response at all.[82] This isn't surprising – women are not a homogeneous group.

A vast amount of this experimental research on pornography was carried out during the seventies and eighties – to review it all would be exhausting. The American social scientist Edna F. Einsiedel summarized the research prior to 1986, for the US Attorney-General's commission. Her conclusions were that there was consistent support for the view that sexually explicit material designed to be arousing *is* arousing;

rapists are aroused by both forced and consenting sex depictions, but college males are only aroused by forced sex if the victim is shown to enjoy it; arousal associated with rape is positively correlated with attitudes to rape and acceptance of rape myths; both of these correlate positively with aggressive behaviour towards women; and laboratory aggression towards women positively correlates with self-reported sexually aggressive behaviour.[83] A pretty damning indictment of porn. However, others have come to more equivocal conclusions – the psychologists Dennis Howitt and Guy Cumberbatch, reviewing the same research evidence in a British Home Office sponsored report conclude that a simple stimulus–response model of pornography and violence cannot be substantiated. The jury is clearly still out on the matter. Despite this, a number of legal commissions in the USA and Canada appear to have taken the experimental research evidence – and the addiction and copy-cat models – on board as 'truth'. Yet can the experimental research be unquestioningly accepted?

Experimental research on sexuality is valuable in providing partial answers to questions about the relationship between pornography and subsequent reactions to women, sexual arousal or attitudes to sexual violence. But it must be viewed with caution. There is always a question over the measurement of sex in the laboratory; we cannot isolate sex as a dependent variable in experimental situations as if it were some simple attribute such as 'reaction time', the classic phenomenon measured by generation after generation of psychology students. Even something as simple as an erection – simple in the sense of being inducible and then measurable – cannot be isolated from the complex psychological and cultural connotations associated with male sexual arousal and performance. We may try to insist that an erection is an erection, nothing more, nothing less, but unfortunately this isn't true. Yet in the laboratory it appears to be read in this way.

Equally, examining the reactions of North American college students to sexual stimuli in a laboratory, when in the main they are aware of the demand characteristics of the situation – that they are taking part in an experiment about reactions to porn – cannot tell us everything we need to know about men and pornography (in the same way that research on *any* complex social behaviour cannot simply be confined to the laboratory). We should also beware of becoming too bogged down in the findings of experimental research, even if we do not question its validity. For the relationship of pornography to sexual violence cannot be purely a cause and effect phenomenon, isolated from all other aspects of sexuality, gender and power. Pornography is as much a *reflection* of a phallic masculine culture, where a narrow model of heterosexual sex is prescribed for all, as it is a simple script which provides an education in degradation of 'woman'. Pornography must be seen as part of the wider sphere of sexual representation which plays a part in shaping what we understand as normal or transgressive sex, as well as what we understand as 'woman' and 'man'. And if we accept the argument that it is difficult to draw a line between the symbolic representation of 'woman' in pornography and those pervading other genres such as art or film and popular culture, we might ask why it is only 'pornography' that is examined in the laboratory. One function of the experimental research is thus to reinforce the questionable view that pornography is very different from other forms of sexual representation in terms of form, content and effects.

Pornography and Sex Offenders

One of the factors cited as confirmation of the link between pornography (at least hard-core) and sexual violence is the evidence that sex offenders report violent sexual fantasies.[84] As much of the hard-core porn that proliferates today depicts or implies violence and degradation, models of associative learning predict that men and women who use porn will come to view the connection between sex and violence as erotic. If men repeatedly masturbate whilst watching images of women being raped they will learn that fantasizing about rape and eventually acting it out is a sexually arousing experience. Ray Wyre, a critic of pornography who works with sex offenders is unequivocal in his belief in the connection between sexual fantasies precipitated by porn and the subsequent acting-out of violent behaviour:

> In my experience fantasy and behaviour are directly connected . . . There
> is also a connection between an escalation in fantasy and extreme forms
> of violent behaviour . . . the more [men] masturbate to pornography, the
> more likely they will be to put the fantasy into practice. Masturbating to
> fantasy is part of the trigger to act out the content of the fantasy.[85]

Ted Bundy, the American serial murderer, attributed his desire for the sexual violation and murder of women to pornography, pathologizing (and thereby potentially excusing) his behaviour as an addiction he couldn't control.

> It happened in stages, gradually, it didn't necessarily happen overnight. My experience with pornography generally, but with pornography that deals on a violent level with sexuality, is once you become addicted to it, and I look at this as a kind of addiction like other kinds of addiction, I would keep looking for more explicit, more graphic types of material. Like an addiction you keep craving something that is harder, harder, something which gives you a greater sense of excitement. Until you reach a point where the pornography only goes so far, you reach that jumping off point where you begin to wonder if maybe actually doing it would give you that which is beyond just reading it or looking at it.[86]

This progressive addiction model predicts that even if men start on the 'soft stuff' they will eventually progress to something harder; this is similar to many (controversial and contested) arguments about drugs. The implication here is that when men are finally satiated with the 'hardest' porn, they will then move on to acting out their fantasies, as pornography no longer fulfils their needs or desires. There may be individual cases (such as Bundy) which fit this model (although Bundy's blaming of porn for his crimes neatly exonerates him). But clearly not all men who read *Playboy* go on to rape or murder women, any more than everyone who drinks a glass of wine becomes an alcoholic, or everyone who smokes a joint becomes a heroin addict. This is a far too simple view of human behaviour.

More common (and on the surface more convincing) is the copy-cat model of the effects of porn – that men see and then imitate what they view and read. One woman who testified to the 1985 Commission on Pornography commented:

> [My daughters] had an experience with an eleven-year-old boy neighbour . . . Porno pictures that [he] had were shown to the girls and to the other children on the block. Later that day [he] invited [my daughters] into his house to play video games, but then tried to imitate the sex acts in the photos with [my] eleven year old [daughter] as his partner; [my other daughter] witnessed the incident.[87]

Diana Russell interviewed over 900 women about their experiences of sexual violence and argued that there was clear evidence of the imitative impact of pornography in a number of cases:

> He'd read something in a pornographic book, and then he wanted to live it out. It was too violent for me to do something like that. It was basically getting dressed up and spanking. Him spanking me. I refused to do it.

> This guy had seen a movie where a woman was being made love to by dogs. He suggested that some of his friends had a dog and we should have a party and set the dog loose on the women. He wanted me to put a muzzle on the dog and put some sort of stuff on my vagina so that the dog would lick there.

> I was staying at this guy's house. He tried to make me have oral sex with him. He said he'd seen some far-out stuff in movies, and it would be fun to mentally and physically torture a woman.[88]

This copy-cat function of pornography has also been reported by women recalling childhood sexual abuse:

> When I was six years old my brother (then fourteen) was given or bought some 'adult' magazines and he used to show them to me when our parents were out. Then he began to sexually abuse me . . . If our parents were out on a Saturday night my brother would invite a few friends around. They'd bring their magazines and sit around joking about women's bodies. Then my brother would make me strip and straddle the bath while one by one they'd sit underneath and look at my genitals.[89]

Yet even if we accept the arguments of the anti-porn critics that pornography provides a clear script for violence and degradation, we cannot say that every man who is exposed to pornography becomes sexually violent. Not every man acts out these fantasies – in the same way that not every man who sees violence on television or every woman who reads romantic fiction goes on to follow this exact script in their lives. The copy-cat model is just too simple. It implies that we believe everything that we read and that there is no negotiation or interpretation of the images or texts – which is clearly not the case, as the earlier examination of girls' reading of magazines illustrates. Those who advocate a copy-cat model would also have to explain why the representation of 'woman' or 'man' in pornography is seen as more 'real' than all the other representations of 'woman' available in the symbolic sphere. Why rape when you could worship?

Equally, men who have been convicted of rape or sexual abuse are not necessarily *typical* men.[90] Rapists may attribute their actions to pornography, as a means of denying responsibility for what they have done. Or they may wish to comply with the models of attribution for their behaviour used by therapists or interviewers working with them, in the way that a patient of a Kleinian analyst will come to see her problems in Kleinian terms, or the patient of a cognitive therapist sees her problems in cognitive terms. Ted Bundy's explanations for his own violence smack of 'therapy speak'; he is espousing a classic textbook model of addiction. Equally, it might be argued that these men are atypical in that they are the few who *do* use pornography as an exact template for their behaviour – in the same way that convicted violent criminals who may attribute their violence to media imagery are not representative of all men who watch violence.

Yet, as further support for this argument that porn *causes* violence, studies which show a positive correlation between increases in sexually violent crimes and increases in the circulation of pornography are cited.[91] It has been argued that the American states that have the highest rates of reported rape also have the highest rates of porn use and that 95 per cent of delinquents have been exposed to pornography.[92] Studies which have shown that half of child molesters and one third of rapists use hard-core porn to prepare for their attacks are cited,[93] as are studies which demonstrate that rapists show a stronger sexual response when viewing sexual violence than non-raping men.[94] However, correlations between porn and violence may be spurious. Both may be caused by a third factor. For example, Denis Howitt has argued that factors such as divorce may act as confounding variables, as a number of studies show a stronger relationship between the number of divorced males in a population and the number of reported rapes, than between porn and rape. He has argued that if we control for the number of divorced men in a population, there is a very low and statistically non-significant relationship between porn and rape. Equally, whilst 95 per cent of delinquents have used porn, so have 87 per cent of non-delinquents; and there is no difference between sex offenders' and non-offending men's use of pornography.[95] There is also some evidence that rapists come from houses where pornography was banned,[96] which stands in contrast to the view that it is early exposure to porn that sets men on a path of sexual violence, and a number of studies show that rapists' response to sexual violence is *less* than that of non-raping men.[97] So the evidence certainly isn't clear-cut.

Pornography as a Factor in Sexual Abuse

One of the most powerful arguments against pornography is that it is used extensively by rapists and sexual abusers in order to undermine the resistance of their victim – to make them see the acts depicted in magazines and films as 'normal' sexual behaviour. Evidence from women and children subject to sexual violence is presented to bear out this view:

> He encouraged me by showing me pornographic magazines which he kept in the bathroom and told me it was not wrong because they were doing it in the magazines and that made it OK. He told me all fathers do it to their daughters and even pastors do it to their daughters. The magazines were there to help me learn more about sex.[98]

A sixty-four-year-old British paedophile, interviewed by Tim Tate, molested several hundred children between the ages of six and twelve and described how pornography played a role in this:

> I used to leave the child pornography just lying around the house, and when the boy saw it he would naturally be interested in it. Then I'd go alongside him and eventually there would be a situation where I could put my hands on the parts I was interested in. From then onwards it was easy. In my case the pornography would invariably be men having sex with young boys, behaving with them as I would wish to with the boy in the room – buggering them. That's often what I ended up doing and I used the child pornography to get the boys more quickly.[99]

This is an argument which is difficult to dismiss or refute – in this context pornography can clearly have a significant detrimental effect. Children who are exposed to pornography as part of a sexually abusive relationship may feel an added sense of guilt and shame at their viewing of this illicit material, particularly if they find the material sexually arousing, as many undoubtedly do. This can add to the sense of self-blame which many children feel. In this context, pornography could very well act as a powerful factor in maintaining the silence of children, allowing sexual abuse to continue for years.

As well as providing a template for sexual behaviour, critics argue that pornography acts as a precipitator of sexual violence through undermining men's internal inhibitions about rape, because women (and children) are dehumanized. One rapist, quoted by Diana Russell, illustrated this by saying 'It was difficult for me to admit that I was dealing with a human being when I was talking to a woman because if you read men's magazines, you hear about your stereo, your car, your chick.'[100] Andrea Dworkin, one of the most vociferous anti-pornography campaigners, is unequivocal in her condemnation of porn in this light:

> Because of [porn] – because it is the subordination of women perfectly achieved – the abuse done to us . . . is perceived as using us for what we are by nature: women are whores; women want to be raped; she provoked it; women want to be hurt; she says no but she means yes because she wants to be taken against her will which is not really her will because what she wants underneath is to have anything done to her that violates and humiliates her; she wants it, because she is a woman, no matter what it is, because she is a woman; that is how women are, what women are for.[101]

So pornography is seen to legitimate the sexual exploitation of women, making it natural and acceptable. It is seen to provide a visual or written representation of violation and degradation allowing men to see their own execution of these fantasies as normal behaviour.

An analogous argument, and one of the reasons visual material has been the main focus of anti-pornography campaigns – why written material is increasingly exempt from both the ascription of the label 'pornography' and from censorship[102] – is that what we see in porn is 'real' for those who are being photographed. Anti-porn campaigners have focused their attention on the most emotive material – that which involves violence or coercion. It is an argument that is difficult to refute, for even if the depiction of forced or violent sex remains in the realm of fantasy for many of those who read porn, it has been argued that, for the women being photographed or filmed in the making of this material, it is actually happening, and that for many, it is abuse. One witness at the 1985 commission on pornography in the USA reported:

> Women and young girls were tortured and suffered permanent physical injuries to answer publisher demands for photographs depicting sado-masochistic abuse. When the torturer/photographer inquired of the publisher as to the types of depictions that would sell, the torturer/photographer was instructed to get similar existing publications and use the depictions therein for instruction.[103]

So it is argued that if in porn a woman is seen to be simultaneously anally, orally and vaginally fucked, that is really happening. If she is tied and bound and fucked with a dildo, whilst being beaten, that is actually happening. And although many of the acts depicted in pornography are illegal (such as rape), in the US the depiction of rape on film is protected under laws protecting free speech. Drawing a parallel between racism and sexism, Andrea Dworkin and Catharine MacKinnon have asked: 'If lynchings were done *in order* to make photographs, on a ten-billion-dollar-a-year-scale, would that make them protected speech?'[104] In the same vein, it has been argued that the sexual abuse depicted in child porn is real – it is almost impossible to simulate sex with a child without exposing the child to sexual abuse. In most instances, the makers of child porn make no attempt to simulate – the attraction is that the 'sex' is real. Children exposing their genitalia, engaging in foreplay, oral sex or intercourse with adults, other children or animals are not 'acting'.

Testimony from women at the harder end of porn has been used to support the case that their taking part in pornography is often the result of violent coercion and control. Many of the women are working in prostitution and claim to have been forced to take part in photographic shoots or in films. These harrowing personal accounts are powerful ammunition in the fight against porn, and difficult to dismiss as 'not true'. For example, Evelina Giobbe, who testified to the 1985 commission on pornography, described how she had run away from home at the age of thirteen and, following a series of rapes and the 'befriending' by an older man, was eventually sold to a pimp. Afraid of the consequences – beatings, rape and being reported to the authorities for selling sex – she became a prostitute, her whole life controlled by her pimp. She also found herself 'starring' in pornography.

One of my regular customers had a vast collection of both adult and child pornography, including photographs of prepubescent children in bondage. He was a theatre producer and had video equipment in his home . . . He made pornographic videos of myself and another woman on average of once a week for a whole year.

I was often sent to an apartment on the West Side. There were usually two or three men there. After I had sex with them, they'd take pictures of women in various pornographic poses. I didn't have the vocabulary to call them pornographers. I used to think that photography was their hobby. Today, I realize that the studio apartment, furnished with a bed and professional camera equipment was in fact a commercial photography mill.[105]

In these critiques women who appear in pornography are positioned as unwilling victims or as having been conned or coerced. One of the most infamous examples of this was the confession and renunciation of porn by Linda Lovelace (a.k.a. Linda Marchiano), who starred in the film *Deep Throat*. The film centred on the story of a woman whose clitoris was in her throat and therefore needed deep oral penetration by a penis in order to achieve orgasm. Her skill was to be able to relax her throat muscles so that she could swallow an erect penis without choking or gagging. The film was a cheap-budget porn flick made in a matter of days for a budget of only $40,000, yet its influence spread far wider than the dirty-mac brigade. By the end of the seventies the film and its associated products (T-shirts, sexual aids, cassettes, bumper stickers) had grossed $600,000,000.[106] It was seen by a vast number of American movie-goers who had never before seen porn. It became chic, the topic of suburban dinner-party conversation. The complicity and enjoyment of Linda Lovelace was used as ammunition against the 'killjoy feminists' who wanted to ban the sex depicted on screen. As Gloria Steinem comments, the smiling, happy face of Linda Lovelace as glass dildos are inserted into her vagina, as yet another penis penetrates her throat, belied any identification with her humiliation: '*She's there because she wants to be. Who's forcing her? See how she's smiling? See how a real woman enjoys this?*' [Russell's italics][107] was the desired female response. Women were reportedly taken to see the film in droves by their male partners, to learn 'what a woman could do to please a man *if she really wants to*.'[108] Oral sex was suddenly fashionable. Linda Lovelace was held up as the ultimate model of a sexually emancipated woman.

But according to Linda Marchiano herself, in her book *Ordeal*, published a decade after the film was released, this could not have been further from the truth. She claimed to have been introduced to prostitution by her husband (and latterly her pimp) Chuck Traynor. Seeing her perform her sexual feats at a party with a group of men had given the director Gerry Damiano the idea for the film. But Marchiano claimed to have been no more a willing participant in the film than she was in prostitution; she claimed to have been coerced and brutally controlled by Traynor for the whole of their time together. She describes how she was regularly beaten, raped and violated sexually, often with a gun to her head. She was gang-banged, forced to do sex films with a dog and never allowed to show any emotion. Her punishments included having water forced up her rectum with a garden hose and such severe beatings and rapes that she suffered permanent rectal damage and injury to the blood-vessels on her legs. She was literally a prisoner, escaping from Traynor a number of times, returning on one occasion because of fears for the safety of friends who were sheltering her, and on two others because of the disloyalty of those who sheltered her. Traynor denied the stories of abuse; when Linda Marchiano attempted to publicize them after she eventually broke free (Traynor having found a new 'model' and actress, Marilyn Chambers), she faced a disbelieving public. Her accusations were seen as the ramblings of a madwoman with an over-active imagination, her charges described by Traynor as 'so ridiculous I can't take them seriously'. She was apparently greeted in a similar way by those who had watched and imitated the celluloid contortions she now described as 'throat rape'. Gloria Steinem has wryly commented:

> One wonders: Would a male political prisoner or hostage telling a similar story have been so disbelieved? *Ordeal* attacks the myth of female masochism that insists that women enjoy sexual domination and even pain, but prostitution and pornography are big business built on that myth.[109]

In the same vein, it is argued that the children taking part in these films, or in photographic shoots, are as 'willing' as many women who take part in violent porn. They are not running away from the camera. They are not crying or screaming. But they have little choice but take part – the alternatives may be worse. A Florida-based child pornographer, Eric Cross, graphically described the reactions of these children to the 1985 US Senate hearings:

> You might wonder what these children are really like. How do they act when they are with a group of men molesting them? Truthfully, they are psychologically manipulated to such a degree that their facial expressions are blank, as though they are thinking, 'Just get it over with.' Do they cry or fight off my advances? Usually not. Remember in the child's mind they are as guilty as I am. They think that other boys and girls don't do this, so they must not be good children. They're overwhelmed by shame most of the time, and simply comply with the wishes of the adult. Can you imagine what must have gone through the mind of little eight-year-old Yvonne as her father would deliver her to yet another strange man who would keep her for hours at a time, molesting her whenever he got the urge to do so? One of my most vivid memories was of Lisa . . . the second time I saw her it was obvious someone in the group of men had brutalized her, possibly raped her. She told me she didn't want to be photographed, and she also said, 'Please don't hurt me. Just please don't hurt me.'[110]

These are powerful and upsetting arguments which are difficult to refute, and have proved to be powerful ammunition for the censorship lobby in the porn debates. It is difficult to contest the voice of a woman or child who has experienced sexual violence, and who says she or he has been coerced into appearing in pornography. But as Anne McClintock has argued,[111] the story of women such as Linda Marchiano is a story of *marital* abuse, not simply of abuse through pornography. Equally, the stories of children coerced into child porn must be seen as stories of child sexual abuse – and understood in the context of the myriad factors which precipitate and condone such abuse (see Chapter Four) – not simply as an indictment of all pornography. We should be able to condemn violent pornography, child pornography and the sexual abuse of women and children without having to exert a blanket censorship over all sexually explicit material, and without positioning any adult woman who displays her body as a victim, a dupe (or a whore).

Soft-Core Pornography: The Defiant Woman?

Women coerced into taking part in pornography are not representative of *all* women who work in the sex industry. Many women claim positively to embrace such work, particularly at the most public, prolific end of the market – the soft-core magazines such as *Playboy*, *Mayfair*, *Fiesta* etc., or the tabloid magazines and newspapers that feature topless girls. Many Hollywood stars have made their names by appearing as *Playboy* centrefolds (Marilyn Monroe, Sharon Stone, Demi Moore, to name a few). In Britain, many of the topless page-three girls who adorn the British tabloids have gained a notoriety which leads to their moving into television work, pop music and marriage to their 'prince' (often a professional footballer). The tabloids themselves maintain the allure of the page-three girl by photographing her at parties and nightclubs with glamorous men. So one would be hard-pressed to find women *literally* coerced or conned into appearing in soft-core porn. As there is an unending supply of repetitive, ultimately boring (at least to my eyes) porn available freely in Europe and North America, there appears also to be an unending supply of women willing to be filmed or photographed.

Many women enter into pornography willingly, arguing that it's just a job or that it demonstrates an openness about sexuality, a lack of inhibition: The ultimate in female sexual emancipation – not only are they happy to express their sexuality and display it to a sexual partner, but they feel confident enough to display it to the world. Annie Sprinkle is one example – a woman who has claimed to have revelled in her starring role in hundreds of porn films, before branching into 'performance art' and the exploration of female sexuality with a female gaze, as was discussed above (p. 147). The popularity of the 'readers' wives' sections in many soft-core magazines may also be explained in this way – women wanting the world to see that they are sexual and desirable, that they too can be a porn 'model'. However, that this self-exposure is a positive celebration of female sexuality is a view which has been vehemently rejected by many critics. Susan Griffin, in a violent condemnation of pornography and pornographers, has argued that:

> The model in a pornographic magazine is not defiant. She has been paid
> to take off her clothing. And she has about her posture the attitude of

one who has been paid to move in a certain way. She is chattel. When she is chained her chains are redundant, for we know she is not a free being. The whole value, the thrill of a 'peep show' or a centrefold depends on a woman's degradation. In this way she plays the whore. For she is *literally* for sale.[112]

The woman's image may be for sale but we have to acknowledge that many of the women themselves don't see themselves as degraded. 'When a woman's best asset is her body, why not flaunt it?' advocates of such material would say. Where do we draw the line between women exhibiting their bodies in pornographic magazines and films, and those whose fortunes are made by their appearance as 'supermodels' or actresses?

As women are sold the message that beauty (and sexuality) is their passport to happiness, from fairy tales through to adult mass media imagery, are the porn 'stars' any different? Is showing their genitalia so perverse? When female performance artists expose their genitalia and define it as 'art', can we still condemn the female porn star? Do women not have a right to explore, or enjoy, what is deemed by the majority to be in the realm of the 'obscene'? Do explicit representations of sex or of women's bodies inevitably position 'woman' as violated victim? As sex itself is often associated with an exploration of issues of power and control – and as gendered power differences are at the centre of the script of heterosexuality – in censoring the representation of such issues are we not censoring sex itself?

Censoring 'Sex'

The pornography debates are not just about representations of sex, they are a critique of sexual relationships and in particular of heterosexuality as it is currently constructed. Implicit within many of the feminist critiques are the questions: What is 'proper' sex? What are the appropriate sexual positions (in every sense of the word) for woman and man? Many anti-pornography campaigners appear to be categorizing sexual activities that involve power differences, dominance and submission, or any element of objectification, as improper, implying that 'normal' sex is a relationship between equals in which no issues of inequality are involved. In this way, as Lynne Segal has argued, in attempting to ban the representation of sexualized power imbalances in pornography, we are implicitly condemning much of heterosexual sex.

The fact that many of the radical feminist porn critiques *are* rooted in a condemnation of 'normal' heterosexual sex is illustrated by the comments of two of the most vociferous critics of pornography, Andrea Dworkin and Catharine MacKinnon:

> Intercourse occurs in the context of a power relationship that is pervasive and incontrovertible. The context in which the act takes place, whatever the meaning of the act in and of itself, is one in which men have social, economic and physical control over women.   DWORKIN[113]

> If sex is ordinarily accepted as something men do *to* women, the . . . question [is] whether consent is a meaningful concept.
>
>   MACKINNON[114]

Those adopting this position will condemn 'pornography' because it represents heterosexual sex (or heterosexual power imbalances), regardless of its explicit violent content. Yet it is not only explicit sex that is condemned. Catharine MacKinnon has also commented, 'What looks like love and romance in the liberal view looks a lot like hatred and torture in the feminist view. Pleasure and eroticism become violation.'[115]

These arguments must be seen as part of the feminist 'sex debates' of the seventies and eighties, in which heterosexuality was positioned as central to man's oppression and subjugation of woman, and women who claimed to 'choose' heterosexuality were described by radical separatists such as Mary Daly as 'dupes', or their sexuality seen as a forced choice because of the dominance of heterosexuality within patriarchy, and therefore not a choice at all. In the minds of many feminist activists it was impossible for a heterosexual woman to be in any way 'liberated'. In 'sleeping with the enemy' she was not only undermining herself but symbolically increasing the oppression of all women. As the Leeds Revolutionary Feminist Group proclaimed in a pamphlet published in 1981:

> Any woman who takes part in a heterosexual couple helps to shore up male supremacy by making its foundations stronger . . . Every act of penetration for the woman is an invasion which undermines her confidence and saps her strength. For a man it is an act of power and mastery which makes him stronger, not just over one woman but over all women.

> So every woman who engages in penetration bolsters the oppressor and
> reinforces the class power of men . . . As no individual woman can be
> 'liberated' under male supremacy, so no act of penetration can escape its
> function and its symbolic power.[116]

This denunciation of heterosexuality led to vociferous debates in the
seventies and eighties and to divisions between lesbian and heterosexual
feminists in both Britain and North America – often described as the
'sex wars'. Many feminists declared that lesbianism was the only way
for women to achieve any form of emancipation. As Charlotte Bruch
commented, 'lesbianism is the key to liberation and only women who
cut their ties to male privilege can be trusted to remain serious in the
struggle against male dominance.'[117] As a result of this, as Sarah Schulman
has documented, 'in the early seventies, one day half the women's
movement came out as lesbians.'[118] Whilst this is probably an exaggeration (and many of these 'political lesbians' later resumed heterosexual
relationships), these critiques of the structure of male–female relationships and the role of heterosexuality in maintaining women's status as
'other' undoubtedly had a considerable effect on the material lives of
many women, who embarked upon relationships with women or
attempted to rework their relationship with men as a result. In recent
years, 'political lesbianism' has become a rare thing. Heterosexual
feminists have rejected the position of 'dupe' and publicly proclaimed
their enjoyment of sex with men and their ability to engage in heterosexual relationships which are not oppressive.[119] Outside radical feminist
circles, lesbianism is more about sex, desire and love than it is about
gender politics.

These debates around heterosexuality are parallel to and underpin
the feminist porn debates. The essence of both discussions is the question
of the 'correct' expression and depiction of women's sexual pleasure
and desire. Undoubtedly pornography which is constructed within a
masculine gaze presents us with a narrow view of female sexuality or
desire: 'Woman' is depicted desiring man (or his penis); any exploration
of autonomous female pleasure (or desire for other women) is invariably
a display for the male voyeur, as we have already seen, as satisfaction
can only be achieved through the intervention of the phallic man –
through woman being fucked. This is in essence a power imbalance –
as the anti-pornography campaigners have repeatedly argued – reflecting

the dominant construction of heterosexual relationships, where the role of 'woman' is created within the script of femininity, with 'woman' taking up a position which is secondary to that of 'man'.

If we accept this as a simple reflection of 'reality', seeing the enactment of sexual power imbalances in either representation or material practice (i.e., during the act of sex) as a reflection of the 'true' oppression of women, then it isn't surprising that both pornography and heterosexual sex are condemned. But as has been illustrated already, representation reflects fantasy as much as 'reality', and women are not simply passive dupes, mindlessly taking up the position of subjugated other to man. As I argued earlier, women may act out the role of 'girl' but this doesn't mean they *are* 'girl'. Heterosexual women *can* negotiate a position for themselves which is positive and empowering, even if this means a partial adoption of a feminine masquerade. As vehement feminist defenders of heterosexuality such as Wendy Hollway and Lynne Segal have argued, being 'straight' does not inevitably mean being in a strait-jacket. There is nothing inherently *bad* about heterosexual sex, and many women like to fuck. As one woman I interviewed commented, 'The power and pleasure I experience during intercourse is like nothing else. It's my greatest release.'

The radical feminist positioning of heterosexual sex or representations of sexual power imbalances as 'bad' is at odds with many women's experiences and, if it is taken on board, may result in feelings of guilt or shame at the pleasures and desires in which they indulge. Or it may result in the absence of any discussion of women's sexual pleasure or desire that runs contrary to the 'correct' political line – in a recent feminist 'reader' on heterosexuality, in which women were asked to account for how they reconciled heterosexuality and feminism, the dominant voice was one of apology. None talked openly of the pleasures of heterosexual sex.[120]

We must also acknowledge that it is not only heterosexual sex that is associated with issues of power. Arguably, *all* desire and sexuality is irrevocably linked to imbalances of power, the unobtainable and the gap between wanting and having – regardless of gender or sexual preference. Lesbian (and gay male) sex is not immune from power games. We can see this played out most explicitly in the recent wave of lesbian erotica, in which women take up positions of power and powerlessness and desire is often premised on the exploration of difference. And this is a reflection of the sexual lives of many lesbians, who have moved away from 'politically correct' vanilla sex towards the exploration of 'bad girl' or 'post-feminist' sex. In direct contrast to many of the lesbian feminist arguments of the seventies and early eighties, men are no longer seen as 'the enemy', and forbidden sexual roles and practices – such as S/M, butch/femme role play, penetration and sexual desire divorced from politics – are being openly explored and celebrated. The increasing ubiquity of representations of these practices has opened up questions of the accepted definitions of 'pornography' and the issue of whether there can be a 'pornography' framed within a female gaze. It is a controversial topic.

Pornography for Women: A Contradiction in Terms?

In the censorship debates there is an implicit assumption that all women will condemn pornography, that a pornography *for* women is a contradiction in terms. Public pronouncements would seem to suggest that this is 'true'. Carol Vance has commented on the marked absence of any women giving a positive view of porn during the 1985 US Senate hearings, which she sat through as an observer. One woman, who attempted to defend her position as a *Penthouse* pin-up, was verbally attacked, her account dismissed. No women talked of the use of pornography in a consensual setting, or of finding it positive or pleasurable – that would have been to court accusations of 'perversion'. So the voices of women that have been represented in the public debates have been predominantly anti-porn. It is assumed that this is the *natural* position of 'woman'.

Research on pornography appears to reinforce this message. The majority of women who have taken part in research which examines their beliefs or feelings about pornography have been reported as saying that it has at best had a negative effect, and at worst a neutral effect on their lives. For example, in a study of women in Canada, the psychologist Charlene Senn found that the majority of women believed that pornography was linked to male violence towards women, that it was harmful and could not be seen as 'just entertainment'. Similarly, in a survey conducted in the British edition of *Cosmopolitan* in the late eighties, of the nearly 4,000 women who replied, only 3 per cent categorized pornography as 'ok', 'not all that bad' or 'fun'. A similar survey in *Company* magazine reported that 98 per cent of the women respondents believed that pornography encouraged violence against women. A survey of 567 women conducted in the north of England in 1990 reported that three quarters believed that soft-core pornography degrades women, two thirds that newsagents should be banned from selling magazines such as *Playboy*, *Penthouse* and *Mayfair*, and 83 per cent that pornography increased violence towards women.[121]

So it would seem that the pro-censorship debate has permeated lay consciousness and that the negative effects of porn are now accepted – by many women at least – as 'fact'. The views of anti-censorship campaigners, or academic feminists such as Lynne Segal, Elizabeth Cowie, Carol Vance and Linda Williams, who have argued that pornography is more about fantasy than reality, appear to have little impact on lay beliefs. Whilst we may question whether the women who take part in surveys on porn are representative (those who would condemn it are more likely to respond) and argue that women who enjoy porn are unlikely to speak out publicly, feeling understandably wary about exposing their own sexual fantasies, there is undoubtedly a trend towards unilaterally condemning pornography amongst women. That is certainly the impression I received when talking to, or interviewing, women about sexuality and pornography over the last few years. There are very few women who have anything positive to say about pornography, and many become extremely angry when it is suggested there may be any ambiguity over its damaging effects. This is the case regardless of whether women have viewed pornography themselves – many who would vehemently condemn it have not actually examined either soft- or hard-core material in any detail (if at all) and condemn it on reputation or on reports of its contents or effects.

Yet not all women feel this way. Many women *do* read or watch pornography, sometimes with their partners and sometimes on their own. Despite the notion that 'good girls' don't like porn, even material produced primarily for men may be erotic for women. As one woman who was interviewed commented:

> 'I enjoy watching porn with my partner before we have sex. It puts me in the right mood, and turns *him* on to watch it with me. Most of what we watch is just couples having sex. Pretty normal stuff. I wouldn't watch anything violent. I like reading the magazines, too. Sometimes they turn me on even more than the films.'

The sex women watch or read about doesn't necessarily remain at the level of fantasy. As many critics of pornography claim, erotic material both shapes and reflects sexual desire and behaviour. But in a consensual relationship, where violence is not the focus of sex, this can have a different meaning entirely:

> 'Of course we sometimes act out what we've been watching. That's part of the fun. It makes me a bit more adventurous than I might be otherwise. It gives us ideas. It also gives me more confidence to ask my partner to do things for me. Mostly he doesn't have to be asked. He can tell what turns me on by my reactions to the films.'

Women who view pornography are invariably discerning viewers. They will often be turned on by very different imagery than men (I have yet to find a woman who admits to finding the classic come shot erotic). They may be more critical of the representations of women in mainstream pornography. As one woman commented, 'Women in porn look like dolls. Or like tarts. They have enormous breasts and skinny waists. Sometimes I think they just look silly, as if they've been pumped up with air.'[122] Many women prefer to read erotic material rather than watch videos or look at magazines. The success of classics such as Pauline Réage's *The Story of O*,[123] the diaries of Anaïs Nin or Nancy Friday's *The Secret Garden*, has spawned a gamut of erotic novels and 'diaries' – aimed primarily at women (such as the Black Lace series in Britain). These books go a step further than the 'sex and shopping' blockbusters of the eighties – less shopping and more explicit sex.

There is a growing body of visual 'pornography' being produced by and for women. In the early eighties a group of female porn stars got together and formed a support group, Club 90,[124] which led to the development of a female production company, Femme, and the beginnings of pornography seen from the perspective of the (heterosexual) female gaze. This is sex beyond the dominance of the phallus. As Candida Royalle, the founder of Femme, has commented:

> Porn was always for men. Now that women are finally allowed to have a sexuality, we are looking for stimulus. Women are saying, 'Okay, now let's look at a film.' Well, now it's time to start making films for women. That doesn't just mean quality and scripts. It means, what's sex all about?[125]

Pornography framed within a female gaze depicts 'sex' in which woman is more than object or hole to be fucked. It allows (or focuses on) depictions of female pleasure and desire rather than simply demonstrating the mechanics of sex or the power and pleasure of man. It allows depictions of women in positions of sexual power. Yet unsurprisingly (given the themes running through romantic fiction, which Anne Snitow has described as 'pornography for women'), themes of dominance and submission are also ubiquitous, reflecting common fantasies of women. As one woman who does use pornography commented, 'I wouldn't admit it in public, but I always have fantasies about being dominated when I masturbate. I read stories about women being punished in order to get turned on.' This woman is not alone. As Lynne Segal has written of her own sexual fantasies: 'I am always passive, objectified, humiliated, and whatever abuse I can imagine to be happening at the time also contains the threat of even worse to follow.'[126] This is reminiscent of the themes running through girls' comics, as we have already seen.

This exploration of sex and desire from the woman's perspective is a direct attempt to counter the masculine dominance of the erotic and to create a space for the development of a woman's voice and gaze in the sexual sphere. As the Canadian collective Kiss and Tell argues:

> Pornography is assumed to be made by men and for men. Sexual images by and for women are never mentioned. It's such a familiar erasure of our lives. It leads to a law where what is assumed to be true about men is by default true about women. A *Penthouse* portrayal of a woman in bondage and a woman's portrayal of herself in bondage are seen as the same thing. There is no difference between a tired old view of the Subordinated Other, and a vulnerable self-exploration.[127]

This very act of producing explicit sexual material by and for women stands as one of the most powerful forms of resistance to the dominance of the phallocentric masculine gaze and the narrow definitions of the sexual positions in which we can imagine 'woman'. This clearly follows in the traditions of feminist artists and film-makers who have framed 'woman' within a female gaze. Yet whilst erotica featuring and aimed at heterosexual women is becoming more common, it is lesbians who have perhaps gone furthest in exploring the erotic and creating 'pornography' within a female gaze. Lesbians are arguably less constrained in defining their sexuality as separate from the phallic sexuality of 'man' and so have more space for the exploration of female sexuality outside the passive reactive position we see in much of art, film and pornography. I would prefer not to follow Monique Wittig, who declared 'lesbians are not woman'[128] because their lives defy the script of heterosexual femininity, but rather to argue that lesbians can provide us with a vision of 'woman' outside the constraints of heterosexuality and show us that it is not inevitable for women to have to 'do girl'. Looking to lesbian erotica and pornography gives us an insight into some of the possibilities of representations of the sexuality of 'woman' framed within a different script. Yet ironically, this genre of representations has received as much condemnation from feminist critics of pornography as pornography framed within a masculine gaze.

Pornography: Do Good Girls Look the Other Way?

Persimmon: Back in the seventies, anti-porn analysis reigned supreme in the feminist movement, and I was a for sure feminist . . . I was a new convert to the adventure of feminism, full of passionate ideas and unexamined arrogance; a born-again lesbian, making right-on art about right-on sex: pure theory. *If what we* don't *like is man-made images of subservient women in lacy underwear, then what we do like must be perfectly naked lesbians, with equal haircuts. If this one's touching that one's cunt, that one had better be touching this one's cunt, at the same time, in the same way, or else it's not True Equality.*

I made a lot of sculptures of women floating in the air, because perfect mutuality was otherwise anatomically impossible.

But nothing is ever that simple. At the same time as I was making theoretical art, my sex life was more complicated. My lover at the time was a retired sex worker who had come out in the sixties . . . sex between us was sweet, terrifying, and wild.

The feeling of our sex was *not* what I was calling up when I made those sculptures. Why didn't I notice that the sex I was having and the sex I was portraying were so different? Why didn't I pay attention to how sex *really felt* when I was making those flying fucks? Shame, I guess. Shame so deep I couldn't look it in the face. *Sometimes even the softest of scenes scared me. Other times rape fantasies turned me on. Sometimes I pretended my lover was a guy.*

Let's be clear about this: it wasn't feminists who taught me sexual shame. I learned it long before, under harder hands. By the time I was a

teenager I had already learned to disconnect from my body. How I felt
didn't matter. Sex wasn't about how I felt. It was about doing what I was
told. Trying not to gag when my gentle boyfriend came in my mouth;
pretending I was turned on when I wasn't or pretending I wasn't when
I was; pretending I didn't see the tied-up naked girls in the porn mag;
pretending I didn't know her, want her, want to be her. *Because if you
want that (they say), you will be telling men that rape is fun (they say), you will
be asking for it (they say). Good Girls look the other way.*

The feminist movement gave me far more than its faults. It gave me
hope, pride, work, a place to stand. But sometimes it seemed no different
from where I grew up. You had to pretend and not notice you were
pretending. You had to shut up and swallow it.   *Kiss and Tell*[129]

The very concept of lesbian pornography arouses strong emotions, as
the extract above demonstrates. I have quoted it at length as it provides
an excellent illustration of the contradiction inherent in lesbian pornography debates. Good girls (or feminists) are not supposed to enjoy
'pornography'. Yet where does that leave women's fantasies and desires?
What if it is the forbidden which turns us on? Does the suppression of
sexual representation not act to repress *women's* desires? Many lesbians
have ignored the critiques, in order to explore what were previously
invisible pleasures and desires.

Lesbian film-makers, and photographers such as Della Grace,[130] Jill
Posner[131] and the Canadian collective Kiss and Tell have captured
women having sex with women or women desiring women in explicit
images celebrating the sexuality of 'woman'. Many of these images
show women gazing at the camera, strong and proud in their sexuality
and their bodies. There is no coyness or feigned resistance here – even
in the images of the archetypal 'femme' women. This is a positive
exploration of female sexuality and desire, with women very much
controlling the gaze. Sexual, erotic and powerful, these representations
explore female sexuality from the point of view of women who feel
no shame or embarrassment about their sexuality or desire. This stands
in direct contrast to the archetypal visions of female sexuality framed
in the masculine gaze; here it is woman who is in control of the gaze
at every level – as photographer or film-maker; as spectator within the
image; and as intended viewer of the image that is produced.

Similarly, lesbian erotic fiction contains scenes between women which centre on women's pleasure and desire outside the constrictions of the traditional script of femininity; these are not stories of women waiting for the mythical prince. Some of this fiction has involved a deliberate attempt to move away from traditional heterosexual positions of power/powerlessness, allowing two women to experience and express their desire for each other without one or other taking up the position of sexual object:

> I stretch out on the bed and she rubs my back, sensuously and slowly like she did that first time. When I turn over, she positions her vulva above my face and begins to lick my labia, darting her tongue into my vagina, causing internal sparks to shoot around my body, along my limbs. I separate her folds and press my lips against her cleft, move my head from side to side. I search out the faint smell of her, draw down the soft liquid, say a prayer of thanks for this blessing, this sacrifice.
>
> She must have a finger inside me from the way I feel all full inside, feel that more generalized pleasure that penetration brings added to the exquisite blaze pulsating from my clitoris. What I am doing to her merges with what she is doing to me, blends with our humming sounds, the feeling of enclosed, protected space. I feel weightless, surrounded by warm loving, peak and relax with a sustained sense of excitement.[132]

Here, women are depicted enjoying sex and pleasuring each other, without fear, dread or denigration – very different from phallocentric images of women's sexuality. It is not the penis, that 'fiery brand' immortalized in romantic fiction, that provides ecstatic pleasure here.

More explicit erotic imagery plays on sado-masochistic themes yet does not position 'woman' as object to be used. Here is an example of the work of Joan Nestle, playing gently on the dominance–submission theme in a way that still celebrates female sexual pleasure and power:

> I push her back, letting her know I will not accept her impatience. Soon her breath quickens and a new sheen of sweat shines upon her skin. I lean forward and lick drops of her body's wetness off her chest, lingering in the hollow of her throat. Now she knows what I will do and all her strength cannot stop me. I stand straight in front of her, close but not resting on her. She senses my certainty, smells my perfume and tenses.
>
> 'You know what I am going to do.'
>
> Her head turns, following the words. Her eyes are still closed.

'Oh Joan, Oh God', she implores. My hand moves down to her hips, to her lower belly, to her thighs. I peel off her pants as I travel, letting them fall to her ankles. She stands naked before me. Her body is arched, hungry, tight. I enjoy all that I see with a deep appreciation for her work and with a delight at what I can bring her. I move closer, my breath touching her. After a silence, a protracted moment of suspended action, I cup her cunt in my hand. Her wetness is already seeping through. My red nails are petals of crimson against her wiry hair. Now she rests in my palm, her smallest muscle is throbbing in my hand. My body moves behind each rubbing, pushing her harder against the wall, pushing her into her own rhythm of want. Suddenly, knowing she is ready, I seize her turned head and with a quick move, enter her, reminding her of the waiting, wanting, softness beneath the bone.[133]

Lust, desire and seduction – but an absence of objectification, and no hint of misogyny. A sexual act that takes on a different meaning from those described in much of heterosexual fiction, because both protagonists are women and the pleasure of the woman seduced is at the centre of the scene. Male authors, using similar language, have often produced a very different set of meanings. For example, take Henry Miller, in *Nexus*, talking of his hero Val and his 'seductive chat' to his friend's wife Ida: 'I like your cunt, Ida . . . it's the best thing about you.' The sex they engage in excites her desire, but it is the *man's* power and pleasure that is at issue, not hers:

I laid her on a small table and when she was on the verge of exploding I picked her up and walked around the room with her; then I took it out and made her walk on her hands holding her by her thighs, letting it slip out now and then to excite her still more . . . It went on like this until I had such an erection that even after I shot a wad into her it stayed up like a hammer. That excited her terribly.[134]

Yet this glorification in the objectification of the female – and the sadistic delight in her desire – is not absent in lesbian fiction. Pat Califa is a mistress of this genre and delights in crossing boundaries in her depictions of 'bad-girl' sex. In one tale, 'The Calyx of Isis,' her heroine, Tyre, comments, 'I don't find vanilla sex particularly effective. I've got nothing against it, anymore than I have against chicken farmers or Halley's comet, but they don't get me off, either.' Her birthday surprise for her lover, Roxanne, is the living-out of a sexual fantasy – a 'bad-girl's' sexual dream:

> I want a gang, a pack, a bunch of tough and experienced top women. I'll leave the exact number up to you, but I don't just want a threesome in warm leatherette. I would rather it not be women Roxanne already knows. And no novices, they would just get in the way. Once you get that group together I want to give them Roxanne, and if she makes me proud I want her to belong to me, wear my rings. If she still wants me. She might decide it's too much, or maybe she'll tumble for one of the other tops. I have to know where she's at before I fall any more in love with her. I want somebody I can perfect with hard, constant training. A living work of art I can show off on Folsom Street as my counterpart. So pretty and alive and responsive to me that it will make all the other tops, boys and girls, gnaw on their arms.[135]

Pat Califa is not alone in her fantasies (which are acted out in minute, erotic detail in her writing). In the nineties, the traditional themes of romantic fiction – of courtly love or forced 'seduction' – are played out in explicit sex scenes in lesbian fiction, film and photography. 'Bad-girl' sexuality, fucking and power games are now celebrated, not derided.

Take the genre of lesbian erotica characterized by magazines such as *Quim* (UK), *Bad Attitudes* and *On Our Backs* (US), and *Wicked Women* (Australia), in which power, pleasure and pain are forthrightly explored. Many visual images and erotic stories portray women engaged in rough sex, sometimes overtly sado-masochistic, at other times engaged merely in devouring or 'seducing' each other. Arguably, these representations subvert the feminine masquerade by showing 'woman' as both active and sexual, capable of taking up the positions of subject and object of desire alternately. There are many representations of women playing at sexual power games – butch/femme, whips and leather – that subvert rather than reinforce phallocentric traditions because these women are knowing actors in these sexual scenarios.

One of the dominant representations here is that of the woman literally taking on the phallus by wearing a prosthetic penis – a strap-on dildo. This often involves assuming an archetypal masculine phallic subject position – yet doing so in clear parody, as an obvious masquerade, because these women are still women and are not 'really' pretending to be anything else. There is no attempt to disguise the material reality of the woman's body – that she has breasts, that her 'penis' is not 'real'. In addition, the woman who takes on a masculine or phallic identification, if only temporarily, is deliberately taking up this position whilst knowing that it is not based on material reality, that it is not immutable. She can stop at any time. She can take off the symbolic phallus – literally – in a way a man never can. In this way the masquerade of both masculinity and femininity is played out and exposed. As Judith Butler has argued in her book *Gender Trouble*,[136] this performance radically undermines assumptions about sex, gender and sexuality by parodying the heterosexual 'original'. The strap-on dildo acts as a fetish, as a play with desire, power and 'perversion'. As Parveen Adams has argued, the themes in lesbian erotica represent a new form of transgressive sexuality, which defies a pathological label:

> There is erotic play and plasticity and movement: she constructs fetishes and substitutes them, one for another; she multiplies and tries them on like costumes. All this is done quite explicitly as an incitement of the senses, a proliferation of bodily pleasures, a transgressive excitement; a play with identity and a play with genitality.[137]

Yet this isn't merely about women taking on the phallus at the level of the symbolic. These pornographic or erotic representations reflect the 'real-life' sexual practice of an increasing number of lesbians, particularly those in the younger age groups. Perfect rubber phalluses are selling like hot cakes. Perhaps this is because many women are finding that they can attain pleasure, power, or just a sense of amusement, through deliberately assuming this aspect of masculinity as masquerade. Or perhaps it is because for many women – lesbian and bisexual, as well as heterosexual – the act of penetration is pleasurable and satisfying.[138] Dildos are only one means of satisfying this particular desire – a symbolic phallus that never fails, as it is always hard. It is in the complete control of the woman who wears it. There is no anxiety; performance is impeccable every time – the perfect phallic fantasy.

As in lesbian erotic fiction, these are representations of objectification *deliberately* played out – women taking control of their female lovers or willingly taking up the position of derided sexual object themselves. This is where this genre of lesbian erotica differs from the traditional phallocentric depiction of the violated woman: Being fucked, or assuming a masochistic role, is a choice or an option, a sexual game that increases desire. It is a deliberate play on the erotic potential of power and powerlessness. Out of the bedroom, in the main,[139] the game stops. In the bedroom, unconscious fantasies, anxieties and forbidden desires are played out and explored. Take this segment of a story from Kiss and Tell, the feminist collective of artists and photographers who explicitly explore themes around female sexuality, desire and pornography in their work:

She stayed where she was. 'You're in charge'.

I caught my breath. 'Yes,' I said. 'Okay.' I let the thought run in my mind. 'Get me a drink of water,' I said.

She brought me a glass of water.

'Okay, kneel by the bed,' I told her. She obeyed.

Amazing. I was trying not to grin, but it was hard. I drank some water and then, on a second's impulse, I threw the lot in her face. She knelt there, water dripping down her neck. She looked very serious and sweet.

'Get on the bed,' I said.

She obeyed. We lay together, kissing and feeling each other, till that terribly lovely pain rose in me again.

'Tie me up,' I said.

She went to my suitcase and pulled out four long leather straps that I had certainly never packed. She stretched me out on the bed, tying my wrists and ankles to the iron bedstead. She lay on top of me, touching my bound body softly, kissing my mouth. I wanted to hold her, touch her, but I was tied to the bed. A wild helplessness filled my chest, like panic, but sweeter.

When I was moaning under her, she got up and went back to my suitcase. She pulled out a knife. 'Don't,' I said. She stopped. I could see the pearly light on her cheekbones, the line of her shoulders, her breasts under the tight T-shirt, her legs spread casually wide.

'No, it's okay,' I said. 'Do it.'

She cut the buttons off my shirt, one by one, and opened it; cut my bra into pieces and threw it on the floor. She slit open my pants and pulled them off. It was a sharp knife. I could tell. I lay there, tied open, exposed. She sat back, her eyes cruising my body. I waited. She waited. My mouth was dry. My heart was pounding, pounding.

'Please,' I said, and she slowly moved toward me. With the back of the knife blade, she stroked my nipples, first one, then the other, over and over. Fear and desire fought in my throat. My body was slick with sweat. My breath came fast and ragged.

She leaned over to the bedside table and pulled out a package of latex gloves . . . she pulled one on. It was shiny silver. Safer sex with style. She untied me, retied me ass up. I could feel her eyes on me. There was no way to hide. The back of her blade caressed my butt, and then suddenly the edge, swift and sharp. I gasped and twisted my tied body so I could see her over my shoulder. Her face was hard and beautiful. She parted the cheeks of my ass and her knife whispered across my crack. Slowly, she slipped a finger up my ass, and then out. My cunt was open, wet, yearning toward her, but she ignored it. Her fingers were slick with lube from somewhere, nowhere. Two fingers now up my tight hot hole, burning inside me, filling me with fire. I couldn't breathe. She pushed into me, slowly, slowly, taking me moaning, crying, tied writhing on the harsh sheets. The impossibly slow strokes, her knife, her mouth. She had me, held me, hurt me. I was hers.[140]

There is no sense here of the sexual object not being a person, an active agent; there is humour in the taking-up of roles and acknowledgement of the beauty of the other. This is a game between equals – a far cry from sexual violence or objectification based on fear, disgust or dread. It is in many ways reminiscent of women's reading of Mills & Boon and Harlequin novels. For whilst the woman here is 'taken', she is revelling in this masochistic role but the action is very much in her control. The 'bottom' in an SM scene always provides the boundaries and controls the action, as the heroine of romantic fiction brings the hero to his knees. This extract illustrates the pleasure in powerlessness, the erotic charge in being willingly 'had'.

Lesbian erotica that plays on sado-masochistic themes has been accused by some of reinforcing 'hetero-patriarchal' power, in that it emulates the objectification of women that often takes place in heterosexual sex, in both representation and material reality.[141] But lesbians who read or view sado-masochistic imagery do not act out these scenarios on unwilling victims. For many women it remains at the level of fantasy, the transgressive nature of the imagery being at the centre of its attraction. It is a play on the power games women have been unable to escape if they in any way want to adopt the feminine masquerade. Here women are choosing to take up the position of object – analogous to that of the powerless, overpowered infant – but often alternating to assume the position of aggressor, switching roles in fantasy in a way that is often impossible in material reality. Both women and men fantasize about being seduced, about being overpowered. It is one of our most basic desires, originating in that early relationship with the mother when we are helpless and dependent on that first woman not to misuse her power, as was argued above. Re-creating those early fantasies, desires and fears is one of the most common erotic thrills. It shouldn't surprise us that when women take up the pen, the brush or the lens it is a fantasy that they too explore, or that the violent passions which underline sexual desire are forthrightly explored.

We shouldn't be surprised that the nineties have seen this exploration of 'forbidden' lesbian sex. It can be seen as resistance to the dominant ethos of the previous generation of lesbian feminists, who argued for the rejection of all that was representative of heterosexuality, including penetration, power games and any notion of violence or surrender, as we have seen. So fucking, power, SM, and the deliberate taking-on of phallic symbolism has become both transgressive and exciting. As Linda Williams has argued:

> The remarkable, but politically incorrect, popularity of sado-masochistic fantasy among many contemporary women does not mean that feminism has retreated and the masculine sadists have won. Indeed, it means that the compulsion for women to be strong necessitates an erotically transgressive release in being dominated.[142]

Perhaps this is why one of the dominant themes within lesbian erotica is of women being 'fucked', sometimes by women, often by gay men. This, perhaps, is as transgressive as you can get – as far from the PC, right-on, radical feminist sisterhood as could possibly be imagined. It is also, arguably, acting to subvert heterosexuality at the same time because it is in no way 'straight sex'. Pat Califa, a mistress of this genre, describes, in 'The Surprise Party', the reaction of her lesbian heroine to the realization that the male cop who is sexually assaulting her in the back of his car is gay:

> Were these two cops faggots? It didn't make sense. Her cunt convulsed. Leathermen were sexy enough – dark knights and princes that she loved

to look at, even if women weren't supposed to touch. By comparison, cops were kings – fuck emperors. In the hierarchy of sex objects, she guessed gay cops ranked next to God.

She is made to 'give him head':

> He held her head still and bucked his hips, rolling the tip of his hard penis back and forth across the spot in the back of her throat that made her gag. Tears came into her eyes, her nose ran, and her mouth streamed with saliva and coughed up mucus. Every now and then, he let her up for air, but as soon as she had taken a deep breath, he seized her again, and filled her throat, and pummelled it. It was deeply and perversely thrilling to be used in this way, with just the right amount of cruelty. She found herself wishing she could taste his cock instead of the bland skin of the condom. And she was proud she had made it hard, not one of the city cops in the front seat. These were dangerous thoughts, but she could not relinquish them.[143]

Dangerous indeed – oral rape might be one of the worst things imaginable in material reality. In fantasy it allows an exploration of the forbidden (for many lesbians) – the penises of men. This isn't always a masochistic scenario: Taking up the position of 'man' and *doing* the fucking is a not uncommon fantasy. In the sex between gay men and lesbians which is an increasingly common practice in the 'queer culture' of the nineties (again, especially in the younger age groups), we see this transgression taken one step further. This is men having sex with women outside of the boundaries of heterosexuality – these gay men and lesbians are *doing* (or parodying) heterosexuality, willingly experiencing any threat to their identity as 'queer' – and exploring another aspect of their own sexual repertoire. As one lesbian I interviewed commented, 'Fucking a gay boy with a strap-on is one of my favourite fantasies.' This is perhaps the ultimate subversion of the traditional position of 'woman', and acts to destabilize or overturn heterosexual hegemony – in the same way that lesbian drag kings and butches, as well as drag queens, in the words of Judith Butler, 'implicitly reveal the imitative structure of gender itself'.[144] This is a woman 'doing' *man*.

We may question whether the naïve outsider (be they straight or gay) who does not know how to 'read' these transgressive acts will see them as anything other than 'normal' sex – or see the drag king or queen as wanting to *be* (rather than *do*) 'woman' or 'man'. As Lynne Segal has argued, 'if "queer" still looks queer, however titillatingly "wild" and deviant, it may mystify and muddle more than threaten and trouble its straight audience.'[145] But as the audience is *not* intended to be straight – lesbian erotica or porn is produced for lesbians, not for men or straight women – *mis*readings are not a problem for the creators of this particular sexualized gaze. It is a problem only for those whose assumptions about *normal* sex or the 'natural' position of 'woman' or 'man' are challenged by these open subversions. It's not surprising that such imagery is invariably banned.

Unravelling the Contradictions in the Porn Debates: Moving towards an Analysis of 'Sex'

The debates about pornography – and about the meanings behind the fantasies of 'woman' framed in the pornographer's gaze – defy simple analysis. On the one hand we cannot deny that the warding-off of the fear of 'woman' through her denigration as sex object or her violation *is* present in much of the material that is designated as pornography. We can also see it in many men's treatment of women, in particular in the whole gamut of ideologies associated with sexual violence. But pornography does not *cause* this. Porn undoubtedly eroticizes sexual violence and presents 'woman' as object, potentially allowing men to legitimate violent actions as part of a normal sexual repertoire. Yet the denigration of 'woman' and sexual violence existed long before pornography. Banning pornography is not the answer to the problem. If it were and we could eradicate sexual violence overnight through censorship, few would oppose it. 'Free speech' is nothing in comparison to women's lives. But it isn't that simple.

The combination of misogyny and masculine insecurity underlying the systematic violation of women goes far beyond pornography. Arguably, porn is as much a symptom as a cause. It reflects sexual fantasies and desires as much as it may act to shape or reinforce them. It was not the pornographer who created the script for phallic sexuality we see in heterosexual porn, where man is active subject and woman object to be fucked. Arguably, both pornography (and other forms of representation) framed within a masculine gaze and men's acting-out of objectification or violence towards women are manifestations of more deeply rooted sentiments – men's fantasies, fears and anger associated with women, their vulnerability in the face of the almost impossible task of living up to what it is to be 'man', and the taking-up of the masochistic position, the traditional role of 'woman', so often assumed (in fantasy, at least) by man.

Those against pornography have rightly criticized the dominant script of 'sex', the negative depictions of 'woman' and the allusions to sexual violence that are contained within many pornographic images and texts. Yet by condemning all explicitly sexual material as 'pornography' under the umbrella of 'protecting women', they are implicitly reinforcing the notion that in heterosexual 'sex' woman is inevitably victimized, objectified and secondary to man. They distract attention from the myriad other factors which precipitate and allow sexual violence. And they leave little (if any) space for the exploration of sexuality and desire from the perspective of women. For if we follow the edicts of many anti-pornography campaigners we will ban overt sexual imagery produced by and for women, including much lesbian erotica/porn. As much of the sexual imagery produced for and by women challenges the traditional position of 'woman' within the script of heterosexual femininity, it is understandable that conservative campaigners would see it banned – it is 'obscene' because of the very fact that it subverts 'family values' and offers a different image for women. But can feminist campaigners live with themselves if they defend this same position? Can they be party to a further suppression and negation of women's sexuality and a reinforcement of the traditional positioning of 'woman' as either asexual Madonna or as whore – the former standing as the 'ideal' state if pornography were banned, the latter the ascription applied to any explicit depiction of female sexuality and, by implication, to those women who admit to enjoying porn.

As we have already noted, pornography is not a unique genre of representation. Similar themes run through art, film and literature and the boundary between 'pornography' and other imagery framed within a masculine gaze is not easy, if at all possible, to define. Drawing boundaries for the censoring of 'pornography' is never an easy task. We may agree that explicit violent, child or animal pornography should be banned – but after that, where do we draw the line? It is always open to question and is always a matter of subjective opinion. The boundaries have clearly changed over the last century – the censorship of *Lady Chatterley's Lover*, or the relics of Pompeii seems laughable in the face of the overt sexual imagery freely available today. Because of its heterogeneous nature, it cannot easily be categorized – as we have seen. Perhaps we should stop using the term 'pornography' – it is a vague umbrella term which has come to stand for too many different things.

There will never be any simple rational answer in this arena – despite the sometimes righteous proclamations of many of the 'experts' who reside within. By its very nature, explicit sexual material is unsettling and emotive. Being faced with forthright representations of the fantasies of others – or with our own repressed desires – is often disquieting or disturbing. It is much more simple to classify it as 'bad'. If we read or view pornography and accept it as a 'true' reflection of how men see women (or of how women should see themselves), it is understandable that many women will reject it. It is inconceivable that women should have to live out the role of 'woman' as described in the pornographic script. If women are *made* to do so, it is a clear case of abuse and should be treated as such. But if we see pornography as a representation of fantasy, it is a different case entirely. Our focus is then shifted to the conditions which provoke such fantasies, and to their relationship with other aspects of the sexual scripts that regulate what it is to be 'woman' and 'man' – to the material consequences of representations of 'woman' and 'sex' on women's lives.

NOTES

1. Williams, Linda, *Hard Core*, London: Pandora, 1990, p. 267.
2. Horney, Karen, *Feminine Psychology*, H. Kelman (ed.), London: Norton, 1967, p. 135.
3. Griffin, Susan, *Pornography and Silence*, London: The Women's Press, 1981, p. 33.
4. Cameron, Deborah & Frazer, Liz, *The Lust to Kill*, London: Polity Press, 1987, p. 381.
5. Sanchez, Linda, *Quim*, 1992, issue 4.
6. This woman is talking about soft-core heterosexual porn. She also told me that she sometimes watched it whilst she did the ironing, to add some interest to what was essentially a tedious activity.

7. I am talking here about heterosexual pornography, aimed at men.

8. Quoted by Williams, 1990, p. 5.

9. Ibid., p. 9.

10. It is arguably the Victorian legacy that has had the widest influence on views of pornography today. See Marcus, Stephen, *The Other Victorians: A Study of Pornography in Mid-Nineteenth-Century England*, New York: American Library, 1974.

11. Foucault, M. *The History of Sexuality, Vol. 1*, London: Penguin, 1976, p. 3.

12. Ibid., p. 17.

13. Ibid., p. 18.

14. Ibid., p. 35.

15. Kendrick, W., *The Secret Museum: Pornography in the Modern Culture*, New York: Viking, 1987.

16. The same criteria for prohibition introduced by the Victorians still exist today to a large extent – with women excluded because of the supposed shock to their senses or their purported disinterest in sex without 'love', and children lest they be morally corrupted. It is men who remain as almost the sole occupants of the commercial world of sex, although censorship debates still focus on the exclusion of 'unsophisticated' men because of the assumed incitement to rape.

17. Russell, D. E. H., *Making Violence Sexy: Feminist Views on Pornography*, Buckingham: Open University Press, 1993.

18. Itzen, C., *Pornography: Women, Violence and Civil Liberties*, Oxford: Oxford University Press, 1993.

19. Today, it is primarily the visual image that is liable to be condemned as 'pornographic'. The printed word is now almost immune from censorship or prosecution: as a 1985 commission concluded, it was seen to need 'for assimilation more real thought and less almost reflexive reaction than does the more typical pornographic item'.

20. Quoted in Kendrick, 1987, p. 233.

21. As would heterosexual porn aimed at women, in which woman is not victimized.

22. Senn, Charlene Y., 'The Research on Women and Pornography: The Many Faces of Harm', in *Making Violence Sexy: Feminist Views on Pornography*, D. Russell (ed.), Buckingham: Open University Press, 1993, pp. 179–93, p. 181.

23. Harriet Gilbert carried out a critique of Andrea Dworkin's novel *Mercy*

(New York: Four Walls Eight Windows, 1990) and argued that it is indistinguishable from what its pro-censorship author would define as 'pornography'. See Gilbert, Harriet, 'So Long as It's Not Sex and Violence. Andrea Dworkin's *Mercy*', in *Sex Exposed: Sexuality and the Pornography Debate*, Lynne Segal & Mary McIntosh (eds.), London: Virago, 1992.

24. It certainly is in Britain, and in a majority of North American states – if not in many European countries, such as Sweden, Holland and Italy. (Although even where it is illegal, it is still available. Pornography is big business, a multimillion-dollar industry, and what is most forbidden or transgressive is always sought after.)

25. See Vance, Carol, 'Negotiating Sex and Gender in the Attorney-General's Commission on Pornography', in Segal & McIntosh, 1992, pp. 29–49.

26. Dietz, P. E. & Sears, A. E., 'Pornography and Obscenity Sold in "Adult Bookstores". A Survey of 5,132 Books, Magazines and Films Sold in Four American Cities', *University of Michigan Journal of Law Reform*, 21 (1&2), 1987–8, p. 11. Cited by Itzen, 1993.

27. The slide-show text was written by Jeanne Barkey and J. Koplin. These examples were taken from Itzen, Catherine, 'Entertainment for Men: What It is and What It Means', in Itzen, 1993.

28. Ibid., p. 34.

29. Or someone adopting a theoretical framework where pornography is seen as simply fantasy.

30. Segal, Lynne, Introduction, in Segal & McIntosh, 1992, p. 6.

31. *For Men*, September 1994, p. 56.

32. *Lipstick*, no. 11, 1993, p. 58.

33. *Fiesta*, no. 6, 1994, p. 99.

34. Lovelace, Linda, *Inside Linda Lovelace*, New York: Four Square Books, 1976, p. 80.

35. Crabbe, A., 'Feature-Length Sex Films', in Day, Gary & Bloom, Clive, *Perspectives on Pornography: Sexuality in Film and Literature*, London: Macmillan, 1988, pp. 144–66.

36. Griffin, 1981, p. 34.

37. Again, pornography aimed at heterosexual men.

38. Horney, Karen, 1967, p. 145.

39. Interestingly, this distinction doesn't simply apply in heterosexual sex. In the cases of male rape reported in American prisons the receptive (buggered) partner is seen as feminine, and as degraded because of this,

whereas the active penetrative partner is viewed not as carrying out an act of homosexual sex (or rape), but acting as 'man'.

40. Arguably, this is also the case with gay male sex.

41. Segal, Lynne, 'Sweet Sorrows, Painful Pleasures. Pornography and the Perils of Heterosexual Desire', in Segal & McIntosh, 1992, p. 69.

42. This may appear to assume heterosexuality. However, the fear and dread of woman is not merely a result of current desire, but is associated with deep-rooted fears arising from early development and from the continuous circulation of 'woman' as sign.

43. Freud, S., 'The Infantile Genital Organization of the Libido', *Collected Papers, vol. 2: Clinical Papers; Papers on Technique*, London: The Hogarth Press and the Institute of Psychoanalysis, 1924. Quoted by Horney, 1967, p. 145.

44. Horney, 1967, p. 145.

45. Cowie, Elizabeth, 'Pornography and Fantasy: Psychoanalytic Perspectives', in Segal & McIntosh, 1992, p. 138.

46. McClintock, Anne, 'Gonad the Barbarian and the Venus Flytrap: Portraying the Male and Female Orgasm', in Segal & McIntosh, 1992, p. 112.

47. Ibid., pp. 112–13.

48. Ibid., p. 112.

49. Benjamin, Jessica, 'Master and Slave: The Fantasy of Erotic Domination', in *Desire: The Politics of Sexuality*, A. Snitow, C. Stansell & S. Thompson (eds.), London: Virago, 1984.

50. Cowie, in Segal & McIntosh, 1992.

51. Stoller, Robert & Levine, I. S., *Coming Attractions: The Making of an X-Rated Movie*, New Haven: Yale University Press, 1993, p. 22.

52. Day, Gary, in Day & Bloom, 1988, p. 5.

53. Crabbe, in Day & Bloom, 1988, p. 61.

54. McClintock, in Segal & McIntosh, 1992, p. 123.

55. Williams, 1990, p. 242.

56. Dollimore, Jonathon. Quoted in Garber, Marjorie, *Vice Versa: Bisexuality in Everyday Life*, London: Hamish Hamilton, 1996, p. 162.

57. Ibid., p. 162.

58. Baker, Peter, 'Maintaining Power: Why Heterosexual Men Use Pornography', in Itzen, 1993, p. 125.

59. Bryant, J., *Testimony to the Attorney-General's Commission on Pornography Hearings*, Houston, Texas, unpublished manuscript, 1985, pp. 128–57.

60. Baker, in Itzen, 1993. p. 130.

61. Ibid., p. 130.

62. Munton, Tony, personal communication.

63. Itzen, Catherine, 'Pornography and the Social Construction of Sexual Inequality', in Itzen, 1993, p. 67.

64. Griffin, 1981, p. 3.

65. Quoted by Sweet, C., 'Pornography and Addiction: A Political Issue', in Itzen, 1993, pp. 179, 180.

66. Morgan, Robin, 'Theory and Practice: Pornography and Rape', in Lederer, Laura, *Take Back the Night: Women on Pornography*, New York: Morrow, 1980.

67. Russell, Diana, 'Pornography and Rape: A Causal Model', in Itzen, 1993, pp. 310–49, p. 321.

68. See Howitt, Denis, 'Pornography: The Recent Debate', in *A Measure of Uncertainty: The Effects of Mass Media*', G. Cumberbatch & D. Howitt (eds.), London: Libbey, 1990; Howitt, D. & Cumberbatch, G., *Pornography: Impacts and Influences*, London: Home Office Research and Planning Unit, 1990; and Itzen, 1993, for reviews of the evidence. Howitt concludes that there is no consistent evidence for a causal relationship between pornography and violence; Itzen concludes that there is.

69. 'The Report of the Commission on Obscenity and Pornography', New York, 1970.

70. Ibid., p. 57.

71. Quoted in Kendrick, 1987, p. 219.

72. *Attorney-General's Commission on Pornography. Final Report*, Washington DC: US Government Printing Office, 1985.

73. *American Booksellers Inc. v. William H. Hudnut*, 771 F. 2d 323, 328–9 (7th civ. 1985). Quoted in Itzen, 1993, p. 584.

74. See Merck, Mandy, 'From Minneapolis to Westminster', in Segal & McIntosh, 1992, pp. 50–62.

75. Ibid.

76. Malamuth, N., 'The Effects of Mass Media Exposure on Acceptance of Violence against Women: A Field Experiment', *Journal of Research in Personality*, 15, 1981, pp. 436–46.

77. Russell, D., 'Sexual Exploitation: Rape, Child Sexual Abuse and Workplace Harassment', Beverly Hills, California: Sage, 1984. The research was carried out by British psychologist S. Rachman at the Institute of Psychiatry in London.

78. Malamuth, N., Heim, M. & Feshbach, S., 'Sexual Responsiveness of

College Students to Rape Depictions: Inhibitory and Disinhibitory Effects', *Journal of Personality and Social Psychology*, 38, 1980, pp. 399–408.

79. Malamuth, N. & Check, J. V. P., 'Penile Tumescence and Perceptual Responses to Rape as a Function of Victim's Perceived Reactions', *Journal of Applied Social Psychology*, 10, 1980a, pp. 528–47.

80. Donnerstein, E., 'Aggressive Erotica and Violence against Women', *Journal of Personality and Social Psychology*, 39, 1980a, pp. 269–77.

81. Zillman, D. & Bryant, J., 'Effects of Massive Exposure to Pornography', in Malamuth, N. & Donnerstein, E., *Pornography and Sexual Aggression*, New York: Academic Press, 1984.

82. See Senn, Charlene Y., 'Women's Multiple Perspectives and Experiences with Pornography', *Psychology of Women Quarterly*, 17, 1993, pp. 319–41.

83. *Attorney-General's Commission on Pornography. Final Report*, 1985, pp. 901–1033.

84. See Itzen, 1993, p. 250.

85. Wyre, R., 'Pornography and Sexual Violence', in Itzen, 1993, p. 243.

86. Interview with Ted Bundy, Associated Press, 25 January 1989, p. 4. Quoted in Sweet, in Itzen, 1993, pp. 191–2.

87. *Attorney-General's Commission on Pornography. Final Report*, 1985, p. 785.

88. Cited by Russell, in Itzen, 1993, p. 327.

89. Woman respondent to a British Magazine survey on pornography, quoted by Itzen, C. & Sweet, C., 'Women's Experience of Pornography', in Itzen, 1993, p. 230.

90. In the abusive treatment meted out to rapists or child abusers in prisons, men convicted for other crimes mark very clearly what they see as their difference from this group.

91. For example, Baron, L. & Strauss, M. A., 'Four Theories of Rape: A Macrosociological Analysis', *Social Problems*, 34, pp. 467–89.

92. See Howitt & Cumberbatch, 1990, pp. 30, 34.

93. Ibid., p. 40.

94. Ibid., p. 38.

95. Ibid., p. 39.

96. Goldstein, M. J., Judd, L., Rice, C. & Green, R., 'Exposure to Pornography and Sexual Behaviour in Deviant and Normal Groups', *Technical Report of the Commission on Obscenity and Pornography*, vii, Washington DC, 1970.

97. See Howitt & Cumberbatch, 1990, p. 38.

98. *Attorney-General's Commission on Pornography. Final Report*, 1985, p. 786.
99. Tate, Tim, 'The Child Pornography Industry', in Itzen, 1993, p. 214.
100. Russell, D., *The Politics of Rape: The Victim's Perspective*, New York: Steine Day, 1975, pp. 249–50.
101. Dworkin, A., 'Against the Flood: Censorship, Pornography and Equality', in Itzen, 1993, pp. 516–35, p. 523.
102. The other reason is that written material is considered to have a less immediate effect, as it requires cognitive processing on the part of the reader. As women are generally acknowledged to prefer written erotica, and men visual erotica, there is an interesting gender difference here.
103. Witness Testimony, *Attorney-General's Commission on Pornography. Final Report*, 1985, pp. 787–8.
104. Dworkin, A. & MacKinnon, C., *Pornography and Civil Rights: A New Day for Women's Equality*, Minneapolis: Organizing against Pornography (distributed by Southern Sisters, Inc., 441 Morris Street, Durham, NC, 27701), 1988.
105. Testimony, *Attorney-General's Commission on Pornography. Final Report*, 1985; reprinted in Russell, 'Surviving Commercial Exploitation', in Itzen, 1993, pp. 38–9.
106. See Steinem, Gloria, 'The Real Linda Lovelace', Ch. 2 in Russell, in Itzen, 1993, pp. 23–31.
107. Ibid., p. 24.
108. Ibid., p. 24.
109. Steinem, G., 'Outrageous Acts and Everyday Rebellions', East Toledo Productions Inc. Quoted in Russell, in Itzen, 1993, p. 27.
110. Quoted in Tate, in Itzen, 1993, p. 215.
111. McClintock, in Segal & McIntosh, 1992, p. 129.
112. Griffin, 1981, p. 111.
113. Dworkin, A., *Intercourse*, London: Secker, 1987, p. 125.
114. MacKinnon, C., 'Feminism, Marxism, Method and State: An Agenda for Theory', *Signs*, 1982, 7(3), pp. 515–44, p. 532.
115. MacKinnon, C., 'Not a Moral Issue', in MacKinnon, Catharine, *Feminism Unmodified: Discourse on Life and Law*, London: Harvard University Press, 1987, p. 149.
116. Leeds Revolutionary Feminist Group, *Love Your Enemy? The Debate between Heterosexual Feminism and Political Lesbianism*, Only Women Press, 1981.

117. Bruch, Charlotte, 'Lesbians in Revolt', in *The Furies*, 1 (1). Quoted by Segal, 1994, p. 50.
118. Schulman, Sarah, *The Sophie Horowitz Story*. (Tallahassee, Fli Naiad, 1984.) Quoted by Segal, 1994, p. 51.
119. See Segal, Lynne, *Straight Sex*, London: Virago, 1994, for a thorough analysis of many of these debates and a reclaiming of heterosexuality as positive for women.
120. *Heterosexuality: A Reader*, Sue Wilkinson & Celia Kizinger (eds.), London: Sage, 1993. As a response to this reader, both Wendy Hollway and Lynne Segal published work which did celebrate heterosexual sex. See Segal, *Straight Sex*, 1994, and Hollway, Wendy, 'Differences and Similarities in a Feminist Theorisation of Heterosexuality'. Paper presented at the annual conference of the British Psychological Society, Blackpool, 1993.
121. Itzen, Catherine & Sweet, Corrine, 'Women's Experiences of Pornography: UK Magazine Survey Evidence', in Itzen, 1993, Ch. 13.
122. Many of the women interviewed also commented that they found women in porn physically unattractive.
123. Réage, Pauline, *The Story of O*, London: Corgi, 1972.
124. See Williams, 1990, pp. 249-50.
125. Candida Royalle, quoted in ibid., p. 229.
126. Segal, Lynne, 'Sensual Uncertainty, Or Why the Clitoris is Not Enough', in *Sex and Love: New Thoughts on Old Contradictions*, Sue Cartledge & Sue Ryan (eds.), London: The Women's Press, 1983, p. 42.
127. Kiss and Tell (Persimmon Blackbridge, Lizard Jones, Susan Stewart), *Her Tongue on My Theory. Images, Essays and Fantasies*, Vancouver: Press Gang Publishers, 1994, p. 80.
128. Wittig, Monique, 'The Straight Mind', *Feminist Issues* 1 (1), summer, 1980.
129. Kiss and Tell, 1994, pp. 6-7.
130. That Della Grace herself is the object of fascination and vilification is not surprising. As with her adoption of a beard and masculine garb in the mid nineties, her imagery poses perhaps the greatest threat to man, as 'woman' is demonstrating not only active sexuality but taking up a blatantly masculine position.
131. See *Nothing But the Girl: The Blatant Lesbian Image. A Portfolio and Exploration of Lesbian Erotic Photography*, Susie Bright & Jill Posner (eds.), London: Cassell, 1996.

132. Tee, Corinne, *Dreams of the Woman Who Loved Sex. A Collection*, Austin, Texas: Banned Book, 1987, p. 44.

133. Nestle, Joan, 'Woman of Muscle, Woman of Bone', in *Tangled Sheets. Stories and Poems of Lesbian Lust*, Rosamund Elwin & Karen X. Tulchinsky (eds.), Toronto: The Women's Press, 1995, pp. 35–40.

134. Miller, Henry, *Nexus*, New York: Grove Press, 1965, p. 183.

135. Califa, Pat, 'The Calyx of Isis', in Califa, P., *Macho Sluts*, Boston: Alyson Publications, 1988, p. 96.

136. Butler, Judith, *Gender Trouble: Feminism and the Subversion of Identity*, London: Routledge, 1990.

137. Adams, Parveen, 'Of Female Bondage', in *Between Feminism and Psychoanalysis*, Teresa Brennan (ed.), London: Routledge, 1989, p. 262. Quoted in Segal, 1994, p. 164.

138. This is in contrast to the assertions of sex researchers such as Shere Hite, who argued that clitoral orgasm provides the greatest pleasure for women, or the comments of early feminists such as Anne Koedt, whose paper 'The Myth of the Vaginal Orgasm' opened up the exploration of female sexual desire in the late sixties. See Segal, 1994, p. 35 for a discussion of this.

139. One of the controversies over SM practice is whether it continues outside of the sexual scenario.

140. Kiss and Tell, 1994, pp. 106–7.

141. See Linden, Robin R., Pagano, Darlene R., Russell, Diana E. H. & Leigh Star, Susan, *Against Sado-Masochism. A Radical Feminist Analysis*, California: Frog in the Well, 1982.

142. Williams, in Segal & McIntosh, 1992, p. 251.

143. Califa, Pat, 'The Surprise Party', in Califa, 1988, p. 219.

144. Butler, 1990, p. 137.

145. Segal, 1994, p. 206.

CHAPTER FOUR

Sexual Science and the Law: Regulating Sex – Reifying the Power of the Heterosexual Man

Rational Truth

The intent of sexual science is to obtain careful observations or measurements of sexual phenomena which, in turn, are expounded in a theoretical structure. Predictions . . . are deduced from these theories, which once again are measured against observations of sexual behaviour. Progress in sexual science is facilitated by the inflating database and the continually reformulated theories.   ABRAMSON, 1990[1]

Law and Truth

Legal reasoning . . . is intellectual and rational . . . the judge can come to know enough about the whole complex of the law and fact to discover enough of the truth to settle wisely disputes before the court . . . It requires an open and cultivated mind.   DERMAN ET AL, 1995[2]

Ideology and Power

At any given time, the more powerful side will create an ideology suitable to help maintain its position and to make this position acceptable to the weaker one. In this ideology the differentness of the weaker one will be interpreted as inferiority, and it will be proven that these differences are unchangeable, basic or God's will. It is the function of such an ideology to deny or conceal the existence of struggle.   HORNEY, 1967[3]

Secrecy

What is peculiar to modern societies . . . is not that they consigned sex to a shadow existence, but that they dedicated themselves to speaking of it *ad infinitum*, while exploiting it as *the* secret.   FOUCAULT, 1979[4]

Saturation

Nothing is less certain today than sex . . . and nothing today is less certain than desire, behind the proliferation of its images . . . In matters of sex the proliferation is approaching total loss. Here lies the secret of the ever increasing production of sex and its signs, and the hyper realism of sexual pleasure . . . No more want, no more prohibitions, and no more limits . . . It is the ghost of desire that haunts the defunct reality of sex. Sex is everywhere, except in sexuality.   BAUDRILLARD, 1990[5]

Regulating the Material Body

Representations of 'sex', and of 'woman' and 'man' do not sit in a theoretical vacuum, of interest only to academics concerned with the symbolic sphere. They have 'real' effects. Phallocentric visions of 'woman' and the conflation of 'woman' with 'sex' directly influence many arenas of material practice, in which the physical body of woman is regulated and controlled.[6] I am not talking here about the actions of individual misogynistic men but about institutionalized practices and procedures sanctioned or condoned by the machinery of the state. Until very recently, it was these material practices that preoccupied the critical attention and political campaigns of feminists attempting to liberate women from the shackles of patriarchal subjugation and control. It is a relatively recent luxury to be able to condemn and resist representations of 'woman' in the symbolic sphere – for centuries women did not have rights over their own bodies or their own lives. In many contexts they still don't. In examining the relationship between representations of 'woman' and 'sex' and the regulation of the body or the person in the physical world, I could have looked at a number of other areas:

Reproduction

Access to contraception, abortion and treatments for sexually transmitted diseases; myths about menstruation, pregnancy and the menopause; the control and treatment of women during pregnancy and childbirth; elective abortion and infanticide of female children; infant mortality rates; edicts and controls of fertility.

Work and Education

Women's rights to education or paid work; the position of women as unpaid houseworkers; women's earnings; women's promotional opportunities; the presence of women in positions of authority and power; sexual harassment in the workplace; women's tax and pension rights; maternity leave and the rights of mothers to work; child-care provision.

The Body

Female circumcision; foot-binding; cosmetic surgery; sexual and gynaecological surgery; witch trials.

Mental Health

Rates and causes of mental illness in women; the conflation of femininity with madness; 'treatments' meted out towards women positioned as 'mad'.

Power

Women's ability to own land or money; the right to vote; custody rights over children; the right and ability to live outside the control of man; women and religious power.

Marriage

Mental health and marriage; physical health and longevity of life span and marriage; domestic violence; 'childbrides'.

Sexuality

Forced child and adult prostitution; prostitution law; forced marriage and polygamy; sexual slavery; dowry murders.

Each of these areas could fill a book in itself – indeed, over the last century, many books have been written, many campaigns to change discriminatory practices run and, in Europe and North America at least, many changes in the material conditions of women's lives brought about as a result (although we still have a long way to go). The same could be said of representations of 'woman' and 'sex' in sexual science and sex law. If we examine the way in which 'sex' is legally and scientifically defined, representations of and official reactions to sexual violence, and theories and treatments for sexual deviancy and sexual problems, we can see how phallocentric images of 'woman' and 'sex' are enshrined and legitimated in the machinery of the state. This has serious and often damaging consequences for the lives of many women (as well as for men who step outside the phallocentric boundaries of sex).

'Sex' is not an immutable, biological, given fact, driving us unthinkingly or instinctively towards pleasure (or pain). What we define as 'sex' is not a simple instinctual or hormonal process – 'vaginal intercourse' may be commonly acknowledged to be 'sex', but are masturbation, nocturnal emissions or the rubbing together of naked bodies? We are not born with a natural template that determines how we desire, how we express our sexuality and what is unequivocally a sexual crime or problem. These processes are determined by social rules and tastes;[7] they differ across cultures and across time.[8] In Anglo-American western cultures science and the law are two of the major social institutions that influence these processes, shaping what we see as 'sex', how we learn to desire, how we experience our sexual selves and how we learn to repress or conceal the sexuality that is currently forbidden. As a consequence this shapes how we experience ourselves as 'woman' or 'man'. The penalty for ignoring the edicts of science or the law is that we become sexual outsiders or outcasts, our sexuality seen as a sign of illness, crime or, to some, sin. This is not merely a process of categorization, a matter of ascription of labels we can discredit or ignore. Scientific and legal edicts have concrete effects in enforced referral for invasive treatment, incarceration or, in extreme circumstances, sentence of death; they constitute a sexual ideology with material and often drastic effects.

For the last two hundred years 'sex' has been exposed to the rigours of the secular gaze, the sexual body scrutinized, categorized and contained within the boundaries of exact measurement and control established by scientists and legal experts. Common law and science act to categorize and classify what is 'other' in the sphere of the sexual; what is outlawed because deviant, or open to clinical intervention because dysfunctional. Law and science combine to define 'normal' sexuality by regulating what is 'abnormal' – under-age sex, incest, anal and oral sex, adultery, homosexuality, rape and sexual abuse and obscenity and pornography. There are clinical classifications and treatments for dysfunction and perversion. Some laws are rigidly enforced; others ignored. Some 'dysfunctions' are tolerated; others carefully treated. Yet in the annals of science and the law the lines of demarcation between normal and abnormal sex are reassuringly clear – no messy uncertainty here.

What science 'knows' about 'sex' and 'woman' is focused almost entirely on the physical body; sexuality is reduced to its bodily components, to instincts and drives, to genetics, hormones and reproductive organs. This is partly a result of the dominant ethos of modern-day scientific endeavour, which follows the philosophy of positivism. This stipulates that the gaze of the scientist is primarily concerned with what is measurable or observable, with what can be experimentally manipulated or tested to see if it is 'real'. The scientist is concerned with facts, not values; with 'truth', not supposition or belief. Concepts such as desire, lust, love, pleasure or misogynistic fear are too nebulous and vague, not easily trapped within an experimental prism; they are material for the philosophers, the poets and the playwrights.

Male sexuality has been reduced to testosterone and androgens, to the functioning of the penis, to erection and ejaculation; female sexuality (if considered at all[9]) is reduced to oestrogen and progestogen or to the biological components of reproduction – menstruation, pregnancy and the menopause, considered almost solely at a biological level[10] – or to heterosexual response, mainly receptivity to the penis in heterosexual intercourse. These easily observed and measured bodily 'realities' are dissected and displayed in order finally to uncover the mysteries of sex. Biological theories are offered as explanations for sexual violence, sexual problems and sexual deviation, as well as for the vagaries of 'normal' sex. Subjectivity, and social or cultural context, is in the main marginalized or denied.

However, the rhetoric of objectivity that dominates in both science and law is itself merely a smokescreen for the acting out of ideologically motivated power and control. Science and law are both gendered and phallocentric.[11] The smokescreen of objectivity acts to conceal the way in which the rule of science and law is intrinsically influenced by the fears and fantasies of 'man'. In this hallowed sphere, the mysteries of woman and the fear she provokes in man can be carefully classified and controlled. An illusion of power serves to ward off the fears of phallic powerlessness, the fear that we really do not 'know' what woman is, or what sex, or sexual desire, is about. Both science and sex law act to reify the mythical power of the phallus by emphasizing the active, powerful sexuality of man in contrast to the passive, receptive (or absent) sexuality of woman. The model reflected in both science and law is heterosexual man.[12] He is the benchmark against which all else is measured. It is his interests which the powerful social institutions act to protect and serve. Equally, the boundaries of 'normal' sexuality established in scientific and legal theory are those of heterosexuality; all that deviates or detracts from this is at risk of categorization and control. So lesbians and gay men as well as women who deviate from the script of femininity become the targets for legislation which is at best biased and discriminatory, at worst misogynistic and homophobic, in many of its dictates and decrees.

Yet whilst science and law may be prime sites for the regulation of 'sex', they are also prime sites for resistance. Both science and law have been laid open to feminist scrutiny and critique. Some have argued that both professions are simply sexist, acting to support the interests of man whilst denigrating or negating the interests of woman;[13] wholesale rejection of legal and scientific theorizing on the subject of 'woman' and 'sex' has been advocated as a result. Others have taken a more moderate stance, recognizing that both science and law contain many contradictions, many dictates supporting male privilege and interest, but others playing a part in the protection and empowerment of women.[14] Here the baby is not thrown out with the bathwater, and both law and science are seen to offer something positive for women. Campaigns to change the more archaic aspects of the law or scientific theory and practice have been executed as a result.[15] In the following two chapters I will examine how the law defines 'sex', sexual deviancy and sexual problems and then examine in detail the phenomenon of sexual violence – in particular the way it is represented and explained in science and law. Each of these issues is not merely a matter of abstract theory; for in the execution of punishment or 'cure', in the legal apportioning of 'blame' for a sexual crime, both science and the law have very concrete material effects on the lives and bodies of women and men.

Most people would agree that we need some legislation on sex, that the boundaries of the law and her sister profession sexual medicine provide safety and security against general debauchery and licentiousness, that we need to control the sexual outlaws, the sexual criminal, the rapist and the abuser. Yet it is not that simple. How do we define a sexual crime? How do we define sexual deviance or a sexual problem? It all depends on our definition of normal sex. We cannot merely accept science or the law as neutral or see the boundaries of 'sex' they police as a reflection of given, somehow natural rules. We must see this institutionalized protection of 'normal sex' for what it is – one of the most powerful means of maintaining heterosexual hegemony and phallocentric constructions of 'woman' and 'man'. The cool and calculated analysis of sex is part of a wider process of secularized control of the body[16] and, through control of the body, control of the person. (Madness and criminality, two other forms of disruptive deviancy, have also been subjected to the 'objective' analysis of these legal and scientific experts.) The mechanisms of this control are a means of convincing us that all the confusing irregularities of human experience can be explained and contained, that anything out of the ordinary, anything not 'normal', can be punished or treated – thereby maintaining our safety and security and giving us reassurance that those deemed 'other' can be clearly categorized and thus controlled. However, rather than providing us with objective knowledge and guidance, examining how science and law regulate the boundaries of sex and sexual deviancy largely demonstrates the power of phallocentric privilege itself; examining anomalies and anachronisms in the practice of law in this area demonstrates how rigidly the dominant institutions define and seek to maintain their privilege and control.

Defining the Boundaries of 'Sex'

Theological and Canon Law: God's Word Made Flesh

> Any Woman who acts in such a way that she cannot give birth to as many children as she is capable of makes herself guilty of that many murders, just as with the woman who tries to injure herself after conception.   ST AUGUSTINE, AD 354–430

> A man with a hundred tongues who lived for a century would still not be able to complete the task of describing the vices and defects of a woman.   *Mahabharata*, Hindu text

> Take her skin from her face and thou shalt see all loathsomeness under it . . . within she is full of phlegm, stinking, putrid, excremental stuff.
> ST JOHN CHRYSOSTOM, AD 347–407

> In pain shall you bring forth children, woman, and you shall turn to your husband and he shall rule over you. And do you not know that you are Eve? God's sentence hangs all over your sex and his punishment weighs

> down upon you. You are the devil's gateway; you are she who first
> violated the forbidden tree and broke the law of God.　TERTULLIAN[17]

Edicts defining and controlling sexuality have been at the centre of
theological law for centuries and have provided the foundations for
much of the common law which defines and controls 'sex' today,
even though theological and common law differed in their aims.[18]
Historically, a main concern of theological law has been the danger of
woman's sexuality, as the extracts above illustrate – the images of
'woman' as temptress, her body an instrument of evil and corruption
for which she must be eternally reviled and punished, of woman
incapable of intellectual thought, childbirth and child-rearing her natural, God-given destiny.

Christian dictates on sexuality have their origins in the Augustinian
creed, which was established in the fourth century AD. St Augustine
was originally a scholar, and adhered to the strict Manichean faith,
which advocated complete celibacy and dictated that sexual intercourse
which led to pregnancy was to be condemned because it caused a soul
to be trapped in another's body, perpetuating a cycle of good versus
evil.[19] In his eleven years as a member of the Manichean faith Augustine
battled unsuccessfully against his own sexual drives. Rather than resolve
what he saw as the conundrum of whether he should confine himself
to a mistress, to prostitutes or to a wife, he underwent a religious
conversion to Christianity and found that he suddenly no longer desired
sexual release.

Augustine's celebration of his new-found celibacy and freedom from
lustful desires for women came to be enshrined in the doctrine and
decrees of the early Christian church. His hostility towards the act of
sexual intercourse led him to declare that nothing was more likely to
'bring the manly mind down from the heights than a woman's caresses,
and that joining of bodies without which one cannot have a wife.[20]
Men were told to worship the spiritual nature of woman but to despise
her bodily reality:

> A good Christian is bound toward one and the same woman, to love the
> creature of God whom he desires to be transformed and renewed, but
> to hate in her the corruptible and mortal conjugal connection, sexual
> intercourse and all that pertains to her as a wife.[21]

Augustine preached that woman could pass into the kingdom of heaven only if her body was cleansed and her spiritual self literally separated from those organs connected to sexual intercourse and child-rearing. In this way she would be 'suited to glory rather than to shame'. This offers a chilling parallel to the sexual murderers of today, many of whom cut out or disfigure women's genitalia whilst claiming divine inspiration for their crimes (see p. 408). The only way for woman to be *truly* spiritual and rational, Augustine declared, was for her to remain a virgin, denying her sexuality and physicality altogether. This heralded centuries of celebration of female virginity,[22] epitomized by the Catholic church's belief in the 'virgin birth', through which Mary is reputed to have given birth to Jesus without having been soiled by carnal desire or sex.

Whilst celibacy became the ideal to which the angels (or their earthly counterparts, the clergy) should aspire, Augustine acknowledged the biblical edict to procreate and so declared that sex could take place, but only within marriage and with impregnation of the woman (not pleasure) as its sole aim (an interesting reversal of his earlier position). All sexual activity outside marriage was considered sinful – as was sexual intercourse not carried out in the appropriate 'missionary' position, with the woman on her back facing the man.

Augustine's decrees were not novel, but merely the continuation of a long-held belief, enshrined in theological law, that active sexuality on the part of a woman was sinful and perverse and, if not avoided, would lead to the downfall of man. As Paul decreed in Romans 1:25– 27, women who 'changed the order of nature' by taking up a sexually active position were evil 'daughters of men' accused of seducing the 'sons of gods'. (In sharp contrast, men who took the *passive* position in homosexual activity were the ones who were deemed degraded and condemned.)[23] So male and female sexual behaviour was closely defined – passive receptivity prescribed for women and proscribed for men. This is the script of heterosexuality we see in women's magazines, romantic fiction, films and pornography, positioned as moral edict in the Christian bible.

Later Christian scholars and theologians extended and clarified the boundaries of what was considered sinful sexuality. St Thomas Aquinas outlined four 'sins against nature' that were to be prohibited and condemned: masturbation, intercourse in an unnatural position, homosexual activity and bestiality. These activities were seen as more serious than adultery, rape or seduction because they were sins against the laws of nature, as set down by God.[24] The punishment for contravention of such laws was ultimately eternal damnation – exclusion from the promise of eternal life in the kingdom of heaven. The fornicator, the adulterer or the homosexual may have enjoyed their sinful pursuits on earth, but always with the knowledge that they would be excluded from everlasting salvation whilst the pure of heart and mind would bask in God's grace as their just reward.

This isn't merely historical anachronism – arguably, fifteen centuries later, the traces of these archaic edicts remain. The Christian belief in the sanctity of marital sex and the sinfulness of all else, still holds in many quarters today – certainly in official religious doctrine. Yet as common law and science took over the regulation of 'sex' in the eighteenth and nineteenth centuries, punishment on earth took the place of threatened punishment to come. Sex outside the boundaries of 'normality' has been brought into the statute-books, turning sexual sinners into common criminals. The scientific expert has moved away from the religious emphasis on sexual iniquity and vice to define clinical categories of sexual problems and 'perversions'. Categories of sin, debauchery and moral turpitude have been replaced by taxonomies of disease, madness and degeneracy.

Scientific Taxonomy and Classification: Categorizing Deviance and Perversion

It was only in the second half of the late nineteenth century that the scientific community saw the publication of a number of key sexological tomes which both spelt out the importance of sexuality for society as a whole and gave an air of respectability to its scientific study through the discipline of 'sexology'[25] Krafft-Ebbing was working in Germany, Magnus Hirsch and Havelock Ellis in England; all were committed to objective, disinterested analysis of both sex and the anatomical body. Sigmund Freud was also an influential pioneer, but his work has arguably had less impact on mainstream sex research, as his methods are positioned as 'unscientific' and his theories 'untestable'.[26]

The dominant model of late-nineteenth- and early-twentieth-century science was of sex and sexuality as biological phenomena, an instinct for reproduction or a drive that somehow must be released. Any aspect of sexuality that could not be explained within this framework was at risk of being deemed a 'perversion'. Since the birth of sexology all manifestations of sexual perversion, delinquency and dysfunction have been clearly classified within the taxonomies of psychiatric illness. This was ostensibly to provide a framework for the development of valid and reliable theory and for the prescription of appropriate intervention. It allowed experts to communicate with each other about specific sexual problems or forms of deviance and to compare across populations to see if their treatments or theories of aetiology were correct. But as is the case with the law, clear ideological judgements about 'sex' and about the status of 'woman' and 'man' underpin all these supposedly objective systems of classification.

One of the earliest sex researchers, Havelock Ellis, catalogued a range of sexual abnormalities – sexual urges which are displaced on to objects outside the 'normal' sphere of desire and arousal. Ellis wanted to move away from the notion of wickedness inherent in the previously ubiquitous term 'perversion' – he was talking of *illness*, not evil or vice – and so he called these categories of abnormality 'symbolisms'. His classifications formed the building blocks for modern-day descriptions of 'paraphilias' and are worth a brief examination. They also illustrate the tight boundaries placed by science and sexology around 'normal' sexual expression (phallocentric heterosexuality) and the strict rules which define what is an 'acceptable' erotic object.

Ellis claimed there were three levels of erotic 'symbolism' – eroticism towards parts of the body, towards inanimate objects and towards acts and attitudes. He defined arousal by hands, feet, breasts, buttocks, hair, secretions and odours as 'normal'; arousal by 'lameness, squinting, pitting of smallpox, paedophile [sic], presbyophila, or love of the aged, and necrophilia' and 'erotic zoophilia' (excitement caused by animals) as 'abnormal'. All arousal by inanimate objects – 'gloves, shoes, stockings and garters, aprons, handkerchiefs, underlinen' – or by 'acts and attitudes' such as 'whipping, cruelty, exhibitionism, mutilation, murder, being whipped, . . . acts of urination and defecation and the coitus of animals' was also categorized as abnormal. Sado-masochistic sex – sex involving the infliction of punishment, pain or injury on a consenting partner – was first discussed as a medical category by Krafft-Ebbing in 1886. He conceived of it as resulting from a 'congenital hereditary tainted constitution', involving a 'pathological intensification of the masculine sexual character [in sadism and a] degeneration of the psychical peculiarities of women [in masochism].[27] It remains as a category of sexual dysfunction (or perversion) today; it may also be categorized as a 'crime'.

The modern-day classification systems have not diverged much from this model. The *Diagnostic and Statistical Manual of the American Psychiatric Association* (*DSM*), one of the most widely used systems of classification, lists exhibitionism, fetishism, frotteurism, paedophilia, sexual masochism, sexual sadism, transvestic fetishism and voyeurism as 'paraphilias'. Homosexuality was only removed from the *DSM* in 1973; before this date it was classified as psychiatric deviance. The *International Classification of Diseases* (*ICD*), an international taxonomic system, includes all of the above, as well as bestiality, transsexualism, disorders of psychosexual identity and homosexuality – although a disclaimer is included with the latter that we should 'code homosexuality here whether or not it is considered as a mental disorder'.[28] Clearly many people still do; *ICD-9* leaves our options open.

Whilst the law condemns those who break laws of consent as sexual offenders, in the taxonomies of sex research child sexual abuse is classified as 'paedophilia'. The *DSM* defines this as 'intense, sexual urges and sexually arousing fantasies, of at least six months' duration, involving sexual activity with a pre-pubescent child'. To receive a diagnosis, the person has to have acted on these urges – or to be 'markedly distressed by them'. Transformed into a clinical disorder, the behaviour of sexual abusers of children is thus contained within a diagnostic category as a list of presenting 'symptoms'.

Interestingly, adult sexual assault or rape is not categorized as a 'sexual disorder' – perhaps it would condemn too many men. Those who are categorized as 'sexual sadists' because they have sexual urges and fantasies involving the physical and psychological suffering of the victim, *may* commit rape, we are informed by the *DSM*. In these cases 'the suffering inflicted on the victim is far in excess of that necessary to gain compliance, and the visible pain of the victim is sexually arousing.'[29] We are reliably told that only 10 per cent of rapists exhibit sexual sadism. Presumably, by implication, the other 90 per cent are 'normal men' who inflict an *appropriate* degree of 'suffering' to gain the woman's compliance. It is also interesting that 'perversion' – with a few notable exceptions – is seen to be a male prerogative:

The extreme forms of symbolism (perversion) are chiefly found in men. They are so rare in women that Krafft-Ebbing stated, even in the late editions of his *Psychopathia Sexualis* that he knew of no cases of erotic fetishism in women.   HAVELOCK ELLIS, 1946[30]

Except for Sexual Masochism, in which the sex ratio is estimated to be 20 males for each female, the other paraphilias are practically never diagnosed in females, but some cases have been reported.

DSM111-R, 1987[31]

As both the early experts and the more recent diagnostic bible inform us, women are rarely 'perverse'. It is only in the case of masochism – ironically, as it is, perhaps, the archetypal feminine position – that female 'perversion' is at all acknowledged. Is this merely a reflection of women's lack of imagination? Or is it because a phallocentric view of 'woman' underpins these diagnostic categories – a view of 'woman' as sexually passive and inactive? Yet as the earlier examination of women's erotica illustrates, women are certainly capable of exploring and experimenting with sexuality in the realm of the 'perverse' – even if sexologists choose to turn a blind eye.

None of these diagnostic categories of sexual disorder are based on incontrovertible 'fact' – there is no reason why arousal associated with hair is 'normal' but attraction to an elderly person is not. It all depends on the social values adopted by those who construct the classification systems. Yet this scientific classification of sexuality as deviance or dysfunction is often seen as reflecting the 'truth' and thus gives a false air of respectability to the theories and the therapies of the sex experts. It sets in stone (or academic tome) and gives a false legitimacy to what are subjective, value-laden judgements of what is abnormal and what is not. It conceals the ambiguities and uncertainties of 'sex' under a cloak of scientific rhetoric. It also pathologizes and individualizes sexual behaviour that deviates from the norm, legitimating the right of the experts to intervene. Yet this is no more objective or rational than the sex laws which define a particular sexual act as criminal in one place and time and legal in another (see below). What is *perversion* in one context may be normal sexual behaviour in another.

Havelock Ellis's classification of 'perversions' was probably of little importance to the majority of people in the nineteenth century; equally, if representations of sexuality in today's pornography are anything to go by, clearly many readers could be clinically defined as deviants – sex with animals, fetish objects, SM and 'water sports' are not uncommon fare in the pornographer's visual diet. These sexual practices may technically be classified as 'paraphilias', but who cares? Only if you come forward to an expert for help will the diagnostic categories be invoked. What's more, the very notion of these acts being transgressive may add to their allure (the recent trend for SM clothing worn as a fashion accessory has been greeted with dismay by serious aficionados of SM sex). Social, cultural, legal and psychiatric judgements are open to resistance. That is, at least as far as the state allows.

Common Sex Law: Anomalies and Anachronisms in Definitions of 'Illegal' Sex

Marriage and adultery

Sex laws in the late twentieth century are a hodgepodge of anomalies and anachronisms, yet they still position phallocentric heterosexuality as the norm and enshrine belief in female sexual passivity with strictures to control the libidinous temptress. There are many contradictions in the law itself, particular sexual activities coming within the jurisdiction of legislators at one point in time and not at others. An act that is illegal in one context may be legal in another; an act that is encouraged or accepted in one context may be criminalized and condemned in another. In fact, the very definition of what constitutes 'sex' can vary greatly within the law. As Gayle Rubin has commented, 'the only adult sexual behaviour that is legal in every state is the placement of the penis in the vagina in wedlock'.[32] Looking at how the law defines and regulates 'sex' and sexual crimes illustrates very clearly the role it plays in defining and regulating what it is to be 'woman' and how, at the same time, assumptions about what it means to be 'woman' or 'man' are irrevocably linked to our very definitions of 'sex'. These are all fluid concepts, open to interpretation and subject to change.

Whilst there is remarkable agreement across legal systems about the criminal nature of sexual assault (although questions of how it can be defined and who is to blame are open to interpretation), there is much disagreement about the boundaries of 'normal' consensual sex – whether homosexuality, adultery, sex with children and the practice of 'perversions' should be criminalized and, if so, what the punishment should be. Historically, as we have noted, 'sex' was only allowed to occur within marriage and was restricted to procreation and the missionary position. Yet whilst adultery may contravene theological doctrine – one of the ten commandments being 'Thou shall not covet thy neighbour's wife' (clearly positioning the man as active agent, the woman as object of his desire) – the majority of people would not view it as a *criminal* offence today – certainly not in Britain. Yet, technically, it *is* a crime in many American states;[33] until 1978 adultery was a criminal offence in Italy; in Greece until 1981. In Saudi Arabia adultery is still very firmly outside the law, with flogging or stoning to death the penalty usually exacted on those caught – often only the woman. When the United Nations attempted to prevent such punishment for adultery in 1980, the president of the Saudi Court of Appeal declared that flogging and stoning were appropriate punishments for 'such a horrible crime that makes men start to doubt if they are the natural fathers of their children' and which causes 'both the family and society to disintegrate'[34] – primogeniture as justification for the annihilation of the lascivious woman.

Saudi Arabia is not unique in punishing women for sex crimes carried out jointly by a woman and a man. Women are punished for adultery because it is seen to be their duty to refuse men's advances and to provide boundaries for male sexuality (the theme of romantic fiction enshrined in law). An assumption implicit within the law is the notion that the male sex drive cannot be contained and that, as a consequence, it is woman's responsibility to refuse or resist. As one British MP, engaging in a debate on sex law earlier this century, pronounced:

> Sex attraction is one of the elemental things in life, and it will be agreed that when you get down to the instincts which move men and women in sex matters, the outstanding *instinct* of the male is pursuit . . . The *instinct* of the female is resistance, reserve, followed, if she is won, by surrender, but broadly speaking she has the reserve, and the resistance . . . and the most potent individual force that makes for sexual morality in a community is woman's modesty [my italics].[35]

The implication here is that the woman who *doesn't* object is responsible for the sexual act that then takes place, as man can't help his 'instincts'; *women* are blamed for adulterous sex (as well as for sexual violence; see Chapter Five). This is also why even in contexts where adultery is not officially outlawed, men who punish their adulterous wives (often with murder) are treated sympathetically by the law (see p. 404).

The Question of Consent

The arena in which the law is most vigilant is sex without consent. The law defines 'sex' as an activity that is only allowed to take place between adults, between those who are deemed mature enough to give or withhold consent.[36] Yet the age of consent for sex varies greatly across cultures and across time, leading to different definitions of what constitutes child sexual abuse and variations in the age at which young girls are deemed 'ready' to receive the sexual attentions of older men.[37] For example, in sixteenth-century England children were betrothed and married well before the age of puberty, invariably because of the financial or political gain such matches would accrue for their parents. In the Elizabethan era the age of consent for girls was ten.[38] In many cases, the boy was not physically able to consummate the union. The marriage of Catherine of Aragon and her first husband Prince Arthur is one notable case, the lack of consummation being the reason that Henry VIII could marry his brother's wife.[39] Up until the late nineteenth century girls could legally engage in sexual intercourse at the age of twelve. This was raised to the age of sixteen in 1885 only because of the increasingly common practice of parents selling their daughters to brothel keepers.[40] A report published in 1882, which prompted the 1885 Act, stated that the desire for young girls was so great that prostitutes in the West End of London had to dress as little girls in order to get any custom.[41] W. T. Stead, then editor of the *Pall Mall Gazette*, caused an outcry when he publicized the fact that he had with great ease purchased a thirteen-year-old girl from her mother for prostitution. The resulting public debates acted to spur on the legislative campaigns of early feminists such as Josephine Butler and J. Ellice Hopkins,[42] creating a climate that facilitated changes in the law of consent. Yet until the 1929 Marriage Act it was still legal in England for girls of twelve to marry and have full sexual intercourse with their husbands but illegal for them to have sex with anyone else. Today, any girl who 'has sex' (defined as sexual intercourse) under the age of sixteen is committing a legal offence. If there is a five-year age difference between the girl and her partner, it is 'child sexual abuse'.

Yet this young age of consent is not merely a historical anachronism. For example, in Bangladesh (which is one of the few countries where at 55.9 women's life expectancy is lower than that of men's, at 56.8) one fifth of women today have given birth by the age of fifteen. Within the United States of America the age of consent varies across states: In Oregon it is twelve, in Missouri, Georgia and Washington fourteen, and in California, Idaho and Wisconsin eighteen.[43] In many cultures there are no laws about the age of consent whatsoever and sexual activities between adults and children occur unchecked and unquestioned. For example, anthropologists have recorded that in the Sambian tribe of the New Guinea Highlands part of the initiation of boys into adulthood involves fellatio (oral sex) between young boys and men, with the young boys ingesting the adult male semen as a rite of passage into manhood.[44] All boys take part in this ritualized activity so they can become strong and courageous warriors. It is not categorized as 'sex'.[45]

So what is considered to be sexual violation of a child in one context is deemed acceptable (or compulsory) sexual behaviour in another. There is no immutable point at which children become sexually responsible and capable of giving consent, no point at which a sexual act 'naturally' becomes legal or acceptable between adult and child, between two adults or between two children. The only physical restraints are the development of the sexual body, which will preclude sexual intercourse or pregnancy on the part of the girl, and the ability to maintain an erection and ejaculate semen on the part of the boy. However, these physical restraints only apply when we conceive of 'sex' as being heterosexual intercourse leading to pregnancy – other forms of sexual activity are not inevitably restricted by biology or physical maturity in the same way. It is *social* laws that define these boundaries and tell us when we are legally allowed to become 'sexual', and these boundaries are variable, as we have seen.

SM Sex and the Spanner Trials

Children are not the only group deemed incapable of giving (or withholding) consent and thus needing protection from the law. The law defines certain sexual acts as being completely outside the rule of consent; there are certain things one cannot consent to at all. In the Spanner Trials that took place in England in 1988 four men were convicted under the 1861 Offences against the Person Act for carrying out acts of consensual sado-masochistic sex. At their unsuccessful appeal in 1993 the Law Lords commented that 'sex is no excuse for violence'[46] (which is ironic given the context of common legal rulings on rape; see Chapter Five). The result of the ruling in the Spanner Trial is that any sexual act that results in injury which is not 'transient and trifling', even if there is consent, can lead to a conviction. The Law Lords acknowledged that technically this meant that the infliction of a 'love bite' – that favoured indicator of teenage romance – could lead to conviction within the law.

The essence of the Spanner case was that the consent of the victim offered no defence to the charges – at least in the case of homosexual SM sex. The summary of the appeal to the House of Lords is telling: 'Consensual sado-masochistic homosexual encounters which occasioned actual bodily harm to the victim were assaults occasioning actual bodily harm, contrary to s.47 of the 1861 Act . . . notwithstanding the victim's consent to the acts inflicted on him, because public policy required that society be protected by criminal sanctions against a cult of violence which contained the danger of proselytization and corruption of young men and the potential for serious injury.'[47]

Here, consent is not possible because of the fear of the homosexual peril – from which 'young' men must be protected (a common belief, see pp. 281–2). That the Law Lords were concerned to stamp out homosexuality as much as SM sex is illustrated by the comment on the current sexual lifestyle of 'K', a fifteen-year-old youth who had willingly taken part in SM sex. It was said that 'it is some comfort to be told, as we were, that "K" has now settled into a normal heterosexual relationship.'[48] Not a normal, non-SM relationship (the issue of the case) – a normal *heterosexual* relationship. Is this a patronizing and heterosexist refusal to acknowledge the rights of young men to engage in homosexual sex, whatever its form? Or is it appropriate protection? Whatever our view in what is ultimately an ideological debate we must recognize the fact that young women are rarely protected from older men's unwanted sexual advances in such a way. During the debates on raising the age of consent from twelve to sixteen that took place in the English Parliament in the 1920s, one MP described the difficulty men have in defending themselves against the seductive powers of young women and argued for the protection of the right of men to have sexual access to girls under the age of sixteen. This was his description of the temptations men are powerless to resist:

> She sets to work to throw allurement after allurement over him. She throws all the artifices of her sex to achieve her object. She gradually sees him being lashed into the elemental and aggressive male, and when that point is reached he is like a runaway horse; his control is gone. He pursues and he succumbs.[49]

This is adult–child sex positioned within the boundaries of romance, something unthinkable if the child is a boy.

Defining Rape: Reifying the Penis as Phallus

'Rape' is legally defined as sex that occurs in the absence of consent. If we examine the definition of rape we have a further demonstration of the ideological assumptions underpinning sex laws and their narrow definition of what we consider to be 'sex'. For example, in England and the majority of states in North America rape is narrowly defined within the law as penetration of the vagina by the penis[50]–anal or oral penetration or assault by objects would be defined as 'indecent assault', a lesser crime in the eyes of the law. (New South Wales, Australia, is one of the few places that has a broader cover definition of 'rape', which includes penetration by objects, as well as the penis, and penetration of the mouth, rather than just the vagina or anus.) In England, where a life sentence can be given for 'rape', ten years is the maximum for 'indecent assault'.

Yet in the same way that women (or men) may engage in many activities other than vaginal penetration with the penis and define them as 'sex' (oral sex; mutual masturbation; sex toys; anal sex . . .), penetration by objects other than the penis or violation of parts of the body other than the vagina may be experienced as a traumatic 'rape'. A woman who is violated with a broom, a baseball bat and a stick – as was the case with a gang rape of a woman which occurred in Glen Ridge, New Jersey in 1991[51] – is the victim of an extreme form of sexual violation. To her it is 'rape'. To categorize this as less serious than rape with a penis is a complete denial of the seriousness of the crime as well as a

274 Fantasies of Femininity

glorification of the power of the penis as weapon. This is 'rape' defined from the point of view of phallocentrism.

Within the law certain groups of individuals appear to be deemed incapable of being raped. Women working as prostitutes or women who are deemed 'promiscuous' may find it almost impossible to bring a successful charge of rape against a man, regardless of the circumstances – as do married women against their husbands. Consent is deemed to be always present in these circumstances (see Chapter Five). Equally, within a model of heterosexuality which positions man as seducer and woman as resistant, 'rape' of a woman by a man has to be extreme or violent to be proven. Or, as is outlined in Chapter Five, it is merely seen as 'sex'. In the same way, gay men are assumed to consent to sex with other men, so 'rape' is deemed less serious – or impossible – when they are the victims. It is only the young boy sexually abused by an older man, or the raped heterosexual man, who are likely to be believed if they claim to have withheld consent. Whilst defence counsel has been known to plead precipitation in cases of the rape of a homosexual man, this would be unthinkable in the case of rape of a heterosexual man for whom 'sex' with a man is unthinkable. In this vein, many people believe that rape is worse for heterosexual men than it is for women, as it is a sexual act which violates the 'normal' boundaries of sexual behaviour. The fact that the defence of attempted rape has been successfully used by heterosexual men in a number of recent murder trials demonstrates the serious way in which the law views rape of a heterosexual man.[52] For these men (and the law), it seems, it is better to kill than to be subjected to rape.

However, consent is often assumed to be present if the victim of sexual abuse or violence experiences any form of sexual arousal or response during the event – a not uncommon finding in both male and female victims of certain forms of sexual assault. This is even more visible and noticeable to the abuser when the victim is male. It is not rare for the man to have an erection or to ejaculate when being subjected to rape.[53] This can cause increased trauma for the man, can be used to infer homosexuality and, by implication, complicity in the 'sexual' act. This 'myth of complicity'[54] is also common in cases of sexual abuse of boys, where abusers have been known to comment on the size of the victim's erection during the attack, positioning the boy as a willing party in what is reconstructed as a purely 'sexual' encounter. Equally, if a boy experiences an erection he may be less likely to categorize the experience as 'abuse', even if force is used, and so be reluctant to disclose.

However, within the law, the very existence of male 'rape' is rarely acknowledged. In England the first prosecution for male rape was brought in 1995, following the introduction of the crime on to the statute-books in 1994 (this first convicted offender was given life imprisonment). A similar position exists in the United States, where few states (exceptions being Michigan and Massachusetts) recognize male 'rape'. In both countries sexual assault by one man on another is categorized as 'indecent assault' and, as a consequence, lesser penalties than those meted out for rape are attached to this crime. As forced buggery between men isn't categorized as 'rape', the cross-examination of the sexual history of the complainant,[55] which has been almost universally banned in male–female rape trials, is allowed.

However, it is not the case that male rape doesn't exist within the law. One of the contexts in which it has been officially recognized is in American prisons. A number of surveys have estimated that at least 14 per cent of prisoners in the USA will experience rape which, given the figure of 1,200,000 men in prison at any one time, means 150,000 male rapes per year.[56] Yet convictions are rarely, if ever, brought. Many young prisoners are subjected to repeated gang rapes, and it has been demonstrated that if men are not sexually dominant in these contexts, engaging in rape, they are at high risk of being positioned as sexually submissive – and violated. This situation may be changing as a result of the 1994 US Supreme Court ruling that prison officials could be held responsible for not protecting a prisoner from sexual violence, which resulted from a number of prominent rape cases being brought to appeal, including the gang rape of a male–female transsexual who was placed in a male prison. This ruling ended what one male rape victim described as 'the Gulag of rape',[57] where prison warders implicitly condoned open and often organized sexual violence.[58]

Under current laws on male rape a transsexual or hermaphrodite cannot, legally, be 'raped' – even if the sexual assault in question involves the penetration of a vagina by a penis,[59] as the law does not recognize a change in sex – born a man, one dies a man. So it is not simply an operational definition which classifies rape, not simply a matter of penis and vagina. It has to be a 'real' man, raping a 'real' woman, in a 'real' vagina – a reconstructed one clearly does not count.

Women as Rapists or Child Sexual Abusers: An Inconceivable Thought

In the majority of countries women cannot be convicted of rape – only of aiding and abetting in a rape, of being accessories, or principals in the second degree. This reflects the phallocentric positioning of 'woman' as sexually responsive rather than predatory (the preserve of 'man') and the difficulty in conceiving of female sexuality outside of 'normal' heterosexual power relations, where man is active and woman is passive (which is also reflected in laws on lesbianism). In the American courts, where a number of such cases have been brought to trial, it has invariably been argued that it is 'physiologically impossible' for a man to be raped by a woman ('If he gets an erection, can it count as "rape"?'), despite medical evidence to the contrary.[60] A number of research studies suggest that a woman *can* rape a man,[61] and that the consequences for men can be severe. Whilst a woman could technically sexually assault or 'rape' another woman with an object (or her fist), this would not be recognized as 'rape' in the eyes of the law. These may be extremely rare cases – men remain the major perpetrators of sexual assault – but that does not mean that they should be ignored or positioned as less serious than rape with a penis.

The law also neglects or negates female perpetration of child sexual abuse. For whilst the majority of research studies suggests that women are by far in the minority as perpetrators of CSA, it is not impossible for women to sexually abuse children. Yet within a legal system which deems 'woman' to be sexually passive, inactive and incapable of sexual crime, it is not surprising that few women are prosecuted or convicted for sexual abuse.

Those women who *are* convicted are invariably seen as doubly deviant,[62] invariably portrayed as monsters, and condemned. Myra Hindley, the British woman convicted of the sexual abuse and murder of three children in 1966, was informed in 1996 that she will never be released from prison. For over thirty years the British press has portrayed her as an evil witch, a danger to society. Similar treatment was given to Rosemary West, convicted of the sexual abuse and murder of twelve women in 1995 (including her own daughter) – that a *woman* could commit such crimes produced incredulity (and horror) in press and public alike. Conversely, in 1989 Hedda Nussbaum was accused, alongside her lover Joel Steinberg, of the sexual abuse and battering to death of his six-year-old adopted daughter Lisa, but freed by the courts on the grounds that she had been beaten and abused by Steinberg herself. The case provoked a feminist outcry that a woman could not possibly commit such a crime.[63] Any recognition of women as sexual abusers of children appears to go against one of our greatest taboos – the image of 'woman' as beneficent, glowing Madonna.

There are great arguments between professionals working in this field as to the actual frequency of child sexual abuse carried out by women[64] – but this is not the issue here. The point is that what we construe as 'sexual abuse' is not an absolute, categorical thing but something affected by socially defined rules surrounding 'sex'. These rules can result in the experience of certain groups of people being ignored – in this case sexual violence carried out by women (but also child sexual abuse where the victim is a boy). Indeed, activities which we clearly acknowledge to be 'sexual abuse' when carried out by a man may be seen as something to boast of carried out by a *woman* on a boy. Many men will brag of their having been initiated into sex by an older woman when in their teens. Looking back on the number of my male school friends who boasted of such 'seductions' when I was thirteen, I can think of no other explanation than that these brags reflected teenage fantasies about the seductive older woman (undoubtedly reinforced by the boys' reading of porn). I am sure now that this supposed sex could not have been happening in such epidemic proportions in a Catholic school in the early seventies, particularly when there was no evidence of these boys having *any* sexual knowledge or experience of sex at all. As adults, many men continue to brag of adolescent sex with an older woman. For example, in a recent issue of the British magazine *Marie Claire*,[65] in an article discussing the number of women men had slept with, one named and photographed man proudly boasted of his sexual conquest of over 200 women, mentioning in passing that he had been initiated into 'sex' by an older woman at the age of thirteen. Would a woman boast of this? It would be viewed as 'child sexual abuse', as 'promiscuous' adult sexuality and evidence of 'acting out'. It would probably also be associated with shame – she would be a 'slag'.

Popular culture celebrates such sexual contact between adult women and boys, supporting its negation within the law. Films such as *The Last Picture Show, Summer of 42, The First Time, The Chapman Report,*

Class, Private Lessons, Weird Science, The Graduate, and the *Tin Drum* present sex between a woman and a boy as 'initiation' rather than 'abuse'.[66] Reverse the gender roles, with male adult and female child, and the picture appears very different (to all but the paedophile). One psychologist who works with male survivors of sexual abuse tells a tale that epitomizes the social reaction to such events. At the beginning of a seminar on female–male abuse he started to describe the nature of the crime – sexual molestation of a boy by an older woman – and a voice from the back of the room shouted out 'lucky dog'. Everyone erupted into laughter.[67] We may interpret this laughter as a defensive reaction to knowledge of a distressing event. But it also reflects the trivial way in which sexual abuse of boys by women is viewed.

Many feminists shy away from any discussion of female perpetration of sexual violence or abuse – to even speak of it is seen as detrimental to women. But we can't have it both ways. If we want to move away from phallocentric models of sexuality and acknowledge that women have a right to a sexuality outside the narrow confines of 'sex' as it is currently defined, we have to recognize that women too can carry out sexual violence and abuse. It may be rare – but it is possible. Equally, many men are traumatized by having been sexually abused as a child – whether by a woman or by a man. The fact that popular culture and the law tend not to recognize these acts as 'abuse' may compound the problem, not alleviate it, as it means it is less likely that the child will disclose – as is the case with much of the sexual violence experienced by women and girls (see Chapter Five).

Policing Deviant Sex: The Case of Homosexuality

Male Homosexuality: The Sin of Sodomy

Laws and scientific theories that regulate and explain homosexuality also reveal the phallocentric bias within science and the law – the fact that both professions reflect the interests and the fears of the 'normal' heterosexual man – and provide further examples of the variable nature of the legal and scientific pronouncements on the rights and wrongs of 'sex'. Arguably, it was in the categorization of homosexuality as 'illness' and sexual crime that the early sexologists had the greatest impact on the lives of individual women and men: It is one of the few forms of 'deviancy' where the sex police come knocking at the door. The homoerotic fantasies we have seen framed in the masculine gaze in art, film and pornography are transformed into material controls of sex as they enter the legal statute-books.

Active homosexual sex between men has been almost universally condemned within theological doctrine throughout the ages – with sodomy being seen as a 'crime against nature' more heinous than murder.[68] In England the act of sodomy was criminalized and made punishable by death under an Act of 1533, promoted by King Henry VIII. The death penalty remained on the statute-books until 1861,[69] when the Offences against the Person Act imposed sentences of between ten years and life.

Historically, the law has been directed as controlling the *act* of homosexual sex, rather than criminalizing the homosexual person – it was the act of sodomy that was outlawed, whether it was 'between man and woman, man and beast, or man and man.'[70] In England, in the years following the 1861 Act that abolished the death penalty for sodomy, the Home Office made attempts to distinguish between the occasional sodomite and the 'homosexual' man – the notion of homosexual identity or orientation having been recently introduced by Victorian sexologists (p. 296). In this vein, Mr Justice Hawkins commented that: 'For the most part that crime [bestiality] is committed by young persons, agricultural labourers etc. out of pure ignorance. The crime of sodomy with mankind stands on a *different* footing . . . [my italics].[71] It was 'different' in that it was almost unequivocally condemned – fucking an animal was clearly more acceptable than fucking a consenting human.

The use of the law on sodomy has been sporadic. As the sexual historian Jeffrey Weeks comments, it is difficult to know how many men were hanged under the powers of the 1533 Act. What is clear from the statistics available is that at particular points in history moral crusades were conducted to rid England of this 'heinous sin'. For example, Weeks reports that in 1806 there were more hangings for sodomy than for murder and in 1810 four out of five convicted 'sodomites' were condemned to death.[72]

In England, the Offences against the Person Act of 1861 was extended in 1885 as part of an act aimed at controlling prostitution, so that any acts of 'gross indecency' carried out between two males, either in public or in private, were made illegal. Labelled a 'blackmailer's charter', it resulted in the ruin and imprisonment of many thousands of men, one of the most infamous being the playwright and poet Oscar Wilde. It remained on the statute-books in England until 1967, when consenting sex between two men over the age of twenty-one, in private, was decriminalized. Whilst in the majority of European countries today the age of consent is the same for heterosexual and homosexual sex – following a recommendation of the Council of Europe in 1981 – in Britain, until 1994, the age of consent was twenty-one for homosexual men, and sixteen for heterosexuals; the former only latterly being reduced to eighteen in a private member's bill.

Male homosexuality continues to be illegal to this day in many cultures – in the mid eighties it was still illegal in Cyprus, Eire, Mexico, New Zealand, the Soviet Union and all Moslem countries.[73] In 1993 it was illegal in twenty-four North American states,[74] with the most severe state penalties being twenty years in jail. Against an appeal brought by gay legal activists in 1986, the Supreme Court upheld the right of the state of Georgia to criminalize adult, consensual, private sex between two men. The appeal concerned the Bowers v. Hardwick case, in which a young man had been arrested in his own bedroom for engaging in 'illegal' sex with another man. Relying on theological dictates concerning homosexuality, the court concluded that homosexuality was a threat to the American family and to the American way of life.[75]

The law on homosexuality highlights many of the contradictions and anomalies that underpin the legislation which frames our sexual lives and exemplifies the invasive nature of the strictures that can potentially condemn our sexual practices. For example, whilst within English law consensual sex between two men over the age of eighteen, if carried out in private, is not illegal, if one of the parties is under eighteen (even by a month), or if another person is present (male or female), even if they are not engaging in any sexual activity, it *is* illegal. If sexual intercourse takes place between two men with another person present, they could be still be sent to prison for life. In contrast, today, individuals engaged in heterosexual or lesbian sex (or even a combination of the two) can enjoy as many partners simultaneously as they wish, and the law of England will say nothing. This particular law against homosexual men is certainly enacted: Each year scores of men are arrested for 'cottaging' – having sex in public toilets – because this is defined within the law as an 'unnatural offence of gross indecency'. Until recently, many police forces placed specially trained officers in public toilets in an attempt to trap such offenders. The voyeurism involved in peeping through pinholes in order to catch men having consensual sex with each other beggars the imagination.

Equally, many men have been convicted for engaging in consensual sex with those under the age of homosexual consent but above the age of heterosexual consent. For example, in 1988 when the age of male homosexual consent in England was twenty-one, twenty-three men were convicted for consensual sex with men over sixteen.[76] The justification for such prosecution and for the differential age of consent for heterosexual and homosexual men is that young boys are deemed open to easy corruption by the seductive powers of older homosexual men. Following discussion of a lowering of the age of consent in the British parliament in 1990, the then Conservative party chairman Kenneth Baker was reported to be appalled, commenting that 'Parents will be shocked to know that this protection for their children could be removed.'[77] Boys are clearly deemed in greater need of 'protection' than girls, who are legally free to choose whomsoever to have sex with after the age of sixteen even though, as the Howard League reports, there is no evidence that boys can be 'converted' to homosexuality. This is an interesting reversal of the belief in 'man' as rational and controlled and 'woman' as vulnerable and easily seduced. (Another legacy of this fear for the corruption of children by supposedly rapacious homosexuals is to be found in Clause 28, introduced by the British parliament in 1988, which made illegal any public promotion of homosexuality as normal or equal to heterosexuality, particularly in schools or places of further education). This was again illustrated by the comments of a conservative MP, Robert Spink, during the 1994 parliamentary debates that preceded the lowering of the homosexual age of consent:

> The public interest is best served by an uncompromising prosecution policy . . . any reduction in the age of prosecution would put teenage boys at danger from the pro-buggery loony. It would be a contempt of parliament for any waiver to be given. The buggery of teenage boys is the only issue on the table.[78]

Today, whilst many aspects of sexual behaviour between men remain
illegal, few convictions are actually brought for consensual sex in private.
This non-application of sex law is not unusual. In 1948 Kinsey remarked
that 95 per cent of American men were regularly engaging in sexual
acts that were technically criminal[79] – yet very few were actually
convicted (or even saw themselves as criminals). For example, whilst
oral sex between consenting heterosexuals is technically illegal in many
US states today,[80] and anal intercourse between consenting heterosexual
adults was illegal in Britain until 1994, under the Sexual Offences Act
of 1956 (s.12 (1)), convictions for these crimes have rarely been brought.
(A sentence of eighteen months was given for the crime of heterosexual
sodomy in 1971.)[81] These are behaviours which the majority of the
population would no longer see as particularly deviant if consensual
and practised in privacy. What this selective application of sex laws
demonstrates is that public consensus on sexual morality (or immorality)
and the law is entwined in a complicated symbiotic relationship. In
many instances public morality changes *prior* to changes in the law
leading to anachronistic edicts lying unused on the statute-books. In
other cases the law (along with medicine and psychology) is strongly
influential in shaping social mores on sex. This is most clearly illustrated
in legal rulings (or refusals to rule) on the subject of lesbianism.

The Horror of Lesbianism

> These moral weaknesses [lesbianism] date back to the very origin of
> history, and when they grow and become prevalent in any nation or in
> any country, it is the beginning of the nation's downfall. The falling away
> of feminine morality was to a large extent the cause of the destruction of
> the early Greek civilization, and still more the cause of the downfall of
> the Roman Empire.[82]

Whilst male homosexuality has been almost universally castigated and
condemned, lesbianism has been remarkably neglected in the statutes
of the law. In English law, there is no age of consent for lesbian sex.
Laws on homosexuality are uniquely applied to men. Theological
doctrine is similarly silent on the subject (one exception being Paul's
epistle to the Romans, concerning the dangers of women turning from
the 'natural into the unnatural' (1:26). Yet whilst women were clearly

romantically and sexually engaging with each other long before the Victorian sexologists categorized them as 'lesbian' (or as female sexual inverts), it would be wrong to assume that women have had the freedom to engage in same-sex sexual activity whilst men have been tortured and hanged for the same. For the fears of Paul outlined in the New Testament, have been enshrined in secular law in a number of different contexts.[83]

For example, in 1260 the Code of Orléans was introduced in France, prohibiting sex between women, stating that whilst for the first two offences a woman would 'lose her member', for the third she would be burned to death. In Italy in 1574 women who were found engaging in sex with other women, if they were over the age of twelve, received the following punishment: 'she shall be fastened naked to a stake in the street of Locusts and shall remain there all day and night under a reliable guard and the following day be burned outside the city.'[84] Burning at the stake was also the punishment for women caught having sex with another woman in medieval Spain, enshrined in the law code of 1256. Particular forms of lesbian sexual activity were deemed more worthy of such punishment. One Spanish jurist argued that 'burning should be mandatory only in cases where a woman has relations with another woman by means of a material instrument.'[85] This edict was repeated in Italy, where it was decreed that if a woman merely made overtures to another woman she should be denounced, if she 'behaves corruptly with another woman only by rubbing', she should be 'punished', yet if she 'introduces some wooden or glass instrument into the belly of another she should be condemned to death.'[86] A distinction between 'vanilla sex' and the heinous crime of phallic masquerade being introduced in the Middle Ages?

Yet perhaps evidencing a foretaste of twentieth-century prudishness (or panic), official secrecy and silence invariably surrounded these particular sexual crimes. A fifteenth-century cleric who declared 'lesbianism' (as we now know it) a sin against God and a crime against nature proclaimed that 'women have each other by detestable and horrible means which *should not be named or written* [Brown's italics].'[87] In the sixteenth century, in Switzerland, the authorities were advised that in the case of those women convicted of same-sex sex the death sentence should be passed, yet the crime itself should not be described, for 'a crime so horrible and against nature is so detestable and because of the horror of it, it cannot be named.'[88] So when one woman was drowned for the crime of sex with another woman in Geneva in 1568, the jurist Colladon recommended that 'it is not necessary to describe minutely the circumstances of such a case, but only to say that it's for the detestable crime of unnatural fornication.'[89]

Sex between women was often implicitly positioned as orgiastic within the law – part of a general absence of libidinous control. For example, the charge of *femina cum feminus* (woman with woman) was often repeated during the witch trials of the Middle Ages, during which thousands of women were condemned for their supposedly voracious sexuality.[90] One of the most famous cases of a woman burned for heresy and witchcraft, that of Joan of Arc, centred around her wearing of male attire and her supposed sexual relationships with other women – all seen as evidence of her criminality.[91] In the fifteenth century it was believed by many that witchcraft (seen here as synonymous with lesbianism), was often the result of the woman's inability to attract and keep a man. As one authority declared, 'A woman usually becomes a witch after the initial failure of her life as a woman; after frustrated or illegitimate love affairs have left her with a sense of impotence or disgrace.'[92] The antecedent of the belief today that all a lesbian needs is a good fuck; she is only a lesbian because she can't get a man. Yet as well as being conceived of as a sad, second-rate activity, lesbianism was also positioned as a licentious sexual act in the annals of witchcraft. One account produced in France in 1460 declared:

> Sometimes indeed indescribable outrages are perpetrated in exchanging women, by order of the presiding devil, by passing on a woman to another woman and a man to other men, an abuse against the nature of women by both parties and similarly against the nature of men.[93]

No wonder the authorities wanted to remain silent on the subject. In England this legal silence has largely continued to this day (in contrast lesbianism *is* named – as illegal – in nearly 50 per cent of US states).[94] It is widely thought that the current absence of any law regulating consensual sex between adult women in England is due to the fact that Queen Victoria refused to allow any mention of lesbianism in the sexual offences acts of the late nineteenth century, on which our laws on sexual consent are based. This was supposedly because she could not conceive of such perverse acts actually being carried out by women –

which is why to this day there is no legal age of consent for lesbian sex in England.[95] A 1904 medical treatise entitled *Woman* appears to reinforce this view, claiming that female homosexuality had never been made a criminal offence because of 'the ignorance of the law-making power of the existence of this anomaly.'[96] This, in fact, was not so. But it appears that even when law-makers knew, they preferred absence of legislation to open acknowledgement of the threat of the lesbian. It wasn't Queen Victoria but the ruling parliamentarians who maintained the silence on lesbianism.

Regulating Lesbianism in English Law

Whilst there may have been no legal age of consent for sex between women, the *concept* of sex (or at least sexual assault) between women was certainly recognized by nineteenth-century legal experts in England. For example, in presiding over one particular case in 1885, a Mr Justice Lopes acknowledged that a woman *could* commit an indecent assault, a previously unthinkable concept; this assault could be carried out by a woman on a man, or could take place between two women.[97] Similarly, official legislation regulating 'indecent activity' between women was discussed in England in 1913, but refused by the then home secretary before it was even brought before parliament, for the reasons discussed above. An uproar was provoked in 1920 by the attempt of the MP Mr Macquisten to introduce a change to the 1885 Criminal Amendment Act, which would recognize in law the crime of 'indecency between women'. If enacted, the change would have placed female and male homosexual sex in an equal position in the eyes of the law, as the wording of the clause to be introduced was: 'Any act of gross indecency between female persons shall be a misdemeanour and punishable in the same manner as any such act committed by male persons under section eleven of the Criminal Law Amendment Act, 1885.'

The reaction to this bill epitomizes traditional reactions to female sexuality that exists outside the boundaries of phallocentric control – disbelief, disgust and, perhaps most strongly, despair. For as the main proponent of the bill, Mr Macquisten, declared to his fellow parliamentarians, 'there is in modern social life an undercurrent of dreadful degradation, unchecked and uninterfered with' [lesbianism]. The notion of 'sex' between women was clearly publicly recognized as a possibility.

But what this 'sex' could possibly involve was still a conundrum; Colonel Wedgwood, whilst agreeing with Macquisten's sentiments of horror and dismay, was driven to comment, 'How on earth are people to get convictions in a case of such a kind?'[98] Arguably, what this sexual activity between women could possibly involve appears to have been so unthinkable to the learned men that two of them, Colonel Webb and Sir Earnest Wild, were driven to declare that it 'was a beastly subject and they did want to pollute the house with knowledge of it.'[99] The latter claimed that lesbianism 'saps the fundamental institutions of society', 'stops childbirth', 'produces neurasthenia and insanity' and 'causes our race to decline'.[100]

The decision of what to do with these female 'perverts' also presented difficulties. Lieutenant Moor-Brabazon suggested three ways of dealing with them: stamping them out with the death penalty, locking them up as lunatics or, best of all, ignoring them – not because they were innocuous, but because they would eventually extinguish themselves, sentiments reminiscent of the eugenics movement that advocated sterilization for 'deviant' men and women. So it was declared:

> [We should] leave them entirely alone, not notice them, not advertise them. This is the method that has been adopted in England for many hundred years, and I believe it is the best method now . . . they have the merit of exterminating themselves, and consequently they do not spread or do very much harm to society at large . . . To adopt a clause of this kind would introduce into the minds of perfectly innocent people the most revolting thoughts.[101]

So, despite its apparent danger, lesbianism remained outside the law. Lord Desart, a former director of public prosecutions who had been involved in the indictment of Oscar Wilde, opposed the bill with the comment:

> You are going to tell the world that there is such an offence, to bring it to the notice of women who have never heard of it, never thought of it, never dreamt of it. I think it is a very great mischief.

The Lord Chancellor, Lord Birkenhead, reiterated these sentiments:

> I would be bold enough to say that of every thousand women, taken as a whole, 999 have never even heard a whisper of these practices. Among

> all these, in the homes of this country . . . the taint of this noxious and
> horrible suspicion is to be imparted.[102]

In the manner of the legal experts down the centuries they were beset
by the fear that if *any* publicity were given to the concept of sex between
women, those women had never previously imagined the existence of
such activities might be tempted to try them. The grave risk was that
they would then forsake their men, as it was feared, in the words of
one parliamentarian, that 'any woman who indulges this vice will have
nothing whatever to do with the other sex.'[103] What fragile male egos
must have promoted such fears. Can the power of the phallus be so
easily superseded?

That women having sex with each other could be such a threat is
undoubtedly testimony to the vulnerability felt by the law-making men
in the face of the autonomous sexual woman, her sexual passivity no
longer confirming man's 'natural' phallic mastery and power, her turning
from the phallus – both as symbol and as embodied sign (in her apparent
rejection of the penis) – acting as the greatest conceivable threat to
'man'. This was perhaps what promoted the apparent blindness (or
lack of imagination?) in generations of law-makers – the inability
(or reluctance) to imagine woman as sexually active and therefore
potentially threatening, as well as the horror evoked by confirmation
that she was capable of being so. For as recently as 1978 the British
government was quoted as stating: 'The question of homosexual acts
by females has never – so far as the government of the United Kingdom
are aware – been generally considered to raise social problems of the
kind raised by masculine homosexuality.'[104]

Legally denying active female sexuality – or the very existence of
woman's rejection of man – can be seen as a defence against the anxieties
and fears associated with 'woman' I have outlined (see Chapters Two
& Three). The above comment reflects the prejudiced fears directed
towards male homosexuality – the threat supposedly posed to young
men by the predatory advances of the rapacious homosexual man
(perhaps concealing a dread many men have of their own homoerotic
desires) – and the narrow definition of 'sex' used within the law
(penetration of vagina by penis); and is analogous to the laws that
narrowly define 'rape' as vaginal penetration by a penis, seeing penetration by objects not as 'rape' and therefore as a lesser crime.

Sexual activity between women *was* implicitly recognized in English law in a number of divorce cases in the late forties, where a woman's 'unnatural sexual relations' with another woman were deemed grounds for her husband to divorce her.[105] The 1956 Criminal Offences Act, ss. 14 & 15 also acknowledged that a woman was capable of carrying out an indecent assault on another woman. But few cases have been brought before the courts. In 1991 Jennifer Saunders was jailed for six years for 'sexually assaulting' her two girlfriends and for impersonating a man,[106] the case being brought after the mother of one of the girls discovered that her daughter had a female lover. Saunders argued in her own defence that both women had known she was a woman and had wanted her to dress as a man in order to conceal the fact of their lesbian relationship. Whether the court was punishing 'assault' (which had been consensual sex at the time it happened), 'lesbian sex' or the audacity of a woman taking on a masculine masquerade is open to speculation.

In other cases when the law on female indecency is invoked there is an implicit assumption that women's sexuality is somehow less than that of men. This was made clear in a 1957 Royal Commission on Homosexual Offences and Prostitution (s. 103), which reported that it had 'found no case in which a female has been convicted of an act with another female which exhibits the libidinous features that characterize sexual acts between males.'[107] This reflects the belief that lesbian sexuality is somehow more benign and innocuous than heterosexual or gay male sexuality (what *do* they do in bed?), an assumption that sits strangely with the converse belief that 'the lesbian' is the epitome of rapacious, rampant female desire. The fact that the British serial killer Rosemary West engaged in 'lesbian sex' appeared to be regarded as unsurprising by both court and media during her 1995 trial for the murder of twelve women. Her defence lawyer revealed his own prejudices in his comments in opening her defence: 'She may be a lesbian, but she's not a murderer.' I wonder which he thought was worse? During the same period, the media was full of salacious reports of the wife of the then Greek prime minister, Dimitra Papandreou, as a result of photographs supposedly showing her engaging in 'lesbian sex' (photographs allegedly of her on a beach embracing another woman). This was seen as evidence of her errant sexuality and threatened her whole reputation (as well as that of her husband) – a 'lesbian' is clearly the antithesis of a 'good woman'.

Yet if the law does not like to think of or mention lesbian sex, it has no compunction in regulating lesbian motherhood. Historically, women in lesbian relationships have been deprived of custody of – or even access to – their children on the grounds of being unfit to be mothers. For example, in the 1981 case of *Dailey* v. *Dailey* the woman's ex-husband argued, 'Your honour, this is the bible belt. This [a lesbian raising her children] might be okay in New York or California, but this is the bible belt.' The woman lost custody of her children, with her access severely restricted, as her husband's attorney argued that in Tennessee the woman was technically a criminal for engaging in lesbian sex.[108] In a similar case in Virginia in 1993 a twenty-two-year-old woman, Sharon Bottoms, was denied custody of her two-year-old son because the judge believed he would grow up not knowing the difference between men and women if he stayed with his lesbian mother. The child's grandmother was granted custody, and commented, 'I don't care how my daughter lives, but Tyler [the child] will be mentally damaged by this. We can take care of ourselves, he can't.'[109] Yet the now consistent body of research on children being raised by lesbian parents has found no evidence that this has any deleterious effects or that the child is any more likely to be homosexual in orientation themselves (the feared outcome of the courts which often prevents custody being granted to a lesbian mother).[110] Encouragingly, in the light of this research, as well as the result of political lobbying, it is becoming increasingly possible for lesbian mothers to be treated fairly in custody hearings after a divorce – so the law does appears to be open to movement. Yet the reactions in parliament of two conservative MPs to a recent British case where joint custody of a child was awarded to two lesbian women are telling:

'I am immensely unhappy when adult sexual behaviour inflicts a distorted lifestyle on children. I believe strenuously that every child deserves a mother and father.' EMMA NICHOLSON

'We don't put children in the hands of the insane. Why should we put them in the hands of the perverted?[111] SIR NICHOLAS FAIRBAIRN

Whilst some sections of the law may be open to change, in many (powerful) quarters, things remain the same.

Condemnation through the Back Door: Army Witch-Hunts and Employment Law

> You can't hardly separate homosexuals from subversives . . . Mind you, I don't say every homosexual is a subversive, and I don't say every subversive is a homosexual. But [people] of low morality are a menace in the government, whatever [they are], and they are all tied up together.
>
> US SENATOR WHERRY, 1951[112]

> The 1950s were perhaps the worst time in history for women to love women.   LILLIAN FADERMAN, 1991[113]

Whilst lesbianism may not be present on the statute-books in the majority of countries of the western world today, this is not to say that it is behaviour that is condoned. Homosexual behaviour – whether between men or women – is still regulated and controlled, kept firmly in the closet, through a form of legislation as powerful as that of criminal law – employment legislation. This is one of the areas in which the law *does* treat gay men and lesbians equally – equally badly.

In England, equal-opportunities legislation covers racism and sexism: It does not cover sexual orientation. In the USA the law varies across states and across professions – it is, again, beset with contradictions. In federal law, a distinction is made between status (*being* gay or lesbian) and conduct (*acting* on it). Under the fourteenth amendment punishment or 'discrimination' cannot be based on status – being gay or lesbian is not proof of conduct. Direct evidence of 'deviant sexuality' is needed before discrimination is allowed.[114] However, this distinction is rarely applied in practice, and being sacked or discriminated against for being gay or lesbian is implicitly sanctioned by the law. In many instances it is explicitly encouraged. If we put the Nazi Germany persecution of gay men and lesbians aside, the most clear case is that of North America in the fifties, when McCarthyite witch-hunts rooted out gay men and lesbians from federal-government posts, purging public positions of the homosexual scourge.[115]

One of the first acts of President Eisenhower when he took office was to sign an executive order investigating and excluding from office any homosexual person in a 'sensitive' position in government, as well as screening all applicants for new positions. Being in the closet with the door firmly locked was the only way to survive. Lie detectors, invasive personal questions and intrusive 'security checks' were carried out to identify those suffering from such 'moral turpitude'. Thousands were dismissed from their jobs, many of whom had no experience of gay or lesbian relationships but were found to have failed the strict tests of 'morality' through actions such as discussing homosexual desires with a therapist or foolishly admitting to occasional homosexual fantasies when questioned by the investigation committees[116] – the thought police in action. The justification was clear: Gay men and lesbians are perverts, their dismissal justified by the 'lack of emotional stability which is found in most sex perverts and the weakness of their moral fibre' – the official party line. This was a misuse of psychological terminology to back up legal persecution – a taste of the modern regulation of sex through psychiatry, medicine and sex therapy. Not just bad, but sick.

At the same time gay men and lesbians were rooted out of the United States armed forces as part of a general witch-hunt which resulted in thousands of military personnel receiving a dishonourable discharge and losing all their veterans' benefits and pensions. Lillian Faderman has documented how the more tolerant attitude towards lesbian sexuality which developed during the Second World War (due to the need to recruit and maintain women as service personnel regardless of their sexual orientation), was replaced by bigoted and prejudiced campaigns to identify and evict the homosexual peril. Women officers in the navy were informed in 1952 that 'homosexuality is wrong, it is an evil . . . an offence to all decent and law-abiding people, and is not to be condoned on grounds of "mental illness" any more than any other crime such as theft, homicide or criminal assault.'[117] But this didn't just apply to women who were actively engaged in lesbian relationships – women who had had isolated sexual experiences before joining the army or women who associated with putative lesbians were also at risk of discharge. They were guilty until proven innocent – something which was nigh on impossible, because fraternization with other 'criminal' (lesbian) women was sufficient proof of guilt. Going to a gay bar could signal the end of a brilliant career.

Stereotypes about the voracious sexuality of lesbians abounded: Lillian Faderman notes, that 'lesbians were presented in the cliché of sexual vampires who seduced innocent young women into sexual experimentation that would lead them, like a drug, into the usual litany of horrors: addiction, degeneracy, loneliness, murder and suicide'[118] –

more than faintly reminiscent of the witch-hunts of the Middle Ages, when autonomous female sexuality was so feared that women were burned. The way to avoid such fearful degeneracy was to adhere to the script of appropriate femininity – army and navy women were sent to lectures informing them that sexual relationships should only take place within marriage and that despite being military personnel they were still expected to behave in a 'feminine way'. This continues in the British Army to this day, where women officers have to dress in 'appropriate' feminine apparel (a dress) in order to eat each evening in the officers' mess. As one army woman I talked to commented, 'I lost a lot of weight living in officer's quarters.'[119] She just wasn't prepared to engage in the masquerade.

In the fifties, in order to identify the sexual outcasts, army, navy and air-force personnel were duty-bound to inform upon each other. Chaplains, psychiatrists and physicians were supposed to report any suspicions of homosexuality.[120] If this avenue failed (for the thousands of lesbians in the army became exceptionally skilled at concealing their sexuality), entrapment was attempted. The marines sent decoys into bars to trap lesbian service personnel and planted informers in women's softball teams, attempting to catch women unawares. If they caught one woman, under interrogation the names of all her friends and associates were extracted. As was the case in the witch-hunts of the Middle Ages, a lesbian under interrogation was vulnerable to sexualized harassment and victimization. One army nurse who was accused with her lover of being a lesbian in 1954 told how the male intelligence officer assigned to investigate their case raped her lover 'to teach her how much better a man was than a woman.'[121]

This isn't mere folk history, a thing of the past or a relic of a less liberal time. Gay men and lesbians are still hounded out of service positions in many countries. When President Clinton attempted to introduce a bill to legalize homosexuality in the US armed forces in 1993, it was greeted with outrage by the conservative right. Is it a coincidence that on the same day that Clinton announced his policy (19 July 1993), the Colorado Supreme Court passed an amendment designed to abolish existing municipal legislation that protected against 'sexual-orientation' discrimination? It also banned any future state or local legislation of this nature.[122]

Even Clinton's failed bill was less liberal-minded than his critics feared. It was not a move towards equal legislation but merely an attempt to enforce the status/conduct distinctions – the 'don't-ask-don't-tell' policy: as long as a conspiracy of silence was maintained gay and lesbian personnel would not be dismissed. (This is a direct parallel with recent debates over 'gay vicars' in the Church of England, where they were officially tolerated if celibate, unofficially tolerated if silent and discreet.) Yet the USA is liberal compared to the British armed forces, where homosexuality is still illegal at the time of writing, although as appeals are being made to the European Court of Human Rights, whether the ban on gay and lesbian service personnel can continue to be enforced in the twenty-first century is doubtful.

Homosexuality: An Offence that Damages Morale

The justification for banning homosexuality in the British armed forces is illuminating, as it continues the centuries-old belief that homosexual activity is immoral, deviant and associated with weakness and degeneracy. Here is the official army line on the matter:

> Homosexuality, whether male or female, is considered incompatible with service in the armed forces. This is not only because of the close physical conditions in which personnel often have to live and work, but because homosexual behaviour can cause offence, polarise relationships, induce ill discipline, and as a consequence damage morale and unit effectiveness.
>
> British Army Guidelines on Homosexuality, 1994[123]

In these guidelines there is no status/conduct distinction to complicate the legislation. 'Homosexuality' is defined as sexual attraction to a person of the same sex – it is *desire* which is policed, not sexual conduct or sexual orientation. For as is clearly stated in a 1994 report which outlines 'policy and guidelines on homosexuality', 'homosexuality is defined as "behaviour characterized by being sexually attracted to members of the same sex".' No problems here on where to draw the line about what constitutes 'sex' (is it kissing, holding hands, fondling, penetration?) – desire is enough. Thoughts and feelings, if admitted, can end a career.

Raids by the military police to find evidence of lesbian sexual activity are still common in the British army. If suspected of such illegal conduct, a woman can have her quarters raided and searched, all her personal possessions examined for evidence of guilt, and her friends interviewed for corroborating information. Personal diaries, letters and photographs will be scrutinized and if a woman confesses to being a lesbian she will immediately be discharged, losing all rights and privileges, including her pension. These investigations have been described by women as akin to rape, and as lesbians in the armed forces live in constant fear of being the targets of investigation, they live their lives within a cloak of subterfuge.

The armed forces make no apologies for this. In the Codes of Conduct circulated to all commanding officers in the British Army in 1993,[124] which start with the declaration, 'The British Army has long held a reputation for high standards, high morale and strict discipline,' the contempt directed at 'civilian society' with its liberal views on homosexuality is made clear. Whilst noting that the army is isolated from the rest of society, it is clearly stated that: 'this relative isolation has, however, meant that the army has been able to maintain high moral and ethical standards largely unaffected by the changes in the patterns of behaviour in society in general.' There is no question here of who is right – the army is positioned as an enclave of respectability, protected from the homosexual menace. This is analogous to the situation in the US, where controversy about gays in the military has been seen not as a debate around the ability or even the 'conduct' of sexual minorities, but the reaction of the reactionary military establishment to the increasing visibility and acceptance of gay men and lesbians in society at large.[125] The army is taking a moral stand to defend the privilege and power of the heterosexual 'norm'.

Demonstrating the strength of the disdain and disgust underlying these army laws, the British Army Codes of Conduct lists homosexuality alongside alcohol and drug abuse, dishonesty, indebtedness, bullying and initiation ceremonies, racial and sexual harassment, adultery and cross-rank relationships as against army rules. It is the only 'offence' (with the exception of drug use) which gives automatic grounds for dismissal. Interestingly, the other 'misdemeanour' which falls into this category is 'single parenthood' [sic], for the Codes of Conduct state that, 'those who become single parents *through circumstances within their control* and who are unable to meet their operational liability will not be retained' [my italics].

This is one of the few 'misdemeanours' which will apply almost solely to women, and reflects an outmoded view of 'unmarried mothers' that has long passed into folk history in civilian Britain, where 31 per cent of births in 1992 took place outside marriage.[126] It acts to criminalize women who choose to have children outside marriage whilst acting to protect army men who are widowed or divorced and left with responsibility for their children, as this was not 'within their control': The old double standard again. As one army woman cynically commented, 'any men left "holding the baby" are always given married quarters, and allowed to have a live-in nanny. I never saw it happen with a woman.'

The 1993 British Army Discipline and Standards paper states very explicitly that 'the strict code of conduct required in the Army is not the continuance of outdated Victorian moral standards or a desire to set an example for society.' Yet the army is a bastion of privilege, its commanding officers drawn from the upper echelons of British society, and whilst it no longer has the power to legislate over public morality (as it could in the colonial power bases, such as British-occupied India) its official values and rules of conduct are a reflection of beliefs held firmly by a majority of those who hold political power. Liberal campaigns may have ensured that acceptance of homosexuality in wider society is slightly greater than it was thirty years ago (although discrimination is still very evident in the workplace). But the army still reflects large sections of public opinion, particularly of those in positions of power, and its treatment of gay men and lesbians provides us with a depressing insight into the narrow, prejudiced views of the appropriate sexuality of 'woman' and 'man' and the heterosexual bias in legislation about 'normal sex'.

The Sick Homosexual

> It was not until 1870 that Westphal published a detailed history of an
> inverted young woman, and clearly showed that the case was congenital
> and not acquired, so that it could not be termed a vice, and was also,
> though neurotic elements were present, not a case of insanity.
>
> HAVELOCK ELLIS[127]

Ellis may have argued that lesbianism was neither vice nor insanity but, arguably, sexual science has consistently acted to reify the notion of homosexuality as perversion – a belief confidently invoked by parliamentarians and public alike today. The early sexologists have been credited with inventing the categories of homosexual and lesbian in the 1850s, their classification of this type of 'sexual' deviance' culminating in the first case histories to appear in scientific literature in the 1870s. Before this date it was merely same-sex behaviour that was legally condemned and controlled.

Krafft-Ebbing, writing in Germany in the late nineteenth century, had initially considered homosexuality as a manifestation of an inherited neuropathic or psychopathic state – later changing his views to position it as more of an anomaly than a disease. Havelock Ellis was more liberal, generously commenting that inverts might be healthy, and normal in all respects outside their special aberration, that he regarded inversion as frequently in close relation to the minor neurotic conditions.[128] He reassured his readers that lots of distinguished people were inverts, but commented that usually only those of the lowest, most degenerate, and sometimes mercenary class were willing to betray their peculiarity.[129] One of the case vignettes he presented was of a physician whose moral traditions had not allowed him to seek the satisfaction of his impulses – an early warning about the importance of staying in the closet which parallels debates concerning homosexuals in the army and the priesthood today. The message was clear: As long as you sin only in mind, not in body, you are exempt from punishment (or treatment); homosexuals were cautioned to resist their inherited perverse desires.

In the writings of the early sexologists women's homosexuality was seen to be irrevocably linked with masculinity. Havelock Ellis commented that:

> Among female inverts, there is usually some approximation to the masculine attitude and temperament . . . the sex organs . . . are sometimes overdeveloped, or perhaps more usually underdeveloped . . . there may be a somewhat masculine development of the larynx.[130]

Krafft-Ebbing contributed a similar view, describing the female invert as having coarse male features, a rough and rather deep voice. These clinical aberrations were put to the test in the thirties in a series of studies carried out under the auspices of the Committee for the Study of Sex Variants in New York City, which set out to determine the characteristics of 'the lesbian'.[131] Women volunteers were interviewed and observed, their bodies inspected. It was concluded that the lesbian could be distinguished from the normal woman on the basis of clear masculine or feminist tendencies, as well as enlarged genitalia. Here are two extracts from the psychiatrist George Henry's reports on two different women:

Rose S

The labia majora are 10 cm long and the minora pigmented in a very pronounced fashion, notwithstanding the general coloration, and they protrude in pronounced, thick preputial curtains. The clitoris is 9 by 4 mm, and very erectile, the hymen worn and gone, admitting one or two fingers.[132]

Frieda

She is a thorough feminist with intense sex bitterness. She will take nothing from any man. She will give herself to a man but only with feelings of contempt for him.[133]

Implicit within these early models of lesbianism was the notion that only aberrant, masculine women could be actively sexual. As sex was inconceivable without the presence of a man (or a penis), a lesbian must have a clitoris which is similar to a penis or, at the very least, take up the position of man. (Similar stereotyped beliefs are clearly still present today, with lesbian – and gay – couples being asked 'Which of you is the man?') At the beginning of the century many lesbians appear to have accepted the theories of the early sexologists with open arms, finding much that was positive in their new official identity and in the notion of being a congenital invert. This gave license to behave sexually in a way that was previously only acceptable for men. One lesbian, Frances Wilder, wrote in 1915 of her strong desire to caress and fondle other women, something she explained as being a result of her masculine mind. If she couldn't help herself, her sexuality could not be castigated – an early example of biological theories being used to support the interests of those otherwise condemned, which we see today in the support of gay men of the attempt to identify a gay gene.

Yet women who were sexual were not only assumed to be masculine, but also deemed sick; in the writings of any early sexual experts the categories of nymphomaniac, lesbian and prostitute were often seen as synonymous – all unnaturally sexual women lumped together in one disparaged diagnostic group. For example, the gynaecologist Carlton Frederick commented in 1907: 'All sorts of degenerative practices are followed by some [nymphomaniacs]. One of the most frequent is tribadism – the so called "Lesbian Love", which consists in various degenerative acts between two women in order to stimulate the sexual orgasm.'[134]

One of his colleagues, Bernard Talmey, commented in 1904, 'it is known that Lesbianism is very prevalent among the prostitutes of Paris.' And the British Psychiatrist Daniel Tuke warned that young girls should be protected against the knowledge of 'lesbic love' lest 'nymphomania itself' set in. At the same time, many physicians drew attention to the supposedly enlarged clitoris of the nymphomaniac and prostitute as well as the lesbian – the apparent sign of their underlying pathology and their possession of a penis-like organ.[135] So the ancient fears and fantasies associated with active female sexuality were now given legitimacy by being spoken through the mouths of venerated medical men.

The establishment of the term 'lesbian', or female invert, in late-nineteenth-century sexology undoubtedly had a dramatic effect on the lives of many women. Sex between women had never been condoned but, as we have seen, the law was reluctant to officially sanction such behaviour and so legal pronouncements on female homosexuality were few. The sexologists had no such scruples. Their writings on the horrors and dangers of lesbianism were widely disseminated in both medical and popular literature, casting suspicion on the motives and morality of thousands of women who had previously been able to engage openly in romantic friendships with other women. Prior to the discovery of lesbianism intimacy between women had generally not been construed as sexual and many women, particularly in the early North American women's colleges, engaged in passionate romantic relationships with each other, which were openly accepted, if not celebrated. This generation of North American women had been influenced by the gains of first-wave feminism and had attempted to achieve a life independent of men. Building a career, eschewing marriage and motherhood, many set up home with a like-minded woman, living together happily for years. But the sexologists caused a cloud of perversion to hang over these women.[136] Those who did not construe their relationships with women as sexual (and even contemporary records make it difficult to gauge whether they actually were) or feared being categorized as lesbians could no longer sustain what had undoubtedly been a positive, supportive life with another woman. It was an effective means of sending these women back to their 'appropriate' feminine position – heterosexual marriage to a man.

It is not a coincidence that the rise in feminism coincided with the publicizing (and castigation) of lesbianism. Both were publicly positioned as abnormalities; both were a threat to the authority of heterosexual man. To be feminist was almost synonymous with being lesbian – a situation which is not very different today (both labels still being used as terms of abuse). As one nineteenth-century expert, Dr James Wier, pronounced, 'every woman who has been at all prominent in advancing the cause of equal rights . . . [has] given evidence of masculo-femininity [viraginity], or has shown, conclusively, that she was the victim of psycho-sexual aberrancy [lesbianism].'[137] Women who argued for women's equal rights or formed strong bonds with other women were deemed abnormal or 'psychologically degenerate'. It is obvious whose interests this served, and whose fears were reflected. Take this comment in an early-twentieth-century medical text, which described the behaviour of girls who are thrown together:

> They kiss each other fondly on every occasion. They embrace each other with mutual satisfaction. It is most natural, in the interchange of visits, for them to sleep together. They learn the pleasures of direct contact, and in the course of their fondling they resort to cunni-linguistic practices . . . After this the *normal sex act* fails to satisfy [them] (my italics).[138]

The fear that normal sex (heterosexual penetration) will be passed over in preference for sex with other girls or women, which has been behind the law's silence on lesbianism for centuries, was clearly also pervasive in the sexology debates.

The Problem of Homosexuality: Researching Deviant Sex in the Twentieth Century

> Homosexuality is a symptom of neurosis and of a grieving personality disorder. It is an outgrowth of deeply rooted emotional deprivations and disturbances that had their origins in infancy. It is manifested, all too often, by compulsive and destructive behaviour that is the very antithesis of fulfilment and happiness. Buried under the 'gay' exterior of the homo-

> sexual is the hurt and rage that crippled his or her capacity for true
> maturation, for healthy growth and love.[139]

> It is not unrealistic to expect a gene or genes influencing sexual orientation
> to be identified within the next few years, since there are at least three
> laboratories in the United States alone that are working on the topic.[140]

In the late twentieth century sexology and scientific research on sex
still serves to position homosexuality as 'other' and thus to defuse
its potential threat to the hegemony of heterosexual man. Take the
comments above from two experts – the former a clinical psychologist,
the latter a biological scientist, both espousing views that have not
changed greatly since the time of their nineteenth-century forefathers
– homosexuality as pathology or as an inherited trait. However, the
majority of today's researchers and clinicians would want to cast themselves in a more liberal light than their predecessors. But what is implicit
in their comments and in those of the many legions of researchers who
proffer similar theories is that sexual behaviour that deviates from the
heterosexual norm is deemed in need of scientific explanation. The
distinction between homosexual and heterosexual states is thus reified;
the notion of the homosexual as an identifiable entity is unquestioningly
accepted and confirmed. And rather than taking this as a step forward
in understanding why some people are homosexual and others are
heterosexual (the bisexual person invariably being completely ignored
– Marjorie Garber's recent book *Vice Versa* being a notable exception),
it is only homosexuality that is opened up to scientific research.

For example, at one recent academic conference on the subject of
sex research,[141] there were at least nine papers presented on research
currently being carried out to investigate the underlying causes of
homosexuality. In contrast, there wasn't one paper attempting to determine the underlying cause of heterosexuality – it is presumed to be the
natural state. Equally, whilst psychoanalysis has for decades theorized
homosexuality, heterosexuality has been positioned as the assumed
norm.[142] This implies that it is the homosexual man or woman who is
somehow abnormal – why else investigate the roots of the 'problem'?
Homosexuality has not been an object of study for reasons of simple
curiosity; it has traditionally been studied in order to provide insights
for prevention or intervention. Until the lobbying of gay pressure-
groups and the impact of gay-pride movements in the seventies resulted

in the removal of homosexuality from the official annals of psychiatry, the attention of sex therapists and many researchers was focused predominantly on providing a cure (recovery being indicated by heterosexuality and 'normal' gender roles being embraced). Therapy ranged from the talking cure, to shock treatment, to threat of bodily injury and brain surgery.[143] Today, as we have seen, the official line is that homosexuality is not an illness – although many researchers and clinicians will privately put forward the view that it is undoubtedly a manifestation of some disorder and, whilst it does not state it explicitly as such, much of the sexological research impetus of today does reinforce reductionist notions of homosexuality as pathology or deviance.

There is a vast amount of funding being pumped into research attempting to isolate the biological causes of homosexuality.[144] Legions of twins and siblings have been studied to attempt to prove a genetic link. Early research carried out in the fifties reported a 100 per cent concordance rate between thirty-seven male monozygotic (identical) twins – if one was gay, so was the other. The rate was 15 per cent for dizygotic (non-identical) twins.[145] Compelling evidence for a genetic cause, or so one might think. More recent work carried out on twins and siblings in North American sex research by Richard Pillard, Michael Bailey and colleagues had reported heritability rates of 50 per cent for both male and female homosexuality. For example, one study of gay men found concordance rates of 52 per cent for monozygotic twins, 22 per cent for dizygotic twins.[146] In lesbians the concordance rate was 48 per cent for monozygotic twins and 16 per cent for dizygotic twins.[147] These findings and others like them have led researchers to suggest that biological factors may play a stronger role in male homosexuality than they do in female homosexuality. For example from a recent study of nearly 5,000 Australian twins, researchers concluded that hereditary factors were important for men whereas environmental influences were more important for women.[148] This raises the question of whether it is meaningful to talk about a 'homosexual' gene at all.

Is it legitimate to categorize together the experiences of lesbians and gay men? Are researchers not continuing the age-old practice of positioning the male as norm, focusing their research attention on male samples and then generalizing to women without examining the question of whether this is valid? The majority of sex researchers, unsurprisingly (they are mostly men), are not interested in lesbians at all. Very little of this biological research has been carried out with lesbians. So 'gay gene' research is really 'gay male gene' research.

One of the criticisms of brain-anatomy studies of homosexuality is that they are even more specific – in the main focusing on gay men who have died of AIDS complications. The widely cited research of Simon Le Vay, published in *Science*, which purported to show that the hypothalamus was smaller in gay men than in straight men, has also been criticized for being based on very small numbers of men and for the lack of incontrovertible evidence about the sexual orientation of those studied – (if sexual orientation is something that can ever be established or fixed)[149] – they were all dead, and therefore could not give any report. Yet in both the popular and academic press, the results are generalized to the whole homosexual population. For example, there have been three studies reporting differences between the brain structure of gay and heterosexual men, each focusing on a different part of the brain: the third interstitial cell of the anterior hypothalamus; the anterior commissure, a bundle of interconnecting fibres of the right and left hemispheres of the cerebral cortex; and the suprachiamatic nucleus region of the hypothalamus. This probably means very little unless one has a biological sciences degree. The important point is that one basic theory of brain difference cannot even be agreed upon amongst the experts. Other suggestions of a biological link have included the 'absence of linkage to micro satellite markers on the X chromosome';[150] actions of the hypothalamic-pituitary-gonadal axis;[151] and steroid 5-alpha-reductase deficiency.[152] Comparative animal research has been conducted, examining the role of steroid hormones in the sexual behaviour of a range of species – including rats, mice and fruitflies as well as reptiles and primates. It is argued that changing hormone levels at certain stages of development changes sexual behaviour. Whether this research can be generalized to human populations where sexual behaviour is not simply mediated by hormonal factors, and whether *behaviour* and sexual identity or orientation are one and the same thing is questionable. But perhaps the most important question is, Why are researchers so desperately searching for this elusive biological marker and what are the implications of their (as yet) fruitless search?

If we can find a simple biological 'cause' for 'homosexuality', so the argument goes, we will have to stop enacting discriminatory practices at a social and legal level. We will have to see homosexuality as 'natural'

– and we can't condemn someone for their inescapable biological make-up. As the *Wall Street Journal* declared in 1990: 'the discovery of definitive biological cause of homosexuality could go a long way toward advancing the gay-rights cause. If homosexuality were found to be an immutable trait, like skin color, then laws criminalizing homosexual sex might be overturned.'[153] It is a familiar argument – taken on in an emancipatory way by early-twentieth-century lesbians who celebrated the notion of congenital inversion, as we have already seen (p. 298). It gave licence to their desire for other women. The downside of this, in the era of DNA tests for genetic 'defects' in the womb, is that parents would have the ability to screen for a homosexual child and may then terminate the pregnancy – no need for anyone to suffer the agonies of a son or daughter 'coming out' and shocking the neighbours ever again.

Yet as with all research which advocates a simple biological cause of behaviour – such as that on mental illness, criminality or aggression – there is both naïvety and politics at play here. Fruitflies or rats may be primarily motivated by biological or evolutionary forces (although environmental factors are also influential there) but humans are far more complicated machines. Our behaviour – sexual as well as any other kind – results from a complex interaction of biological and social factors. Genes or hormones may be one part of the jigsaw but they are not the only one. To attest that a simple biological cause for any behaviour is proven is more a reflection of the ideological motives of the researcher than of the truth. To be fair, many of the scientific experts who work in this field assert that biology must be examined in its social context, stressing that genetic or hormonal factors may provide a potential or propensity for homosexuality. For example, whilst advocating the exploration of genetic factors, Pattatucci and Hamer[154] argue that in their view no single factor, be it genetic, physiological or environmental determines a given person's sexual orientation; rather, they believe that several factors may contribute to the development of an individual's sexual orientation.

Yet before we get too embroiled in this nature–nurture debate we should ask the question whether this argument about the true biological cause of sexual orientation is nothing but a red herring. For what it assumes is that there is this simple distinction between heterosexuality and homosexuality, that gay men or lesbians are a homogeneous group of people identifiably different from the heterosexual man or woman, that homosexuality is an absolute state, not expected to differ throughout life, that it is something we are born with – like red hair or blue eyes. Even a cursory examination of those who assume the category of gay or lesbian, as well as those who engage in same-sex sex, tells us that it is far more complicated than this.

There are very few people within the gay or lesbian continuum who have had a uniquely homosexual sexual life. The majority of people have sexual relationships or engage in sexual acts with people of the opposite sex at some time in their lives. This doesn't mean a great deal in a social milieu where heterosexuality is almost 'compulsory', as the American writer Adrienne Rich suggested in the early eighties. This behaviour could be explained away by peer pressure or attempts to assume a 'normal' sexual role. Many people have argued that their 'true' sexual identity is only realized later on in life when they 'come out' and take on a gay or lesbian identity. Their former heterosexuality is then rejected, as they adopt their natural role. As one lesbian I interviewed commented, 'I really found myself when I stopped having relationships with men, and became involved with another woman. I now think I just didn't realize that I was a lesbian when I was growing up.'

Yet as Marjorie Garber has argued, the notion of a true or real sexual identity or orientation is questionable. In talking of the shifting from male to female lovers and back again in the lives of the two women painters Frida Kahlo and Georgia O'Keefe, she comments that no one relationship, no one orientation, was for them the real one. What was real was what they were doing at the time.[155] She also quotes Jonathon Dollimore, the cultural theorist who co-founded the Sexual Dissidence course with Alan Sinfield at Sussex University, and who after many years of living with a male partner is now living with a woman, as saying:

> We don't want a new hierarchy . . . that claims . . . you are either one thing or the other . . . What I would not tolerate . . . is people who embrace that sort of thing in the exclusionary identity politics mode, saying 'I am now gay' as if their whole lives before that were a lie or don't count. I just don't think desire works like that.[156]

Equally, we could ask how we can 'truly' categorize the legions of women and men who have sex with people of the same sex but don't define themselves as gay or lesbian. One of the insights AIDS has brought into focus is the high percentage of 'heterosexual' married men who regularly engage in gay sex, but don't categorize themselves as 'gay'. What about the married 'heterosexual' women who have female lovers? Or the girls and boys for whom 'sexual exploration' between peers is a normal part of adolescent experience (English boarding schools being a notorious example)? What about the men in prison for whom sex with other men is a common part of prison life, yet who would never identify as 'homosexual', particularly if they take the active role in the sexual act? Or the men in traditional Mexican culture who are considered 'macho' if they engage in the active, insertive role in anal intercourse with other men, not 'homosexual', unlike those who engage in the 'passive' insertive role?[157] What about the 'political lesbians' of the seventies who rejected heterosexuality because of feminist principles, in many cases becoming intimately involved with women because of their rejection of men? What of those 'lesbians' within this group who have never had sex with a woman? Or those who are celibate yet would eschew any description of themselves as heterosexual? Or those who categorize themselves as 'gay' or 'lesbian' yet still sometimes engage in 'heterosexual' sex? What about the growing number of people who describe themselves as bisexual: some because they are actively engaged in relationships with women and men, some because they desire both women and men, and some because they have at some time in their lives had a relationship with both a woman and a man?[158] What about those who appear to *change* their sexual orientation halfway through life? And those who change back again? Where do they fit in?

I could go on. But the point has been made. Before we start to look for explanations of *why* homosexuality occurs we need to be clear about what this form of categorization means. It is not a simple issue. Making a primary distinction between heterosexual and homosexual identity or behaviour is a social decision, not a biological given. In many cultures both same- and opposite-sex love and sexual intimacy are accepted as a normal part of life. The men of Ancient Greece who engaged in sexual relationships with young boys, prostitutes and their wives are the most often quoted example. The young men of the Sambia, who are separated from women for many years and regularly ritually ingest the semen of older boys and men as part of their initiation into adulthood do not take up a 'homosexual' identity.[159] They may incorporate fantasies about fellatio into their sexual repertoire. But after the rite of passage to become a courageous warrior is complete they marry a woman, and the majority cease engagement in same-sex activity. In Sambian culture the notion of a homosexual *identity* is unknown.

This is not to say that 'homosexuality' does not exist; that there is no difference between the 'heterosexual', 'bisexual' or 'lesbian' identified woman, or between the 'gay' and 'heterosexual' identified man. It is to question these very simple distinctions and to draw attention to the fact that in many cultures this is not a line used to distinguish and divide people. It is the dominance of phallocentric heterosexual ideologies that dictates the narrow boundaries of sexual behaviour or desire for (and between) women and men which results in the obsession (and fear) of 'homosexuality' and 'homosexual sex'. As Garber has argued, the public adoption of one sexual label or another is not 'a *description* of a sex life, but an *event* within it . . . to narrate a sex life is itself a sexual performance.'[160] It is the social context which gives this 'performance' meaning, which makes the description of oneself as gay or lesbian (and to a lesser extent, bisexual), a transgressive, risky act.

So is it not more important and interesting to ask why the hetero-sexual/homosexual distinction has become so important and to examine its impact on the lives of individual women and men than to root around looking for a faulty gene? It is ironic that it has often been the gay community that has most vociferously defended the biological research and most strongly asserts the notion of difference between heterosexuals and homosexuals. In a world where being gay or lesbian means being an outsider, it is not surprising that gay communities are fiercely protective of their boundaries; that gay identity is celebrated and often very visibly defined. But this must be seen in the context of the dominant heterosexual culture, which ascribes minority-group status on those who deviate from its norms. If the majority of the population were gay and heterosexuals were the minority 'out' group, being 'heterosexual' would probably no longer be a state assumed to be natural and women and men would want to signify their heterosexual status to like-minded others the same way that gay men and lesbians do today. There would be 'straight' bars and clubs, people would march for 'straight rights' and discuss the merits or otherwise of 'coming out' to your gay or lesbian boss as straight: 'Should one pretend to be gay in order to get on? What does this mean in terms of compromise and liberty; in terms of the fear of being found out?'

A silly fantasy, you might say. In fact, the world is filled with straight bars and clubs, 'straight' fashions, and solidarity between those in the heterosexual majority. It is just that 'straight' clubs and bars are not advertised as such – it's the default option. Equally, it is such an accepted part of our social world that few heterosexuals recognize or actively identify their shared heterosexual status; like being white in North America or Europe, the dominant group never examines its status. Ask a heterosexual woman or man what the most important aspects of their identity are and very few will mention their sexual orientation. Ask a self-identified gay man or lesbian and few will miss it out. Those who are in a same-sex relationship, yet refuse to categorize themselves as gay or lesbian protesting that they 'just happen to have fallen in love' (or lust) with someone of the same sex, are not taking for granted their sexual orientation, they are actively *rejecting* a homosexual identity (even whilst they embrace homosexual sex). There isn't some biological predisposition which causes those who engage in same-sex relationships to identify more strongly with their sexual orientation than those who engage in opposite-sex relationships – either embracing or rejecting 'homosexuality' as an identity, but rarely ignoring it. It is social factors that make it so.

Researchers and clinicians who ignore these social pressures and the social construction of sexual identity may position themselves as 'rational scientists', but in one sense they are merely supporters of phallocentric heterosexual hegemony. By neglecting analysis of heterosexuality and putting only homosexuality under the microscope, they reinforce notions of pathology; of the dysfunctional gene to be discovered; or the deviance to be explained. They implicitly reinforce the hegemony of the script of heterosexuality, which provides the boundaries of masculinity and femininity, and therefore defines our experience of what it is to do 'woman' or 'man'. They police both behaviour and desire.

Science Defines 'Normal' Sex

Normal Sex: A Heterosexual Intercourse

If homosexuality is positioned as the epitome of deviant or perverse sex, its antithesis is heterosexuality. Heterosexual intercourse within marriage is the only sexual act to be universally legal (and universally recognized as 'sex'), and the legally (and religiously) sanctioned relationship of 'marriage', seen to provide the bedrock of social order, is a relationship that can take place only between a man and a woman.[161]

The law frames heterosexual intercourse as normal and legal; science positions it as 'natural'. In common with their theological forebears, the early sexologists positioned sex primarily as an instinct for reproduction, with heterosexual intercourse, the man in control, and the woman acquiescent, being seen as a biologically driven act. For example, take the comments of Havelock Ellis – who was widely acknowledged to be one of the more liberal and reforming sex researchers,[162] on the subject of courtship.

A Biological Phenomenon

Courtship, properly understood, is a biological process which can be found throughout the bisexual animal world. It represents the psychic aspect of the slow attainment of tumescence, the method of securing contrectation.[163]

On the Modesty of Woman

The modesty of women, which, in its most primitive form amongst animals, is based on sexual periodicity, is, with that periodicity, an essential condition of courtship . . . modesty may be said to be the gesture of sexual refusal by the female animal who is not yet at the period of *estrus*.[164]

On the Sexual Priming of Man

Without the reticence and delays of modesty, tumescence could not be adequately aroused in either sex, nor would the female have time and opportunity to test the qualities of the candidates for her favours, and to select the fittest male.[165]

Here we have the masquerade of femininity – woman's charade of feigned resistance to the sexual attentions of man – elevated to a biologically *necessary* process which acts to further the reproductive potential of the species. The script of courtship laid out in romantic fiction and teenage magazines is reified as a 'natural' biological process. Phallocentrism was also dominant in the early theories, the penis being seen as the most important component of sex. As Ellis argued: 'tumescence and detumescence are alike fundamental, primitive and essential; in resting the sexual impulse on these necessarily connected processes we are basing ourselves on the solid bedrock of nature.'[166] Evolutionary development was believed to have led to the gender roles men and women occupied; as Ellis concludes, 'Woman breeds and tends; man provides; it remains so even when the spheres tend to overlap.'[167] So 'woman' was conceived of as a modest, reticent creature, whose role was reproduction and the resistance of the male sex.

Prior to the nineteenth century female sexuality had not been so clearly distinguished from men's – well into the late eighteenth century both sexes had been seen as potentially passionate, lewd and lascivious[168] – but the Victorian sexologists elevated the myth of 'woman' as Madonna or whore into scientific dogma. Working-class women, prostitutes or women from 'immigrant' populations (especially African-American women) were positioned as 'naturally' promiscuous and sexually unrestrained because of their lower position on the evolutionary ladder, whilst that archetype of femininity, the middle-class Victorian maiden, was assumed to be less sexual than man. As William Acton declared in 1870:

> Many of the best mothers, wives and managers of households know little of or are careless about sexual indulgences . . . a modest woman seldom desires any sexual gratification for herself. She submits to her husband's embraces but principally to gratify him; and were it not for the desire of maternity, would far rather be relieved from his attentions.
>
> There can be no doubt that sexual feeling in the female is in the majority of cases in abeyance, and that it requires positive and considerable excitement to be roused at all; and even if roused (which in many cases it never can be) it is moderate compared with that of the male.[169]

In respectable society, the phallocentric view positioned man as actively sexual and woman as sexually responsive to man. Ironically, this laid the blame for women's sexual *unresponsiveness* at the feet (or hands . . .) of men, giving us a foretaste of the pressure to perform many men feel today. As Havelock Ellis commented:

> The chief reason why women are considered 'frigid' lies less in themselves than in men. It is evident throughout that while in men the sexual impulse tends to develop spontaneously and actively, in women, however powerful it may be latently and more or less subconsciously, its active manifestations need in the first place to be called out. That, in our society, is normally the husband's function.[170]

At the same time man was warned of the risk of the woman who was *too* sexual. For as Krafft-Ebbing cautioned in 1886, 'woe unto the man who falls into the meshes of such an insatiable Messalina, whose sexual appetite is never appeased.'[171] The powerful sexuality of the 'nymphomaniac' was seen to pose a danger to the whole of civilization and, as a consequence, extreme 'treatments' were prescribed – clitoridectomy, ovariectomy, blood-letting, cold baths and enforced bedrest all being used as 'cures'. The 'symptoms' that precipitated such extreme forms of intervention included masturbation, excessive desire for marital sex, lesbianism and uncontrolled sexual feelings towards strange men. Carol Groneman has described one case, of 'Mrs B', who referred herself to the American gynaecologist Dr Horatio Storer in 1856 because of 'lascivious dreams'. 'Mrs B' was reported to have sexual thoughts whenever she met any man, although she insisted she would not respond to any 'improper advance'. She enjoyed intercourse with her husband 'greatly' and had sex nightly for the seven years of their marriage. Storer's recommendation in this 'Case of Nymphomania' was that the afflicted woman restrict her intake of meat and brandy, take cold baths and regular enemas, swab her vagina with borax and replace her feather pillows with those of hair to reduce her sexual drive and cool her passions. He warned that if she could not curb her desires 'it would probably become necessary to send her to an asylum.'[172] If a man had been showing such 'symptoms' he would not have been deemed in need of psychiatric or medical help; he would merely have been demonstrating 'normal' masculine drives. Conversely, a woman showing *any* desires for another woman could be categorized as a sick nymphomaniac and subjected to these myriad 'cures'.

'Sex' as Biological Response

This view of sex as a biologically based 'impulse' different for women and men is not a historical anachronism. Following in the path of these early sex researchers many psychiatric and medical texts dealing with sexuality in the late twentieth century still work on the assumption that both 'normal' and 'abnormal' sexuality are primarily instinctual or hormonal phenomena:

> Our sexual behaviour is controlled by phytogenetically ancient parts of our brain and therefore is best understood at the level of instinct, within the concepts of ethology and sociobiology. In fact, the 'reproductive imperative' is the ultimate principle underlying all human behaviour, since animals survive in proportion to their breeding success.
>
> WILSON, 1988[173]

> The cycle of sexual response, with orgasm as the ultimate point in progression, generally is believed to develop from a drive of biologic-behavioural origin deeply integrated into the condition of human existence.
>
> MASTERS & JOHNSON, 1966[174]

> Given the explosive rate at which the fields of molecular genetics and neurobiology are expanding, it is inevitable that the perception of our own nature, in the field of sex as in all attributes of our physical and mental lives, will increasingly be dominated by concepts derived from the biological sciences.
>
> LE VAY, 1993[175]

> The exact role of female sexual motivation in modulating female sexual behaviour is unclear. The resolution lies in understanding the role gonadal hormones play in regulating the female's ability to mate and her interest in mating.
>
> WALLEN, 1995[176]

These biological theories fall into three major camps: evolution-based theorists, who focus on the 'selfish gene' and the instinct to reproduce; endocrinologists, who measure 'sex hormones'; and clinically orientated researchers, such as Masters and Johnson, who focus on the actual workings of the physical body – on the mechanics of sexual response. And whilst many scientists who advocate biological theories of sexual behaviour *do* present us with a sophisticated analysis which acknowledges the importance of social or cultural factors (even if these are often seen as secondary influences),[177] in many instances these are narrow biological theories which implicitly position the script of phallocentric heterosexuality as 'natural' because it is biologically driven and see 'sex' as simply a physiological response.

Take, for example, the comments of the psychologist Glenn Wilson, who has justified male promiscuity and men's attraction to large-breasted, small-waisted women on the basis of 'parental investment theory', which means that the goal of the male is 'to impregnate many females simultaneously, hence his interest in multiple mates of breeding age.'[178] We are informed that men are programmed to seek 'physically attractive women', those with 'proportionately large breasts and hips . . . and [a] narrow waist', which gives a clear indication to man that the woman is 'fertile ground in which to plant their seed'.[179]

On the same lines, we are told by the anthropologist Donald Symons that 'nubility cues' are what are attractive to men: youth, light skin colour and high 'waist to hip ratio' (the hourglass figure – Marilyn Munroe would be the ideal). He argues that evolutionary theory provides the most plausible explanation for the type of woman represented in pornography – young, with large breasts and bright eyes – as men are biologically programmed to find this image erotic. When women wear cosmetics, fashionable clothing or engage in diets, exercise or cosmetic surgery, they are actually attempting to 'manipulate age and parity cues in order to enhance their sexual attractiveness'.[180] This argument may be used to justify as 'instinctual' the constraining rituals of the feminine masquerade, the 'beauty' rituals women's magazines sell as 'pleasure'. Yet how evolutionary theory explains the changing fashions in what is deemed sexually attractive, or differences across cultures, is not clear. The flappers of the twenties, the skinny models of the sixties and many of the 'supermodels' of the nineties, had *no* waist to hip ratio. Are these icons of female beauty not attractive to men? And why are distended ear lobes, facial scarring, elongated necks or distorted lotus feet attractive in other cultural contexts? Would evolutionary theorists suggest that African or Chinese populations have evolved differently? Surely the reproductive imperative is the same everywhere?

Women, on the other hand, are primarily interested in protecting their offspring, 'and hence the coyness of the female and their need to build relationships'[181] – or so we are told. Women are primarily 'seeking evidence that a man is superior breeding material which means physical strength and skills relevant to defence and provision and willingness to share the burden of child-rearing'.[182] Given the evidence that women still take on the burden of child-rearing even in 'egalitarian' couples,[183] they are obviously going wrong somewhere. Ironically, it is those men who are *least* like the stereotypical caveman painted in the sociobiologists' theories who are most likely to take an equal role in the home – the almost mythical new man, whose main goal in life is not muscle growth and macho power.

Traditionally, evolutionary theory positioned women as being relatively passive in this process, their primary function being to attract men and to 'accommodate male sexual initiation'. In recent years, it has been widely acknowledged that 'females' do actively initiate sexual activity, leading one proponent of evolutionary theories of sex, Kim Wallen, to comment, 'the notion of the sexually passive female is, one hopes, dead, as convincing evidence of female sexual initiation has now been reported in a range of mammalian species.'[184] Indeed, as it has been suggested that females are *more* active that males in 'mate choice', feminist evolutionary theorists, such as Dorothy Einon, have claimed that this is a model of sexuality which can be seen to be empowering for women.[185] Yet if we look at how these theories have passed into lay discourse, we find that it is the very traditional (and phallocentric) view that is dominant.

Biological theories of sexuality have, undoubtedly, had a striking influence on lay beliefs about what it is to be 'woman' and 'man'. They certainly formed the dominant views of male–female sexuality entertained by many of the men I interviewed. The belief that men are biologically driven to have sex (whereas women are not) was seen as 'true', as one man commented:

> 'I think men have a great sex drive . . . this is probably going to sound awful, but I don't think women actually need sex as much as men do. Because obviously men have got that biological thing, a greater sex drive . . . you can see it in the animal kingdom . . . I don't think women need to feel that satisfied or they don't have that kind of tension, perhaps.'

A corollary to this view is that whilst women might enjoy sex and that women and men both have a right to express sexuality, their drive can never match that of men:

'I don't think it's wrong for a woman to be sexually active or take a dominant position when making love or whatever. But I don't think the need is as great. Women can enjoy sex, and when they enjoy it it's beautiful. They need to do it, but it's not as great as men's kind of anxiety.'

Others had long believed that women had *no* sexual desire:

'One of the things I grew up with was finding it hard to believe that a woman in any circumstances could have any sexual desire, that was possibly the way my circle of friends worked, it was the men, the boys, constantly doing the playing, the sexual role, whereas the girls were the ones who played the role of the object of their desire.'

Men also argued that women were more selective than men, a fact related both to their passivity in sex and to their greater 'emotional needs':

'Women are a bit more selective . . . there is an emotional need for women to become emotionally attached to somebody before they have sex . . . but it's not totally necessary for men.'

'Men tend to be more overt in physical things – men are probably thinking of sex more than women . . . whereas women are in the receiving position and they tend to be a bit more removed and be a bit more considered and tend to assess the personality of the person.'

Whilst many of the men I interviewed did acknowledge women's desire and arousal, echoing Ellis and Acton, it was always assumed to be less than men's. If a woman's desire was greater than theirs, she was often positioned as having a problem:

'My long-term girlfriend wanted sex more than me. She needed sex, to fill some need in her. I'd put it down to insecurity. It may very well not be. Anyway, very often it became a confrontational area. So I'd have sex whenever just for an easy life.'

These men positioned the differences they perceived in male–female sexual behaviour as simply a biological issue; these were all 'natural' differences that we couldn't do anything about. This sociobiological view may give pseudo-scientific credence to man taking a controlling role in sex, and, at the same time, it reifies the beauty myth and positions male promiscuity as 'natural'. So Glen Wilson, again, waxes lyrical on the biological basis for 'the tendency for males to be sexually recharged by novel females',[186] which he tells us has been observed in most mammals:

> [This] is another manifestation of their reproductively optimal 'promiscuity strategy'. This presents a problem, for men especially, over the course of a long marriage and is responsible for a great deal of adultery. Progressive 'contempt due to familiarity' (at least as regards sexual excitement) is an almost inevitable outcome of sexually exclusive marriage. It is not unusual for sex therapists to see men who are unable to achieve erection with their wives but perfectly capable of stud-like prowess with their new secretary. Once again, what is observed is not a *disease* but a *normal biological phenomenon*, and realistic solutions must be sought [my italics].[187]

This distinction between 'disease' and 'normal biological phenomenon' is interesting, given the tendency of many sex researchers to position sexual dysfunction and 'disease' as biological. Wilson is presumably referring to the statistical frequency of such behaviour, suggesting that men would all like to have sex with their secretaries, given half a chance, and therefore that it is a 'normal biological phenomenon'. The advice that 'realistic solutions must be sought' for man's inability to maintain an erect penis in the presence of his wife, yet to be able to do it every time with his 'new secretary' is tantalizing. Should secretaries have this written into their job descriptions – resuscitation of the flagging apparatus of the boss?

Those who examine the mechanics of sex itself frequently advocate similarly reductionist views. For example, Simon Le Vay has described sexual intercourse as such a simple behaviour that 'one hardly needs a brain to do it.'[188] His description of the 'basic components' of 'coitus', as he coyly calls it, say it all. It could be a recipe book for sex as conceived by the (phallocentric) scientist. Here it is, step by step:

> (1) erection of the penis; (2) engorgement of the walls of the vagina and the labia majora, lubrication of the vagina by glandular secretions and transudation, and erection of the clitoris; (3) insertion of the penis into the vagina; (4) pelvic thrusting by one or both partners; (5) elevation of the uterus, with a consequent forward and upward rotation of the mouth of the cervix; (6) ejaculation of semen into the vagina; and (7) orgasm,

the intensely pleasurable sense of climax and release, often accompanied by increases in heart rate, flushing of the skin, muscle spasms, and involuntary vocalizations.[189]

A typical heterosexual encounter? How easy it sounds (or how boring, depending on one's own sexual proclivities). Le Vay *may* be seen to be egalitarian – at least he *recognizes* female response. But within this definition he reinforces the notion of 'coitus' as penis-focused, with erection of the penis always coming first; as well as implicitly negating any other form of sexual stimulation, or desire, which may be a necessary component of 'sex' (ironic, given that he is gay himself – yet as we have already seen, he advocates a biological root to homosexuality as well).

Desire *is* acknowledged in one of the formative scientific models of sex: Masters and Johnsons' Human Sex Response Cycle Model. It has been highly influential in shaping our understanding of both 'normal' sexuality and sexual problems and forms the basis for the categorization of 'sexual disorders' in the *DSM*. The four stages of the cycle are described within the psychiatric manual as (1) appetitive (fantasies about sexual activities and a desire for sex); (2) excitement (a subjective sense of sexual pleasure accompanied by physical changes); (3) orgasm (peaking of pleasure with a release of tension); (4) resolution (general relaxation, well-being). Seeing sex as a closed energy system, a series of 'physiologic reactions', a cycle that repeats itself, again and again, Masters and Johnson provided a model of 'normal sex' by which generations of couples would come to judge themselves (through the 'sex guides' and sex manuals influenced by Masters and Johnson's approach):[190] Given the appropriate stimulation, the body was expected to respond, the man with erection and ejaculation, the woman with vaginal engorgement and orgasm. We might see this as an advance on the theories of many of their predecessors' positioning of 'woman' as inevitably sexually passive. We may even go so far as to claim it is emancipatory for women, according their sexuality the same status as that of men. But this would be premature.

Masters and Johnson reached the majority of these conclusions about female sexuality from controlled experimentation that took place in a laboratory. Due to the difficulties in persuading women to take part in sex research in the fifties, Masters and Johnson used female prostitutes in many of their pioneering studies.[191] The techniques learned from these women were central components of their 'clinical research programs' carried out on 'normal' couples. In order to test their hypotheses about the 'human sexual response cycle', 'vaginal pulse amplitude', women's orgasmic responses and the female arousal cycle were observed in a neutral, detached manner in the laboratory. This is a model of research which continues to 'dominate in sexology to this day.'[192] Take these recent experimental studies on female sexuality: in one, the response of women reading neutral or sexually arousing passages whilst wearing masks impregnated with androstenol or a placebo were measured;[193] in another, the responses of pre- and postmenopausal women viewing a neutral or erotic film whilst sexual arousal and vaginal pulse amplitude and lubrication were being recorded were examined, with oestradiol, testosterone and luteinizing hormone also being collected. In others, vaginal photoplethysmography in response to sexually arousing or anxiety-provoking narratives was collected;[194] and vaginal erotic sensitivity was measured in 'coitally experienced' women, by means of systematic digital stimulation of both vaginal walls.[195]

In these experiments female sexuality is reduced to the status of abstract experimental variable – the woman herself invisible behind the attention given to carefully selected aspects of her body, which are dissected and discussed. The vibration of her vaginal walls is of interest; her subjective experience of being 'woman' or the social construction of sexuality is ignored. Whether these intrusive experiments are meaningful or justifiable may be questionable, but the fact that this genre of research forms the bulk of scientific research on female sexuality is evidence of the denial of subjectivity at the expense of exact experimentation in mainstream sexology. Take this introductory paragraph in an academic paper on female sexual response, entitled 'Infrared Vaginal Photoplethysmography: Construction, Calibration, and Sources of Artifact':

> During the past five years, several basic and clinical researchers have conducted physiological assessments of female sexual arousal using novel instrumentation approaches (reviewed by Hoon, 1979). One of the most promising approaches is based on the principle of reflected light from the vaginal capillaries . . . Several studies have shown vaginal photoplethysmography measures to be sensitive and valid analogues of sexual arousal

> . . . However, there is still controversy concerning sensitivity of the AC
> versus DC coupled signal . . . and it is still not yet known precisely which
> vaginal haemodynamic processes are represented by these signals.[196]

That these researchers are interested in the sexuality of *women* is
impossible to gauge from this text. Indeed, it is the vagina that they are
interested in, or 'sexual arousal', rather than the woman herself.

To understand why this is not an unusual depiction of the sexuality
of 'woman', we have to look to sex research as a discipline. Sex
researchers are preoccupied with the legitimacy of their field – preoccupied with notions of second-class citizenship and with the stigma of
working in a 'kinky' research area. One prominent sex researcher has
commented that 'sexological research is stigmatized as slightly unsavoury
and verging on pornographic.'[197] Another has claimed that the risks
include 'rejection by peers . . . vilification . . . threats . . . and FBI
listings'.[198] As feminist sex researcher Leonore Tiefer has commented,
it's not surprising that sexologists have doggedly stuck to the most
traditional 'hard' methodologies of positivistic science, whilst rejecting
all that is political or ideological for fear that it add even more of a taint
to their serious endeavours. So serious sex researchers attempt to achieve
legitimacy through adopting the methods of 'rigour' and 'objectivity'
and focusing on what can be observed – the physical body. They
distinguish themselves from what have been described as 'sexophosists',
those who are 'not impartial but value-laden, ideological and judgemental', those interested merely in the 'philosophy of sex'.[199] So sex-
research conferences are invariably closed affairs, which only 'legitimate
scientists' or those specially invited can attend.[200] There are, however,
the signs of the beginning of change. Subjective experiences of sexuality,
and the views of individual women and men are becoming more
legitimate topics for sex research. Yet the legacy of the very reductionist
viewpoint lives on, with the focus of sex therapy being primarily on
bodily response.

Female Sexuality: A Problem of Response

Whilst the nineteenth-century sex researchers confirmed the prejudices
of their theological predecessors in conceiving of female sexuality as
passive or inactive, reinforcing archetypal myths about 'woman', sex

researchers in the latter half of this century have taken a slightly different view. For whilst the pioneering sex researchers of the fifties, such as Masters and Johnson, or Kinsey, concentrated on physical response, they did at least acknowledge that the sexuality of women was as important as that of men. Echoing liberal feminist theories of sexuality, Masters and Johnson claimed that, 'In a comparison of male and female sexual function, it should be emphasized that in sexual response it is the similarities of, not differences between, the sexes that therapists find remarkable.'[201]

Hailed by some as the instigators of the sexual revolution, Masters and Johnson were seen as emancipatory because of their recognition of the importance of clitoral stimulation and the existence of the clitoral orgasm (prior to this it was only the vaginal orgasm that was acknowledged as 'normal'). Yet they still considered female sexuality within the confines of heterosexual marriage, where the woman was expected to experience sexual pleasure and orgasm during heterosexual intercourse and to be aroused by the man (or by anticipation of penetration of penis).

> In essence, the vaginal barrel responds to effective stimulation by involuntary preparation for penile penetration. Just as penile erection is a direct physiologic expression of a psychologic demand to mount, so expansion and lubrication of the vaginal barrel provides direct physiologic indication of the obvious psychologic mounting invitation.
>
> MASTERS & JOHNSON, 1966[202]

Female sexuality was positioned as vaginal *response*, in contrast to male sexuality, which was framed in terms of performance. Sexual 'problems' were thus manifested differently in women and men – a legacy which continues to this day.

The *DSM* categorizations of female sexual dysfunction illustrate this most clearly. The two most common disorders are anorgasmia and disorders of arousal – both positioned as disorders of heterosexual response. The estimates of prevalence of anorgasmia in the general population range from 29 per cent[203] to 4 per cent[204]; as most women don't report such problems (or even categorize them as such) it is impossible to know the exact numbers. The way in which these disorders are classified by the *DSM*[205] is outlined below:

Diagnostic Criteria 302.72: Female Sexual Arousal Disorder

A. Either (1) or (2)

   (1) persistent or recurrent partial or complete failure to maintain the lubrication-swelling response of sexual excitement until completion of sexual activity

   (2) persistent or recurrent lack of a subjective sense of sexual excitement and pleasure in a female during sexual activity

B. Occurrence not exclusively during the course of another Axis 1 disorder (other than a Sexual Dysfunction), such as Major Depression.

Diagnostic Criteria 302.73: Inhibited Female Orgasm

Persistent or recurrent delay in, or absence of, orgasm in a female following a normal sexual excitement phase during the sexual activity that the clinician judges to be adequate in focus, intensity and duration. Some females are able to experience orgasm during non-coital clitoral stimulation, but are unable to experience it during coitus in the absence of manual clitoral stimulation. In most of these females this represents a normal variation of the female sexual response and does not justify the diagnosis of Inhibited Female Orgasm. However, in some of these females, this does represent a psychological inhibition that justifies the diagnosis. This difficult judgement is assisted by a thorough sexual evaluation, which may even require a trial of treatment.

So whilst the nineteenth-century woman who showed too much sexual drive was at risk of being defined as deviant or dysfunctional (as a 'nymphomaniac'), in the late twentieth century it is women who are *unable* to experience desire or orgasm who are at risk of being categorized as 'ill'. But today this categorization is as dubious as the view that the nineteenth-century woman was 'naturally' asexual. Both are value-laden judgements, reflecting our changing social definitions of what 'normal sex' is (and normal sexual roles for 'woman' and 'man').

Take the case of inhibited female orgasm, diagnosed if a woman cannot achieve orgasm through intercourse, but not if she cannot achieve orgasm through masturbation. This clearly defines orgasm during vaginal penetration as the normal experience for women. A woman's ability (or willingness) to give herself autonomous pleasure is not deemed an issue for clinicians, unless she is being taught to masturbate as part of a programme of therapy. If the clinician judges the sexual activity to be 'adequate in focus, intensity and duration', then the woman should reach orgasm – although how the clinician will glean this information without observing the sexual act is not obvious. If the sexual activity is 'adequate', and the woman doesn't reach orgasm we are ominously informed that she will be subjected to 'a thorough sexual evaluation, which may even require a trial of treatment'. This implies that her body will be examined – not her feelings about sex, about men, or about the pressure to respond to vaginal penetration. Perhaps it is the fear of being classified as sexually dysfunctional which results in the high numbers of women who report faking orgasm during heterosexual intercourse (as well as their desire to protect the egos of men).

The *DSM* recognition that many women cannot experience orgasm during intercourse 'without clitoral stimulation' is interesting. A number of surveys have reported that a high percentage of women rarely or never achieve 'unassisted' orgasm during intercourse – up to 80 per cent in one study.[206] It is a relief to know that the *DSM* doesn't deem this deviant or pathological but merely part of the 'normal variation of the female sexual response'. And if the findings of the earliest sexual surveyor, Alfred Kinsey, are in any way correct, women's need for extra stimulation isn't surprising: he reported that 75 per cent of men ejaculate (and therefore terminate intercourse) after only two minutes of penetration. Most women require more than two minutes of vaginal penetration to achieve a vaginal orgasm (if penetration is the only form of stimulation they are getting). Yet two minutes are seen to be enough to please by many experts. The sex researcher, Martin Cole, comments:

> *Naturally*, more responsibility falls upon the male than upon the female in relationship formation . . . moreover, to add to his problems, the male needs to get an erection at least a minute or two before ejaculation in order to, as he sees it, 'have sex' and 'please his partner', [my italics].[207]

This shouldn't surprise us. Within the phallocentric view of sex perpetuated by sexologists it is *naturally* man's climax, his arousal and orgasm which act as punctuating marks of the sexual encounter. The woman merely follows him (by necessity very quickly). This is why man's inability to control his response is a problem; it doesn't allow woman to be pleasured sufficiently. As Kaplan has written:

> A man's ability to control his ejaculation is crucial for proficiency in
> lovemaking . . . The effective lover must be able to engage in sex play
> whilst he is in a highly aroused state in order to bring the woman, who
> is usually slower to respond, especially when she is young, to a high
> plateau of excitement and orgasm.[208]

In an era when women are expected to enjoy sex and to be 'pleasured'
by men the biological difference in men and women's sexual responses
is inherently problematic. It can result in frustration and sexual dissatisfaction for both parties if the man cannot control his ejaculation (particularly if 'foreplay' is not brought into the sexual repertoire). Even if a
man *can* control his own sexual responses, this is invariably at the cost
of splitting off his own pleasure and desire for the sexual act he is
engaging in. According to Anthony Crabbe:

> A man learns, or is taught, that, in order to avoid being a selfish
> lover, he must often distance himself from the sex act. His biological
> capacity to be satisfied more quickly is a liability for which he must
> compensate by concentrating on his performance. Sex manuals make
> this clear.[209]

One man I interviewed said, 'I try to think about football, or about
inane things like cabbages when I'm having sex. It makes me last longer.'
As we have already seen, men often split sex from love as a result of
fears of dependency and vulnerability; yet, arguably, the pressures to
perform sexually and to 'fight' bodily responses reinforce this more
deeply rooted psychological splitting. It also reinforces the notion of
male and female sexuality being different. As Crabbe writes, '[Men]
know that they do not express their sexual pleasure as demonstratively
or for as long as women can.'[210] In a world where it is *men* who are
supposed to be sexual, the realization that women's sexual pleasure is
potentially greater (or at least longer lasting) than men's – that women
can enjoy 'sex' without having to distract themselves with thoughts of
football or cabbages – can clearly bolster feelings of envy or resentment
towards women on the part of men.

The *DSM* categorization of female sexual arousal disorder is also
interesting. It focuses attention primarily on the physical mechanics of
sexual response, yet also acknowledges the woman's feelings and the
importance of the absence of subjective excitement. Well and good,

we might say. At last, the psychological level is being acknowledged. But the woman is implicitly pathologized – technically, she is suffering from an illness because she doesn't respond to a man. Being willing to perform certain sexual acts has also been pathologized. For example, we are told in a recent textbook on sex therapy that an aversion to fellatio is the most common 'sexual phobia' in women. This is described as 'an aversion in women to semen and of course oral sex, when the woman takes the penis into her mouth.'[211] Is semen *really* that erotic? Should a mouth full of semen be woman's greatest erotic desire? The experts seem to think so. Like many other things in life it's a matter of personal preference. Women shouldn't be seen as phobic for declining to fellate. Given that a recent survey suggested that the majority of men are not overly concerned with genital hygiene (only one in four change their underwear every day; one in ten change it once a week), is it surprising that many women prefer not to get too close? Yet as fellatio is generally acknowledged to be one of the sexual activities on the top of the list of sexual preferences of many men (it certainly is in pornography), it is clearly very convenient to position as 'ill' the woman who won't play this particular game.

A similar argument could be made about 'inhibited sexual desire', a disorder which can be experienced by men, but is much more commonly reported in women.[212] It is manifested by 'persistently or recurrently deficient or absent sexual fantasies and desire for sexual functioning'. This could imply that a woman who does not desire her partner (or any man) is somehow ill (a critique which would equally apply to men who don't desire women). This unambiguously refers to a pathology within the woman rather than looking to her partner or the relationship for reasons for her disinterest, or looking more critically at this narrow definition of 'sex', which many women find limiting, boring and inappropriate for their own sexual needs. As these women I interviewed told me:

> 'I'm certainly not interested in an overabundance of pumping penetration, you know it just seems to me that it is possibly one of the ways in which the whole world has been pumped off its axis, if you know what I mean. It's just not necessary at all, this, like, emphasis on performance, it's just such a waste of time.'

*

'Men who are skilled lovers can have any women they want because they're so rare. The thing that depresses me about sex is how grateful we are as women for such minimal pleasure and excitement. If a man's half decent in bed we think he's great.'

As 'sex' is synonymous with heterosexual intercourse, it is perhaps not surprising that those disorders which impede this activity – vaginismus and dyspareunia – have received the greatest amount of attention from researchers and clinicians. Vaginismus is the term used to describe 'recurrent or persistent involuntary spasm of the musculature of the outer third of the vagina that interferes with coitus'. This prevents 'sex' (defined as intercourse) from happening or, if the man perseveres, can result in extreme pain for the woman. Dyspareunia is the diagnosis given to pain experienced by the woman (or man) during intercourse, and may include vaginal pain or more general symptoms such as nausea. Whilst positioned as physical problems, both have a clear psychological component and have often been described as a 'sexual phobia'.[213] The symptoms include anxiety, profuse sweating, nausea, vomiting, diarrhoea or palpitations, often precipitated by an act such as a hug or a kiss, which suggests a progression to sex. Certainly an extreme reaction, by anybody's standards.

Vaginismus is a rare disorder – reported to affect 1–4 per cent of women.[214] One obvious reason for the attention given over to it by researchers and clinicians is that it provides a more amenable and obvious focus for research and intervention than other aspects of female sexuality, as it is more easily identified and measured. This is what the 'real' scientist is interested in – something which can be easily observed. Changes in arousal or absence of orgasm are not so easily measured (at least outside the experimental laboratory where there are a gamut of machines to measure female sexual response in tow). Vaginismus may also be deemed more problematic within a phallocentric frame, as it interferes very directly with a man's ability to penetrate the woman, whereas absence of desire or anorgasmia does not. It is also something that men will very obviously notice – thus precipitating treatment – whereas absence of arousal or orgasm can be ignored (or its presence pretended).

Yet the fact that some men will ignore this 'problem' and endeavour to 'have sex' anyway is illustrated by this recent description of dyspareunia and vaginismus in a text on sex therapy:

Dyspareunia in the female (pain in the vagina during intercourse) and vaginismus can be viewed as similar problems with varying degrees of intensity. They range from a dyspareunia of mild discomfort, through serious and perhaps intolerable pain, to vaginismus, where the reflex contracture of the peri-vaginal muscles effectively prevents penetration by the penis. In more serious cases, any attempt to touch or approach the vagina leads to powerful reflex adduction of the thighs, thus precluding even the possibility of attempted penetration.[215]

That penetration *could* be attempted in such circumstances seems startling. Yet it is obviously not uncommon given the comment above – and appears implicitly to be condoned by the researcher. The language here is telling. That this is a description of a woman who cannot (or does not want to) have sexual intercourse could easily be overlooked in the discussion of peri-vaginal muscles and reflexes of the thighs. It is the parts of her body which are of interest, not her subjective experience.

Many of the aetiological theories put forward to explain women's sexual problems reinforce the very definition of sex as a bodily phenomenon. Illnesses such as epilepsy, cancer, heart disease, diabetes, cystitis, pelvic pain, spinal-cord lesions or arthritis are seen to be major causes of sexual problems, or they are seen to be associated with the woman's reproductive life cycle (which by implication is pathologized or positioned as a narrow hormonal event), with menstruation, pregnancy and childbirth, or with the menopause.[216] Social or psychological theories *have* been suggested – cognitions, sexual abuse, personality, anxiety or depression being seen as possible causes of women's sexual problems[217] – and there *is* a move towards multifactorial models in sex research and therapy, in which social, psychological and biological factors are seen to interact to produce the problems under investigation.[218] John Bancroft's 'psychosomatic model of sex' is one of the most well known.[219] This move is to be commended. But the majority of researchers and clinicians ignore the social construction of sexuality and the way in which both 'sex' and 'sexual problems' are defined; it is extremely rare for any question of what it means to be 'woman' (and the implications this has for 'sex') to be raised or any questioning of the 'normality' of heterosexual intercourse.

Phallic Performance as 'Normal Sex'

So despite the claims of sexologists to be neutral and objective observers of human sexuality,[220] we can see in their categorization of sexual dysfunction a strong adherence to a narrow, ideologically motivated model of 'normal' sex. In descriptions of female sexual problems it is assumed that the woman's partner is a man and the focus of attention is heterosexual intercourse. Monogamous marriage is advocated as necessary for sexual health; in her critique of popular sex manuals Meryl Altman has described Masters and Johnson's *The Pleasure Bond* as 'a marriage manual in the most unironic sense',[221] for whilst it explores alternatives to heterosexual marriage it concludes with proof that they are 'unworkable and damaging'. In the sexologists' version of the fairy tale, the 'dream-team' couple Masters and Johnson take up the difficulties of the sexually dysfunctioning man and woman in order to reunite and 'cure' them. As they walk into the proverbial sunset, they are 'fully functioning' sexually.

And this isn't just the woman – within a phallocentric model of heterosexuality, the pressure is on the man. As one sex researcher commented:

> Few sexual problems are as devastating to a man as his inability to achieve or maintain an erection long enough for sexual intercourse. For many men the idea of not being able to 'get it up' is a fate worse than death.[222]

Where 'sex' is reduced to the biological workings of the body and focused on the actions of (or response to) the penis, it isn't surprising to find that male sexual problems are signified by a dysfunctional penis. For with the exception of 'disorders of desire', where the problem is manifested by absence of interest or aversion to sex, the workings (or not) of the penis are the issue at stake. So the *DSM* classifies male sexual problems as categories of male erectile disorder, inhibited male orgasm and premature ejaculation. As the ability to 'do' sex is so central to what it means to be 'man' it's not surprising that men feel anxious or afraid when they can't 'get it up' (and in); they have 'failed' as real men.

The *DSM* classification system appears to reinforce this very notion. For example, one of the criteria for male erectile disorder (diagnostic category 302.72) is the '*failure* in a male to attain or maintain an erection until completion of the sexual activity' (my italics).[223] Premature ejaculation (category 302.75 in the *DSM*) is also an emotive subject. Its clinical description is 'persistent or recurrent ejaculation with minimal sexual stimulation before, upon, or *shortly* after penetration and before the *person* wishes it (my italics)'.[224] As we have already seen, the pressure to perform sexually and to live up to the myth of the phallic hero is a major cause of anxiety for men. In defining the boundaries of 'normal' performance the *DSM* doesn't necessarily allay fears. For how do we define 'shortly' after penetration, in the description above? If a man wishes to keep an erect penis for two hours and can only manage it for one is his ejaculation 'premature'? What if his partner wants him to go on for longer – can she count as 'the person'?

Yet it is the inhibited male orgasm (category 302.74,) that most clearly reveals the heterosexual bias and the pressure for men to 'do' sex in the classification of dysfunctional sex. It is described as:

> Persistent or recurrent delay in, or absence of, orgasm in a male following a normal sexual excitement phase that the clinician, taking into account the person's age, judges to be adequate in focus, intensity and duration. This failure to reach orgasm is usually restricted to an inability to reach orgasm in the vagina, with orgasm possible with other types of stimulation, such as masturbation.[225]

The classification acknowledges the (little discussed) fact that with increasing age male potency diminishes markedly. So orgasmic problems in an older man are a normal part of aging rather than being 'dysfunctional'. It is younger men who must be able to maintain an erection, enjoy it at the same time and then reach a climax of pleasure. If they can only do this with another man or with their hand they are at risk of being classified as ill, because the vagina is deemed to be the appropriate place for male orgasm to occur (regardless of what hard-core porn suggests).

Given this focus on the penis as central to 'sex', it's not surprising to find that physical interventions, such as penile implants, are one of the most common treatments for erectile problems in both Britain and the United States.[226] These devices consist of a plastic or silicone rod surgically implanted in the penis, with an inbuilt hinge so that the now permanently erect organ can be 'stored' against the body device[227] (up or down, whichever your preference), or an 'inflatable prosthesis', a device which can produce an erect penis on demand by use of a squeeze-bulb device, which fills inflatable silicone cylinders in the erectile tissue of the penis, with saline.[228] The ultimate phallic fantasy – the ever-ready penis. It's reminiscent of the strap-on dildo we see in lesbian porn, yet here minor surgery is part of the price to be paid. Thousands of men undergo such surgery each year.[229]

Male impotence or erectile problems are a serious matter, particularly in a culture where the penis, and successful achievement of sexual intercourse, is how 'sex' is defined. But it is a sorry indictment of medicine that the means of addressing such a difficulty is increasingly seen to lie with prosthetic aids. Can sex *really* be reduced to the successful achievement of a tumescent penis? It does not take much cynicism to ask whose view of sex this is – particularly when very few of the outcome studies examining the effectiveness of these penile implants even think to ask the man's female partner if she is satisfied with the device.[230] The woman is implicitly positioned as passive object, penetration of her waiting body the assumed aim of the sexual game. The irony is that if this really were the aim, the man could do worse than use other parts of his body – his fingers perhaps – and provide satisfaction for the woman who enjoys penetration, as many lesbians (as well as teenagers engaging only in 'foreplay') have long known.

It doesn't take too much of a leap of the imagination to ascertain *why* sex therapists don't advocate such courses of action for men – it could make the penis redundant. Echoing the comments of the legions of legislators who would eschew any mention of lesbianism for fear that women would catch on to the notion and take up the infamous practice, sex experts have advised men not to penetrate the woman's vagina with anything *but* the penis. Certainly not with the fingers. As one sex manual explains:

> Many men who realize the need of preliminary play tend to overdo it. This is not advisable from the medical viewpoint, particularly when the fingers are inserted deep into the vagina, for it may cause infection. The use of fingers should be limited to the entrance of the vagina. Fingering the cervix or the vaginal wall should be avoided for another reason: the woman may develop *deeper satisfaction* from these caresses than from vaginal intercourse itself [my emphasis].[231]

Does this mean that there is nothing essential about the male that provides sexual satisfaction for the female? Could fingers be more stimulating? Masters and Johnson reassure us that the majority of women don't think so, and that this deeper pleasure can only be obtained by the woman pretending that the penetrating fingers are a penis:

> There is usually little value returned from deep vaginal insertion of the fingers, particularly early in the stimulative process. While some women have reported a mental translation of the ensuing intra vaginal sensation to that of penile containment, few had any preference for the opportunity.[232]

A high percentage of the women I interviewed reported intense enjoyment during digital penetration of the vagina. The main complaint, from heterosexual women at least, is that few men could do it well. That they saw it as 'foreplay', with penile thrusting being the main focus of sex. Lesbians tell a different tale; as we have already seen, their sexual repertoire is not limited by emphasis on one part of the body which always has to 'work' for 'sex' to occur. Sex therapists and sex researchers could learn much about the sexuality of women if they widened the scientific gaze to examine lesbian sex. It is rare for them even to acknowledge that it exists (outside of theories of pathology). This means that many aspects of women's sexuality are marginalized or ignored in mainstream sex research – such as female ejaculation, or the changes in sexual response and desire across the menstrual cycle – issues which are as important for heterosexual women as they are for lesbians. It appears to be the case that if an aspect of female sexuality is not immediately noticeable or constituted as an issue within a phallocentric model of 'sex', it is simply left out of the frame.[233]

Female Sexuality and Madness: The Dangers of the Reproductive Body

Science and medicine have not stopped at sexual problems as a means of containing both 'woman' and sex. One of the more insidious means of denigrating both female sexuality and what it is to be 'woman' has been the centuries-old association between sexuality and madness, now seen as a hormonal connection within the mainstream endocrinological analysis of sex. Traditionally this connection between biological lability and ill health was represented by theories associated with hysteria and anorexia. Today, the reproductive syndromes of premenstrual syndrome (PMS), postnatal depression (PND) and the menopausal syndrome have taken on the same connotations: the association of women's madness with the wandering womb.[234]

The association of female reproduction with insanity assumed scientific legitimacy in the nineteenth century and formed the basis for the present position of the reproductive body as a source of illness and vulnerability. As two medical experts claimed:

> The monthly activity of the ovaries . . . has a notable effect upon the mind and body; wherefore it may become an important cause of mental and physical derangement . . . It is a matter of common experience in asylums, that exacerbations of insanity often take place at menstrual periods.   MAUDSLEY, 1873[235]

> Every body of the least experience must be sensible of the influence of menstruation on the operations of the mind. In truth, it is the moral and physical barometer of the female constitution.
>
>   GEORGE MAN BURROWS, 1828[236]

The very fact of reproduction was seen to be an insufferable burden, from puberty to menopause. Thus, as one learned doctor declared, 'mental derangement frequently occurs in young females from amenorrhoea' and treatment in the form of 'an occasional warm hip-bath, or leeches to the pubis' was advocated in order to 'accomplish all we desire'.[237]

It was the medical categorization of hysteria that reified the ancient superstition about the 'wandering womb' as illness. From the time of the Ancient Greeks it had been believed that the womb travelled throughout the body, leaving illness and madness in its wake. In the nineteenth century hysteria, designated recently as 'the joker in the nosological pack',[238] became the source of attribution for a myriad ailments and symptoms supposedly associated with 'woman'. As Sydenham commented in 1848:

> The frequency of hysteria is no less remarkable than the multiformity of shapes which it puts on. Few of the maladies of miserable mortality are not imitated by it. Whatever part of the body it attacks, it will create the proper symptom of that part. Hence, without skill and sagacity, the physician will be deceived; so as to refer the symptoms to

some essential disease of the part in question, and not to the effects of hysteria.[239]

Women's sexuality was firmly connected with both the curse and cure of hysteria and a woman's reluctance (or inability) to bear children was perceived by many authorities, continuing a view first put forward by Plato, to be at the root of this pathology:

> The womb is an animal which longs to generate children. When it remains barren too long after puberty, it is distressed and sorely disturbed, and straying about in the body and cutting off the passages of the breath, it impedes respiration and brings the sufferer into extreme anguish and provokes all manner of diseases besides.[240]

It was believed that 'this disturbance continues until the womb is appeased by passion & love',[241] and so the 'cure' was clear – heterosexual sex, motherhood and marriage, the message of romantic fiction traced back to Plato. Yet it was not only madness but also moral turpitude that was seen to be associated with female reproduction. As Maddock wrote in 1854, 'the reproductive organs . . . are closely interwoven with erratic and disordered intellectual, as well as moral, manifestations.'[242] The sexologists took this long historical connection between badness and the womb and reworked it into a clinical categorization of sexual deviance or perversion. Today, female reproduction and madness are linked irrevocably through the reproductive syndromes – PMS (named late luteal phase disorder in the *DSM*), PND and the 'menopausal syndrome' – the heirs to hysteria and the fear of the wandering womb. The sophistication of the categorization may appear to have increased yet, arguably, the process is the same. Women are at risk of being unstable and in need of treatment because of their reproductive bodies. The whole reproductive life cycle has been pathologized – from puberty to menopause – within the modern reproductive categories. Any symptom, any complaint, any ailment, any abnormality can be neatly fitted into the nosological categories which both describe and dismiss women's behaviour. As Elaine Showalter has argued in *The Female Malady*, hysteria worked wonders as a means of denying women's frustration and anger in the nineteenth century, as a means of categorizing together a cornucopia of complaints. This process is alive and well today.

Take PMS. According to recent studies, up to 40 per cent of women are said to suffer from PMS to such an extent that it seriously affects their lives. The medical profession has taken note. A range of different biochemical aetiological factors has been proposed, from oestrogen and progesterone to dopamine, pyridoxine or prostaglandins imbalances.[243] A similarly wide range of biochemical treatments has been proposed, with women taking oestrogen, progesterone, lithium, fluoxetine or dygesterone, as well as the vitamin B6 (currently most popular) to cure the many symptoms with which they flock to their doctors. However, as there have been suggestions of a placebo effect of 20–80 per cent, and many of the treatments produce marked side effects (which can be worse than the original symptoms), this is actually a very disquieting practice. As the 'faulty hormone' at the root of PMS has not been identified, and the majority of researchers and clinicians are now acknowledging that there isn't one single 'cause' of PMS, treating women as if we 'know' the biological cause of their problems merely perpetuates the clinical physical and mental classification of women's bodies. At a recent conference I attended on the subject of PMS, at which a whole range of theories and therapies had been suggested, a member of the audience asked the expert speaker, 'Is there any guaranteed cure for PMS?' 'Hysterectomy', came the answer – given with no sense of irony at all. This is using a hammer to crack a nut, analogous to conducting a lobotomy to cure depression. Most clinicians, thankfully, are more humane; offering counselling or a range of drug treatments to the women who come forward for help. But few of them question the legitimacy of 'PMS' as a syndrome; few question the notion that it is reproduction which causes disturbance or distress. As I have argued elsewhere,[244] there is considerable evidence to suggest that symptoms women experience in the premenstrual phase of the cycle – or after the birth of a child or during the menopause – are as much to do with social and psychological factors as they are to do with the body. The symptoms are also irrevocably linked to what it is to be 'woman', with reproduction for centuries having been seen as a liability or a cause of dysfunction, and continue to serve as a legitimate source of attribution for women's distress today.[245]

Equally, since the male obstetricians wrested control of childbirth from female midwives as early as the sixteenth century,[246] childbirth has been construed as a technological accomplishment on the part of

the expert – the woman herself is positioned almost as a passive participant. The (until recently) ubiquitous stirrups in which she was strapped
helpless and splayed symbolizing her position as vessel to be relieved
of its burden. The hospital setting maintained women's alienation, their
sense of being sick, or stupid,[247] and of pregnancy and childbirth as an
illness. As Adrienne Rich commented:

> We were, above all, in the hands of male medical technology . . . The
> experience of lying half-awake in a barred crib, in a labour room with
> other women moaning in a drugged condition, where 'no one comes'
> except to do a pelvic examination or give an injection, is a classic
> experience of alienated childbirth. The loneliness, the sense of abandon-
> ment, of being imprisoned, powerless, and depersonalized is the chief
> collective memory of women who have given birth in American hos-
> pitals.[248]

Is this a coincidence? Or is the positioning of female reproduction
as illness or liability not another reflection of the envy of women's
power to reproduce?

Science Explains Sexual Violence

The Biological Basis of Rape and Sexual Abuse

> Some sex offenders, in spite of their behaviour, may not be evil or bad
> people . . . the key to better understanding of sex-offending behaviour
> may be tied more to biology than to theories of evil or moral corruption.[249]

Given the fact that 'sex' is positioned as a bodily phenomenon in much
of sexology and scientific research, we shouldn't be surprised to find
that sexual violence is treated similarly. The law acts to categorize and
condemn sexual offences – science explains the offender's behaviour.
The law inflicts punishment; science, through the professions of psychology and medicine offers treatment. Here he is not evil, but ill; he
is not a monster, but mad or misunderstood. Or perhaps he is merely
a man whose body is to blame, a man who is acting in the manner in
which he is genetically primed, his hormones or bodily parts driving
him out of control. For one of the most influential bodies of scientific
research would appear to suggest that the man can't help it – his biology
is to blame.

One 'fact' that has to be addressed and explained by science is that it is overwhelmingly men who execute sexually violent crimes. Women, regardless of circumstances, rarely behave in a sexually violent way. So scientists have looked for the reasons for this. Evolutionary theory has provided one of the most simple explanations: Men are simply 'born that way'. Like sex itself, sexual violence has been seen as an evolutionary adaptation, which protects the male's biological interests – his need to plant his fertile seed and serve the interests of his 'selfish gene'.

For example, one evolutionary theorist, John Archer, claimed that 'those who initiate violence do so typically where there is some means to the end of fitness to be gained.'[250] Competition for woman – or in this case access to her womb – is deemed 'natural'. Archer continues, 'Unmated males of many species . . . challenge conspecific males who are guarding the fertilizable female (the limited resource for male fitness), and in such cases (for example, many hoofed animals) success in violent contests is highly predictable of mating success.'[251] Here we have an evolutionary explanation for men fighting each other for women, and unquestioned parallels being drawn between animal and human behaviour. All are explained simply as the natural urges of 'unmated males' who are desperately searching for a mate.

This notion has passed into lay consciousness as an explanation for sexual violence, where we see the stereotype of the lonely man who is driven to 'seduce' forcibly (rape) a woman because of his deep bodily drive – a myth perpetuated by both the courts and the media (see Chapter Five). Yet as the majority of rapists and sexual attackers are in relationships with women,[252] this explanation just doesn't wash. It also fails to explain why a man would attack the woman he already 'owns' – his girlfriend or wife. But evolutionary theory can explain that as well, for men enact violence in this way in order to 'deter a wife from pursuing courses of action that are not in a man's interests' – his *biological* interests, that is. Archer continues with what might appear to be an exoneration of wife-battering:

> The use of violence against wives is ubiquitous. But the contexts in which husbands commonly assault wives are remarkably few: in response to a wife's sexual infidelity (or cues thereof), or a wife's unilateral decision to terminate the relationship (or cues thereof), as well as to 'discipline'

a 'too independent' wife, and in response to other factors (perhaps his own infidelity or paranoia) that activate *male sexual jealousy mechanisms* [my italics].[253]

Here, sexual jealousy (and by implication sexual violence) is framed as some inescapable bodily 'mechanism', which has an adaptive purpose (for man).

> We propose that the particular cues and circumstances which inspire men to use violence against their partners reflect a domain-specific masculine psychology which evolved in a social milieu in which assaults and threats of violence functioned to deter wives from pursuing alternative reproductive opportunities, which would have represented substantial threats to the husbands' fitness by misdirecting parental investment and loss of mating opportunities to reproductive competitors.[254]

A woman doesn't need to exert violence to 'keep' her man. She has got his seed or can seek another more 'dominant' male if he strays in order to fertilize her waiting womb. The greatest threat to her from a fitness perspective, we are told, is rape (not the threat of death). Raped, she will lose the

> opportunity to choose who is likely to sire her offspring, thereby depriving her of the opportunity both to have her children sired by a man with desirable phenotypic qualities and to have her children benefit from the time, effort and resources of a father.[255]

Does this suggest that we should merely advise women to take the contraceptive pill? Then rape will not deprive them of this 'choice' of mate. This is faintly reminiscent of the comments of many assailants who believe that the woman cried rape only because they left her after the 'sex' (see p. 398), of the myth that a woman will put up with anything as long as she gets her man (or in this case, his sperm).

Rape, within evolutionary theory, has been positioned as 'a very effective means of controlling the reluctant victim',[256] it is also given legitimacy by being positioned as an act which improves his 'fitness potential'. Man is primed to have sex with and attempt to 'fertilize' as many women as he can in order to maximize his chances of reproducing his genes. As Archer comments:

The fitness costs of any act of sexual intercourse have always been less for men than for women, which suggests that the evolved sexual psychology of men is likely to be less discriminating regarding choice of partner for a single sexual opportunity than that of women.'[257]

This reifies the notion of the promiscuous male, who will have sex at any available opportunity. Rape is simply an extension of this, a practice which has evolved.

Another *design feature* of male sexual psychology which is relevant to the occurrence of rape is the apparent disregard of women's unwillingness as indicated by the use of coercion to achieve copulation. The ability of the male to remain sexually competent in such circumstances presumably reflects the past fitness benefits of pursuing and achieving copulation in the case of female resistance [my italics].[258]

The fact he is 'sexually competent' even though she is screaming in terror, or crying with pain, is deemed proof that rape is biologically primed, that it is a design feature of masculinity. How rape involving bottles, broom handles or fists is explained within this model I do not know. Or rape of men or young children, who have no 'reproductive potential' at all.

This version of evolutionary theory appears implicitly to condone sexual violence, elevating the assailant to the status of anti-hero; he is primitive man, or super-macho man, a warrior hero, merely following in the footsteps of his primitive ancestors. As Archer concludes, 'The competent use of violent skills contributes quite directly to male fitness: both successful warriors . . . and successful game hunters . . . have converted their success into sexual, marital and reproductive success.'[259] The myth of romantic fiction – every woman loves a dominant aggressive man – is also elevated to scientific 'truth'. As two earlier sex researchers commented, 'Normal aggressiveness in the male appeals to the female,'[260] and 'the normal woman likes to feel herself conquered. A masterly touch in her lover is invariably pleasing.'[261]

Serial sex killers have used the hunter metaphor to serve their own ends.[262] The American 'co-ed killer' Edmund Kemper declared, 'I was the hunter and they were the victims'; Ted Bundy, speaking of himself in the third person, says, 'what really fascinated him was the hunt, the adventure of searching out his victims'; David Berkowitz wrote to the press with the boast, 'I love to hunt, prowling the streets looking for fair game – tasty meat . . . I live for the hunt – my life. Blood for Papa.' Evolutionary theorists would presumably argue that these men are merely acting out all that is repressed in our politically correct age, the urges the 'new man' has to deny.

Animal Observation and Experimentation: Proof of Biological Truth

> Humans are primates, and human sexuality is primate sexuality.
>
> PAVELKA, 1995[263]

Comparative research on animals has been used as a powerful tool to reinforce arguments about the biological roots of human behaviour. The fact that sexual aggression can be observed in a range of primate species, including baboons, spider monkeys, macaques, chimpanzees and mountain gorillas has been put forward in support of the argument that rape is instinctive.[264] Animal experiments reinforce this view. For example, in evaluating evidence on sexual aggression in chimpanzees, orangutans and gorillas in laboratory experiments where the male has free access to a female, one researcher, Ronald Nadler, calmly concludes:

> Male dominance over the female and the inability of the female to avoid and/or escape from the male within the confines of the laboratory cage were the major factors that permitted the males to behave in a sexually aggressive manner.[265]

Merely being in the presence of a female apparently incites a male to violence – this is reminiscent of the comments of defence lawyers in rape trials on the provocation presented by women who hitchhike alone (see Chapter Five). Nadler has described the Free Access Test (FAT), in which primates' 'mating' behaviour is observed in the lab, concluding that orangutans show the 'most conspicuous examples of male sexual aggression in the great apes':

> In this species, the male immediately pursued the female at the start of the test, quickly caught the female, and wrestled it [sic] to the floor of the cage. The female initially struggled and resisted but was subdued by the larger and apparently stronger male, which then forcibly positioned the female for copulation. In 3 of the 4 pairs tested, moreover, this pattern

of forcible copulation was carried out by the males on every day of the cycle![266]

Nadler's (somewhat tasteless) exclamation at the end of this quote refers to the fact that the male could not have been mounting the female for purely reproductive reasons, because she was not in the fertile phase of her oestrous cycle. So his behaviour was clearly *aggressive*, not motivated by the interests of his 'selfish gene'. Rape is therefore not simply about an attempt to achieve forced pregnancy.

Given the fact that primates (along with many other animals) are subjected to many arcane and often invasive practices in the name of biological science, one probably shouldn't shudder at the thought of the female orangutans being subjected to repeated acts of sexual aggression, or even question the motives and reactions of the scientists observing this daily rape. As every other aspect of female sexuality is placed under the probing and prying microscope, as we have seen, it is probably thought unfortunate by some that ethics would not permit human rape to be experimentally manipulated and controlled.

The fact that sexual aggression can be observed in animals is generally not used crudely to argue the case that sexual aggression is inevitable, or a simple biological drive. Not all men are sex offenders. Many men do baulk at women's resistance, despite their supposed biological priming. But authors such as Nadler conclude that 'the *potential* for male sexual aggression is inherent in our species and that such aggression is likely to be expressed under a variety of conditions unless society and individuals take specific measures to preclude it.'[267] Arguably, this serves to absolve the individual man – it is his innate drive to sexually violate a more vulnerable female who cannot escape which is to blame. The implication here is that if 'society' doesn't put preventative practices into place, then man cannot help himself and will rape. This suggests that *all* men are vulnerable to being driven to rape or abuse, given the circumstances, because they're all similarly programmed. An extremely nihilistic view of men – strikingly close to the radical feminist view of all men as (potential) rapists; but also in accordance with the findings of social psychologists such as Neil Malamuth who reported the high percentage of men who would rape if they knew they would get away with it (see p. 368).

Experimenting on Men: Measuring the Penis

It is not only animals that have been subjected to experimental scrutiny of tendencies to sexual violence. A similar line of enquiry has been adopted by researchers who are intent on discovering whether sex offenders have deviant physiological responses. Men's sexual reactions are measured using the 'penile plethysmograph', a device which measures duration, diameter and degree of hardness of erections. It has been used to measure men's reactions to sexual material and has led researchers to claim that rapists can become sexually aroused only in the presence of violence.[268] Abel et al. developed

> a series of audio-taped descriptions of sexual interactions between an adult male and an adult female in which the level of aggression was varied over three levels: mutually consenting sex, rape, and non-sexual aggression . . . rapists and non-rapists could be differentiated on the basis of their sexual arousal to stimuli describing the rape of an adult woman.[269]

Perhaps this is the closest that sex researchers can actually get to the experiments carried out by their colleagues who research primates. Whether the exposure of rapists and non-rapists to repeated experiments involving the depiction of rape – aurally or visually – deserves ethical approval is something open to question. Showing convicted rapists explicit and violent material could, arguably, reinforce the erotic connotations of such material – particularly if being strapped into an 'infernal machine' is erotic in itself (as one might imagine it must be – why else would so many men volunteer to take part in such experimental studies?). Equally, showing such material to non-abusing men, such as college students (the favourite subjects of psychology experiments), could have a considerable effect on their perceptions of both violence and women. It may introduce many men to material they have previously had no exposure to, material which denigrates and objectifies women and in many instances appears to celebrate sexual violence.

This research has some value – if measuring penile strength or width is seen as an important aspect of sexual response or proclivity to violence. What is worrying is the status such measurement has been given in sex research, often being seen as one of the few 'real' indicators of sexual response. It gives the researcher something he [sic] can quantify – how big, how long, how hard. Sitting at a recent sex-research conference, paper after paper presented data from penile plethysmograph experiments with no comment on the irony that subjective measures of arousal were rarely included. They would be seen as less reliable or valid (the benchmarks of a 'good' scientific tool). Yet, as men can manipulate their reactions in experiments in which they are wired up to the penile plethysmograph – engaging in competing thoughts means that they can control their arousal when presented with sexual stimuli – the validity of this 'reliable' measure is itself in doubt. Is its continued use merely an extension of many men's obsession with their own penis size, here displaced on to the repetitive measuring of the size and behaviour of the penises of other men?

A slightly different tack is taken by those who would argue that men who rape or sexually abuse children are somehow biologically different from other men, or that sex offenders are 'born that way'. Grotesquely paralleling (or perhaps parodying) some of the heated debates around homosexuality (Is it a choice? Is it genetic?), sexual violence has been positioned as 'sexual orientation':

> Men who are sexually attracted to children are not this way because they *decided* that they wanted to be so. Rather, in growing up they *discovered* this was the nature of their sexual orientation . . . thus it seems difficult to see how a person could be considered blameworthy because he is sexually attracted to children.[270]

How can anyone be born with a 'sexual orientation' that demands expression through violence and oppression? And how is 'discovery' of this orientation supposed to take place? In a child's bedroom? Lurking outside the school playground? In an era when we are all expected to be able to fulfil our sexual desires, when sex is positioned as a right or as a necessity of living, does this mean that men who are sexually attracted to children have the right to exercise their wish to consummate their desires, which are not at all 'blameworthy'? The men themselves certainly seem to think so, for the learned theorist who expounds upon this particular case informs us that he 'has treated a number of "sex offenders" with anti-androgenic medication, who, prior to such treatment, contended that they sometimes could not resist succumbing'.[271] Others confirm the biochemical roots of sexual sadism, claiming that:

The adrenal axis of the endocrine system might be important in sexual sadists and nonsadistic sexual aggressors. The weak androgen, DHEAS, was found to be elevated in sexual aggression . . . [and] there was a trend for cortisol to be higher and prolactin lower.[272]

These researchers go on to generalize beyond the specific group of sexual sadists they studied to conclude that single case studies and uncontrolled group studies 'suggest that temporal lobe pathology is important in sexual anomalies'.[273] Many studies have been carried out to examine testosterone levels in convicted sex offenders – the result being that well-regarded scientists have claimed a causal relationship between testosterone and aggression – in both sexual and non-sexual contexts.[274] Yet this is not a simple and incontrovertible conclusion. Finding high levels of testosterone in sex offenders does not mean that testosterone *caused* their violent behaviour – the raised levels could be one of the *consequences* of their behaviour. Continuous expression of anger, which may result from many different factors, or engagement in competitive behaviour, can actually act to increase levels of testosterone.[275] Equally, sex differences in aggressive behaviour are found well before puberty, when levels of circulating testosterone in boys and girls are similar. Simple hormonal explanations for aggressive behaviour of a sexual or non-sexual nature just don't stand up. But this hasn't stopped physical treatments – such as castration – being offered as a 'cure'.

Biological theories of sexual violence concur on one thing: Whilst sexual violence may be pre-programmed or biologically driven, it is not 'normal' behaviour. Even proponents of the biological-drive theories consider paedophilia an 'aberrant' expression of that drive. This positions the sex offender in the realm of the medical or psychiatric experts, in the annals of illness, the corridors of compassion, leading naturally to 'cure'. And as reductionist theories of madness have, down the ages, led to the development of physical treatments, ranging from psycho-surgery, to ECT, to ever more complicated cocktails of drugs,[276] so is sexual violence as 'illness' physically contained.

Chemical Castration for Sexual Violence

Whilst female 'castration', through clitoridectomy or the more wide-spread 'circumcision' has been a common means of regulating female sexuality for centuries, only in the case of sexual violence have men been subjected to such invasive procedures. Women were circumcised in the nineteenth century to control or curb what were then seen as aberrant desires – 'nymphomania', masturbation or other 'unfeminine ways'.[277] In the countries where circumcision is still practised today, it is (ostensibly) in order to make women marriageable. In none of these cases across the centuries have women committed a sexual crime – apart from being 'woman'.

Yet men are castrated only when their behaviour reaches extremes of sexual violence. And even here it is a relatively anodyne operation, usually involving chemical controls. In contrast, female 'circumcision' involves women being subjected to the total removal of clitoris, labia major and labia minor, often without anaesthetic, and with little thought for infection, pain or future sexual anaesthesia. It goes without saying that it is not a reversible operation. This is an interesting irony of naming: Male 'castration' sounds so extreme, yet it invariably involves reversible drug treatment; 'female circumcision' sounds so anodyne, yet it involves the surgical mutilation of women's genitals. Here are two examples:

> Female circumcision consists merely in the removal of the clitoris . . . The operator, who is generally a barber by profession, rubs ash on his fingers, grips the clitoris, draws it to its full length and shears it with a single razor stroke. Ashes are then sprinkled on the wound to staunch bleeding.[278]

> [Female circumcision involves] excision of the entire clitoris, labia minora and parts of the labia majora. The two sides of the vulva are then fastened together in some way either by thorns . . . or sewing by catgut. Alternatively the vulva are scraped raw and the child's limbs are tied together for several weeks until the wound heals (or until she dies). The purpose is to close the vaginal orifice. Only a small opening is left (usually by inserting a sliver of wood) so the urine or later the menstrual blood can be passed.[279]

We don't have to ask who is doing the naming and, again, whose interests it serves. Castration of men for sexual offending is not a common treatment, but it has been executed on many thousands of men. In a recent review a Canadian forensic psychiatrist summarized the results of studies reporting castration carried out on over 4,000 men.[280] Rates of recidivism of 5–80 per cent are reported. Whilst some men are 'cured', others continue to commit sexual crimes even after having been surgically castrated. This isn't a surprise for those of us who would not locate sexual violence – or 'normal' sex for that matter – in biochemical components of the body. It isn't simply androgens that motivate sexual violence. It is interesting that these terrible raging hormones – in every other instance the scourge of women (PMS, PND, the menopause . . .) – are espoused as motivators of men only in the case of sexual violence. Outside this sphere men are seen as active, agentic creatures, not at the mercy of the labile body at all.

The Pathological Rapist

Not all men rape, so science still has to explain why some do and some don't, given their similar biological make-up. Seeing the individual rapist as a psychological deviant provides some explanation; here it is not his body but his mind that is at fault. Many different personality theories have been proposed: that rapists are timid, passive and immature;[281] that they have a 'fixated passive personality';[282] an antisocial personality, or are alcoholics;[283] or that they are sociosexually underdeveloped.[284] Others have suggested that men who batter their wives are less educated than their partners and, as a consequence, feel powerless; or that their violence has been rewarded in previous relationships – analogous to the school bully who rules the playground.[285] Or that men who are violent towards women have a restricted range of emotions, with anger as one of their only emotional outlets – demonstrating anger acts temporarily to short-circuit their feelings of vulnerability.[286] It has also been suggested that rapists are more likely to have psychosexual problems, including erectile and ejaculatory difficulties;[287] feelings of sexual inadequacy;[288] or unsatisfying sexual relationships.[289] A number of researchers have blamed the women in violent men's lives, suggesting that rapists have mothers who are either rejecting or over-protective[290] (covering all options), resulting in a 'submissive, passive individual'; or 'aggressive, efficient, masculine and sexually frigid wives' with 'a strong need to control the relationship'[291] – a woman who has rejected the feminine masquerade and provokes her man to violence: This is blaming women for male violence, an idea first proposed by Mendelssohn in 1956, which examines 'the potential of victim receptivity' in rape[292] – the idea that women who are raped have given signals which provoke the attack, or that at some level these women want to be raped. This is an argument which can unfortunately reinforce women's own guilt and self blame, and draws attention away from the commonalities which occur in cases of sexual assault, instead focusing on the individual woman and man.

Whether positing biological or psychosocial explanations for the deviant and dysfunctional manifestations of our sexuality, sexual science and the law in the main focuses on the individual. The sexual criminal may be mad, bad or dangerous, but it is *he* that must be treated or punished, or his own particular social environment seen as having been to blame. The child abuser is ill or perverted. He is punished, condemned or clinically controlled, always seen as different from other non-abusing men. The rapist is either a mad monster or misunderstood, a man motivated by uncontrollable biological drives or who simply got it wrong, confused over the issue of consent or trapped by the machiavellian evil of woman. Condemn him, sentence him or experiment on and treat him – he is still seen as separate from the non-raping man. This positions the sex offender as 'other' and implicitly exonerates all other men. It means we can avoid having to examine how masculinity is constructed, and it detracts from the fact that sexual violence is pervasive across classes, across cultures and within a myriad different family structures. We can no more identify the 'deviant-type family' of the rapist or the abuser, than we can legitimately identify the pathological-personality type of faulty hormonal mechanism which motivates such a man. There is no one theory that can explain it all. All male rapists share testosterone. They also share a masculine sexual identity and the need to live up to the role of 'man' in a phallocentric world.

Understanding Sexual Violence: Looking at What It is to be 'Man'

Not all sexual scientists advocate a narrow reductionist view of rape. As a result of two decades of feminist critiques, there is increasing recognition that in understanding sexual violence, we have to look at what it is to be 'man' and how this man is positioned in relation to 'woman' within the script of heterosexual sex. This means that we have to look beyond the individual to the constructions of masculinity and femininity and to the relation of 'man' to 'woman' in a phallocentric sphere. We also have to look to the fears and fantasies associated with *man* as sexual other to man – fears associated with homosexuality in particular, as women are not the only targets of the anger, fear and sexualized violence of man.

Sexually violent men are not all perverts; they are not all mad. They share much with non-violent men – a fear of women; a fear of the feminine side of themselves; a fear of homosexual desire; a fear of closeness in emotional relationships which makes sex or physical contact with children the only arenas in which they can make contact with another person. Given the way in which vulnerability and subordination are eroticized, it's not surprising many men cross the barrier and turn this closeness into 'sex', regardless of the consent of the woman or child.[293] Sex becomes the arena within which men are supposed to satisfy all their own emotional needs, it is the only place that they are able to be vulnerable, given the dominant constructions of what it is to be 'man'. Yet for many men, the very closeness that sex can bring is threatening to their sense of themselves as 'man' and so violence or sexual aggression becomes their knee-jerk response.[294] It's not surprising – 'man' is expected to be powerful and in control; when he is having 'sex' he is supposed to know what to do and to do it well. An impossible double bind is created in which neither women nor men win.

Positioning the rapist or child abuser as 'other' prevents us from recognizing the continuities between sexual violence and 'normal' heterosexual sex. The desire to dominate, the desire for power, the use of the penis as weapon of phallic power and the subordination of 'woman', are embedded in dominant constructions of masculinity, as we have already seen. They underlie representations of 'woman' and 'man' in art, film, pornography and the mass media; they are rooted in man's fantasies and fears about women, his fears that he is not 'man'. Arguably, sex offenders merely adopt a rhetoric in line with phallocentric conceptualizations of what it is to be 'man' in explaining their crimes. As these convicted rapists commented:

> 'Rape was a feeling of total dominance. Before the rapes, I would always get a feeling of power and anger. I would degrade women so that I could feel there was a person of less worth than me.'[295]

> 'Rape gave me the power to do what I wanted to do without feeling that I had to please a partner or respond to a partner. I felt in control, dominant. Rape was the ability to have sex without caring about the woman's response. I was totally dominant.'[296]

> 'Seeing them lying there helpless gave me the confidence that I could do it . . . with rape I felt totally in charge. I'm bashful, timid. When a woman wanted to give in normal sex, I was intimidated. In the rapes, I was totally in command, she totally submissive.'[297]

If 'man' is positioned as having to be in control of sex and to have to 'pleasure' a woman, it isn't surprising that he feels anxiety and dread. This adds to the dread and fear of woman which, arguably, goes back to early experiences with women, to the early fantasies and fears of the mother. Sexual violence is an arena in which man can absolve himself of responsibility for giving pleasure to a woman, in which he can guarantee that he is in control. She cannot reject him here; she will not laugh at him – she is too afraid of death. Or if she is a child, she is completely vulnerable and in his control; she has no previous experience of sex with which she can compare his performance. As one interviewee commented:

> 'For my own experience I wouldn't feel satisfied if a woman wasn't satisfied. I mean it's almost like giving a performance and sort of saying if you don't get applauded what's the hell point of doing it, you don't feel very good about it yourself.'

The man who rapes doesn't have to wait for the applause (or fear that a woman will discuss his performance with her friends, another common fear). Equally, she *cannot* say 'no' and so he avoids the risk of rejection. As one man I interviewed said, 'Women have the real power

because they have what no man likes and that's the "no" response.'
Given the current constructions of masculinity and femininity and the
way they intersect with constructions of 'sex', perhaps we should be
asking why *more* men don't carry out sexual crimes.

Not all men rape. The majority, thankfully, deal with their fears and
desires through other means. Yet in the extreme cases, sexual murderers
desecrate and destroy the objects of their dread and desire. Millions of
women are raped and sexually assaulted every year. Indeed, so are many
men. Despite what sexual science might suggest, these are not the acts
of madmen or monsters. We should be looking at what it is to be 'man',
not positioning those few who are caught as deviant perverts. We
should be looking at the fantasies and fears about 'woman' that underlie
man's misogyny and dread. We should be looking at the continuum
of violence in women's lives[298] and the connections between sexual
harassment, rape and child sexual abuse. We should be looking to the
fear and dread of homosexuality and to the way in which that fear is
sometimes projected outwards on to other men. We should be looking
at the systems which implicitly condone such abuse, seeing it as trivial
or as a product of the malicious imaginations of those who are abused.
We should be looking to the way in which sexual violence is used to
keep women down – as it is women who are the main targets of the
sexual violence of men.[299] This is not to reinforce the notion of the
penis as weapon, seeing heterosexual sex as analogous to rape and
therefore as the worst violation of women. It is not the penis which is
at fault, it is the malevolent man who wields it as weapon. It is man
who positions the penis as phallus and it is man, in the extreme case of
sexual violence, who wields it as a tool of destruction. Psychologists
and sociologists may help us in understanding some of the psychosocial
factors which are commonly associated with such violence, but they
cannot explain it all. Not the mass rapes in war, rape in marriage,
acquaintance rape, rape on college campuses or in the minority cases
of 'real' rape (real in the eyes of the law) by a stranger in the street.
There are many factors which precipitate these acts of rape. As Alexandra
Stiglmayer says of the rapes during the war in Bosnia:

> A rape is an aggressive and humiliating act, as even a soldier knows, or
> at least suspects. He rapes because he wants to engage in violence. He
> rapes because he wants to demonstrate his power. He rapes because he is

the victor. He rapes because the woman is the enemy's woman, whom he wishes to humiliate and annihilate. He rapes because he despises women. He rapes to prove his virility. He rapes because the acquisition of the female body means a piece of territory conquered. He rapes to take out on someone else the humiliation he has suffered in the war. He rapes to work off his fears. He rapes because it's really only some 'fun' with the guys. He rapes because war, a man's business, has awakened his aggressiveness, and he directs it at those who play a subordinate role in the world [of war].[300]

Substitute the word 'world' for 'war' and we have an eloquent description of the complexity of rape. It is about man proving that he is 'man' and lashing out at those who challenge and threaten that certainty. It is not a coincidence or an arbitrary fact that 'woman' is the target of both man's anger and fear as it is she who provokes both his desire and his dread. The way in which sexual violence is represented and dealt with by the mass media, science, and the law tells us more about the institutionalized acceptance of phallocentric fantasies about 'woman' than any other subject in the sphere of sex. It is also an arena in which misogynistic myths have the most marked material effects – in providing a script which positions rape and child sexual abuse as 'sex' and a legal framework which exonerates the behaviour of sexually violent men. So it is to the subject of sexual violence against women that I will now turn.

NOTES

1. Abramson, P. R. 'Sexual Science: Emerging Discipline or Oxymoron?', *The Journal of Sex Research*, 27, 1990, pp. 147–65, p. 149.

2. Derhan, D., Maher, F. & Wallar, L., *An Introduction to the Law*, North Ryde, NSW: The Law Book Company. Quoted in Naffine, Ngaire, *Law and the Sexes: Explorations in Feminist Jurisprudence*, London: Allen & Unwin, 1995, p. 24.

3. Horney, Karen, *Feminine Psychology*, H. Kelman (ed.), London: Norton, 1967, p. 116.

4. Foucault, M., *The History of Sexuality, Vol. 1*, London: Penguin, 1976, p. 35.

5. Baudrillard, J., *Seduction*, New York: St Martin's Press, 1990, p. 66.

6. Foucault has referred to this as control of the 'useful body', in contrast to control of the 'intelligible body' through representation.

7. For example, in the nineteenth century Jeremy Bentham described homosexuality as an 'imaginary offence', which was dependent on changing concepts of taste and morality. See Weeks, 1981, p. 242.

8. For an excellent discussion of the relationship between biological and cultural factors in sex, see Abramson, P. R. & Pinkerton, S. D., *Sexual Nature, Sexual Culture*, Chicago: University of Chicago Press, 1995.

9. See Ussher, Jane, 'The Construction of Female Sexual Problems: Regulating Sex, Regulating Women', in Ussher, Jane & Barker, Christine, *Psychological Perspectives on Sexual Problems: New Directions in Theory and Practice*, London: Routledge, 1993.

10. See Ussher, Jane, *The Psychology of the Female Body*, London: Routledge, 1989.

11. See Eisenstein, Z. H., *The Female Body and the Law*, California: University of California Press, 1988, for an analysis of the law as phallocentric.

12. Many would argue that this is a white, middle-class, heterosexual man.

13. See MacKinnon, Catherine, 'Feminism, Marxism, Method and State: An Agenda for Theory', *Signs*. vol. 7, no. 3, 1982, pp. 515–44; and MacKinnon, Catherine, 'Feminism, Marxism, Method and State: Toward Feminist Jurisprudence', *Signs*. vol. 8, no. 4, 1983, pp. 635–58, for a discussion of these issues in the law. See Harding, Sandra, *Whose Science? Whose Knowledge? Thinking from Women's Lives*, Milton Keynes: Open University Press, 1991: and Keller, Evelyn Fox, *Reflections on Gender and Science*, New Haven, Connecticut: Yale University Press, 1985.

14. See Smart, Carol, *Women, Crime and Criminology: A Feminist Critique*, London: Routledge & Kegan Paul; and Harding, 1991. For an excellent review of the many debates in feminist legal theory, see the two edited volumes: Frances E. Olsen (ed.), *Feminist Legal Theory I: Foundations and Outlooks; Feminist Legal Theory II: Positioning feminist theory within the law*, New York: New York University Press, 1995.

15. See Lees, Sue, *Carnal Knowledge: Rape on Trial*, London: Penguin, 1996.

16. See Foucault, M., *The History of Sexuality, Vol. 1*, New York: Pantheon, 1976.

17. Tertullian, in a letter to his wife. Quoted in Tong, R., *Women, Sex and the Law*, New Jersey: Rowman & Allanheld, 1987, p. 99.

18. For example, Weeks, Jeffrey, *Sex, Politics and Society, The Regulation of Sexuality since 1800*, London: Longman, 1981, p. 243, states that 'the

Wolfenden Report . . . argued that the purpose of the criminal law was to preserve public order and decency, and to protect the weak from exploitation. It was *not* to impose a particular pattern of moral behaviour on individuals.' This is following a long-held pattern within law.

19. See Dynes, Wayne R., *Encyclopaedia of Homosexuality*, London: St James Press, 1990, section on Christianity, p. 22.

20. Ibid., p. 222

21. Quoted in Tong, 1987, p. 100.

22. Virginity is not a universal ideal for women. Anthropologists have reported that in other cultural contexts (such as Central Africa) fertility is the goal to which women aspire, and notions of virginity – or the regulation of female 'promiscuity' – are alien. See Caldwell, J. & Caldwell, P. 'The Demographic Evidence for the Incidence and Course of Abnormally Low Fertility in Tropical Africa, *World Health Statistics Quarterly*, 36, 1983, pp. 2–34.

23. Johannsson, Warren, 'Law: Major Traditions in the West', in Dynes, 1990, pp. 682–5, p. 683.

24. Dynes, 1990, p. 222.

25. The history of sex research has been well documented by a number of recent critics, most notably the social historian Jeffrey Weeks. See Weeks, 1981, Ch. 8; and Foucault, 1976.

26. Sigmund Freud has, arguably, had the greatest impact on our understanding of sexuality in the humanities and in most therapeutic practice, as well as on popular culture, through his identification of the important role sexuality plays in the whole of our psychic lives. However, from the earliest inception of psychoanalytic theories and therapy, the world of *real* Science (with a capital S,) has dismissed Freud almost totally as a prejudiced charlatan, as a man who based all his theories on his analysis of middle-class Viennese women, studied in a way that was simply 'unscientific' – 'his theories cannot be objectively proven – or disproven – so have little weight in the scientific world.' It is a line still fed to generations of psychology undergraduates today, who are taught to forget all their lay perceptions of Freud as a 'great man' of psychology. Freud's place in the academy of 'real' science, including sexology, has been almost completely dismissed.

27. Krafft-Ebbing *Psychopathia Sexualis*, F. S. Klaf (trans.), New York: Bell, 1886, p. 133. (ICD indicates the *International Classification of Diseases*).

28. ICD-9 classification listed in *DSMIII-R* (*DSM* indicates the *Diagnostic and Statistical Manual of the American Psychiatric Association*) p. 462.
29. *DSMIII-R*, p. 287.
30. Ellis, H., 'Sexual Deviation', in Ellis, H., *Psychology of Sex*, London: Heinemann, (first published in 1933), 1946, p. 130.
31. *DSMIII-R*, p. 281.
32. Rubin, Gayle, 'Thinking Sex', in *Pleasure and Danger: Exploring Female Sexuality*, Carol, Vance (ed.), London: Routledge & Kegan Paul, 1984, p. 291.
33. Perkins, R. M., *Criminal Law*, 2nd edn., London: Macmillan, p. 378.
34. 'Howard League Working Party Report', *Unlawful Sex: Offences, Victims and Offenders in the Criminal Justice System of England and Wales*, London: Waterlow, 1984, Section 2:15, p. 11.
35. Parliamentary debates in the House of Commons, 3 March 1921. Quoted in Jeffreys, S., *The Spinster and Her Enemies. Feminism and Sexuality 1880– 1930*, London: Pandora, 1985, p. 84.
36. Foucault, 1976, has argued that it was only in the seventeenth century that the 'pedagogization' of sex occurred, with sex play between children coming to be seen as problematic or deviant and consequently regulated or controlled. However, laws concerning the age of consent have existed in Anglo-American contexts for centuries.
37. For it is girls who are primarily affected by the heterosexual age of consent. There are few cultures where young boys are married to older women.
38. As the risks of pregnancy and childbirth at such an early age were recognized by some parents, it was not unknown for a 'marriage' to take place, but for the wedded couple to be housed separately and not expected to consummate the union.
39. He later attempted to divorce her on the grounds that her first marriage *was* consummated, allowing him to argue that his own marriage should be annulled.
40. 'Howard League Working Party Report', 1984, Section 2:14, p. 10.
41. *Personal Rights Journal*, 15 September 1882. Quoted in Jeffreys, 1985, p. 54.
42. Butler and Hopkins spearheaded a 'social purity movement' and advocated celibacy for both women and men. They were not concerned merely with the dangers of sex for young women but the dangers of sex for everyone. See Jeffreys, 1985, for a discussion of this.
43. 'Howard League Working Party Report', 1984, Section 2:14, p. 10.

44. Herdt, Gilbert, *Ritualised Homosexuality in Melanesia*, Berkeley: University of California Press, 1984.

45. Herdt, Gilbert, *The Sambia: Ritual and Gender in New Guinea*, New York: Holt, Rinehart & Winston, 1987.

46. Lord Templeman, R v. Brown, 11 March 1993, *All England Law Reports*, p. 84.

47. Held by Lord Templeman, Lord Lowry and Lord Jauncy of Tullichettle. Ibid., p. 75.

48. Ibid., p. 82.

49. Quoted in Jeffreys, 1985, p. 84.

50. Two exceptions are the states of Massachusetts, and Michigan, where a gender-non-specific definition of rape includes penetration by objects other than the penis. See MacKinnon, 1983, p. 647. See 520a[h]; 520b.s.

51. In re B. G., 589 A.2d 637, 640–41 (NJ Super. Ct. App. Div. 1991). See *Fordham Law Review*, vol. 63, October 1994. Panel discussion: Men, Women and Rape. Donald Dripps, Linda Fairstein, Robin West and Deborah W. Denno, p. 129.

52. Toolif, Kevin, 'A Queer Verdict', *Guardian Weekend*, 25 November 1995, pp. 14–22.

53. See Morgan-Taylor, M. & Rumney, P., 'A Male Perspective on Rape', *New Law Journal*, 144 (6669), 1994, 1490–93.

54. See Gerber, P. N., 'Victims Become Offenders: A Study of the Ambiguities', in *The Sexually Abused Male, Vol. 1, Prevalence, Impact and Treatment*, M. Hunter (ed.), Lexington, MA: Lexington, 1990, pp. 153–76.

55. Morgan-Taylor, 1994.

56. See *Fordham Law Review*, vol. 63, October 1994, p. 129.

57. Stephen Donaldson, the man who brought the case against prisons to the US Supreme Court, who was gang raped in prison in 1973 after being jailed for refusing on principle to pay a $10 fine following a non-violent resistance action against the Vietnam war.

58. It has repeatedly been demonstrated that power over weaker inmates is routinely maintained by organized gang rape in prison.

59. See *Corbett* v. *Corbett*, 1971, p. 83; *Cossey* v. *UK*, 1991, 2 FLR 492.

60. For example, see *People* v. *Liberta*, 474 n. e. 2d 567, 577 (NY, 1984). See also Sarrel, P. M. & Masters, W. H. 'Sexual Molestation of Men by Women', *Archives of Sexual Behaviour*, 117, pp. 117–31.

61. See 'Female–Male Assaults', in Rumney, Philip N. S. & Morgan-Taylor,

Martin P., *The Legal Problems Associated with Males as Victims of de Facto Rape* (forthcoming).

62. See Lloyd, Ann, *Doubly Deviant, Doubly Damned. Society's Treatment of Violent Women*, London: Penguin, 1995.

63. Lloyd, 1995, pp. 17–19.

64. See Mendel, Matthew Parynik, *The Male Survivor. The Impact of Sexual Abuse*, London: Sage, 1995, for a thorough review of the arguments relating to this debate, as well as a discussion of a number of case studies.

65. July 1995.

66. See Trivelpiece, James, 'Adjusting the Frame: Cinematic Treatment of Sexual Abuse and Rape of Men and Boys', in Hunter, 1990, pp. 47–72.

67. See Mendel, 1995.

68. See *Encyclopaedia of Homosexuality*, pp. 682–98, for a discussion of law on homosexuality across cultures and across history.

69. Weeks, 1981, p. 99.

70. Ibid., p. 99.

71. Public Record Office HO 144/216/A 49134/2. Quoted in Weeks, 1981, p. 119.

72. Weeks, 1981, p. 100.

73. 'Howard League Working Party Report', 1984, Section 2:16, p. 11.

74. Rivera, Rhonda R., 'Sexual Orientation and the Law', in *Homosexuality: Research Implications for Public Policy*, Gonsiorek, J. C. & Weinrich, J. D., London: Sage, 1991, pp. 81–100.

75. *Bowers* v. *Hardwick*, 478 U.S. 186 (1986) at 191. Cited in Rivera, in Gonsiorek & Weinrich, 1991, p. 83.

76. Poulter, J. S., *Peers, Queers and Commons: The Struggle for Gay Law Reform from 1950 to the Present*, London: Routledge, 1991, p. 253.

77. Ibid., p. 253.

78. *Guardian*, 28 March 1994.

79. Kinsey, A., Pomeroy, W. & Martin, C., *Sexual Behaviour in the Human Male*, Philadelphia: Saunders, 1948, pp. 389–93.

80. See *Sex Codes of California*, Sarah Senefeld Beserra, Nancy M. Jewel, Melody West Matthews & Elizabeth R. Gatov (eds.), Public Education and Research Committee of California 1973, pp. 163–8.

81. See Honore, 1978, p. 24.

82. Parliamentary debates in the House of Commons, 1921, vol. 145, 1799. Quoted in Jeffreys, 1985, p. 114.

83. See Robson, Ruth, 'Legal Lesbicide', in Jill Radford & Diana Russell

(eds.), *Femicide: The Politics of Woman Killing*, Buckingham: Open University Press, 1992, pp. 40–5, for a discussion of these cases.

84. Crompton, L., 'The Myth of Lesbian Impurity', in *The Gay Past: A Collection of Historical Essays*, J. Licasta, & R. Peterson (eds.), New York: Howorth Press, 1985, p. 16.

85. Quoted in Faderman, Lillian, *Surpassing the Love of Men*, London: The Women's Press, 1985, p. 36.

86. Brown, J., *Immodest Acts*, Oxford: Oxford University Press, 1986, p. 14.

87. Ibid., p. 19.

88. Monter, W., 'Sodomy and Heresy in Modern Switzerland', *Journal of Homosexuality*, 6 (41), 1981.

89. Ibid., p. 43.

90. See Ussher, J. M., *Women's Madness: Misogyny or Mental Illness*, Hemel Hempstead: Harvester Wheatsheaf, 1991.

91. This is not to say that Joan of Arc was a lesbian, but her refusal to dress and behave as a woman, and her refusal to take up her expected place within a heterosexual relationship were central to her being burned at the stake.

92. Baroja, J., *The World of Witches*, Chicago: University of Chicago Press, 1973.

93. Evans, A., *Witchcraft and the Gay Counterculture*, Boston: Fag Rag Books, 1978, p. 76.

94. In 1991, same-gender sexual contact was illegal in twenty-four American states. See Rivera in Gonsiorek & Weinrich, 1991, p. 82.

95. Sex with a girl under sixteen could fall under the general laws protecting against child sexual abuse.

96. Bernard Talmey, quoted in Faderman, Lillian, *Odd Girls and Twilight Lovers: A History of Lesbian Life in Twentieth-Century America*, London: Penguin, 1992, p. 50.

97. See Edwards, Susan, *Female Sexuality and the Law*, Oxford: Martin Robertson, 1981, p. 43.

98. Ibid., p. 44.

99. Ibid., p. 44.

100. Quoted in Edwards, 1981, p. 44.

101. Parliamentary debates in the House of Commons, 1921, vol. 145, 1977. Quoted in Jeffreys, 1985, p. 114.

102. Hyde, Montgomery, H., *The Other Love: An Historical and Contemporary Survey of Homosexuality in Britain*, London: Mayflower Books, 1972, p. 200.

103. Parliamentary debates in the House of Commons, 1921, vol. 145, 1977. Quoted in Jeffreys, 1985.
104. *Gay News*, 2–14 June 1978, p. 3.
105. *Gardner* v. *Gardner*, 1947; and *Spicer* v. *Spicer*, 1945. Both cited in Edwards, 1981, p. 45.
106. See Smyth, Cherry, *Lesbians Talk. Queer Notions*, London: Scarlett Press, 1992, pp. 23–4.
107. Edwards, 1981, p. 45.
108. *Dailey* v. *Dailey* 635 SW2d 391 (Tenn. Ct App. 1981). See Rivera in Gonsiorek & Weinrich, 1991, p. 95.
109. *Guardian*, 9 September 1993, p. 11.
110. Golombok, S., Spencer, A. & Rutter, M., 'Children in Lesbian and Single-Parent Households: Psychosexual and Psychiatric Appraisal', *Journal of Child Psychology and Psychiatry*, 24, 1983, pp. 551–72. See also Burns, Jan, 'The Psychology of Lesbian Health Care', in Nicolson, P., & Ussher, J. M., *The Psychology of Women's Health Care*, London: Macmillan, 1992.
111. Reported in the *Guardian*, 30 June 1994.
112. Quoted in Faderman, 1991, p. 143.
113. Ibid., p. 157.
114. *Creighton Law Review*, 1994, vol. 27, p. 385.
115. See Faderman, 1991, Ch. 6, for a more complete discussion of these homosexual witch-hunts.
116. Ibid., pp. 142, 145.
117. Quoted in Faderman, 1991, p. 151.
118. Ibid., p. 151.
119. This was an ex-army officer, who is also a lesbian.
120. Discharge of Homosexuals, Air Force Regulations 35–66, Department of Air Force, Washington, DC, May 31 1956.
121. Tilchen, Maida, & Weinstock, Helen, 'Letters from My Aunt', *Gay Community News*, 12 July 1980, pp. 8–9. Quoted in Faderman, 1991, p. 153.
122. Evans & Roher, p. 2 1270, Colo. 1993, cert. denied, 62, USLW 3220 (US Nov. 1 1993). See *Creighton Law Review*, 1994, p. 384.
123. Armed Forces Policy and Guidelines on Homosexuality, distributed on 21 March 1994, to all commands home and abroad from the Ministry of Defence.
124. The Disciplines and Standards Paper, distributed on 21 October 1993, from the Ministry of Defence, Whitehall.

125. *Creighton Law Review*, 1994, p. 473.

126. *Social Trends*, London: Central Statistical Office, 1995.

127. Ellis, 1946, p. 191.

128. Ibid., p. 194.

129. Ibid., p. 205.

130. Ibid., pp. 199–200.

131. Terry, Jennifer, 'Lesbians under the Medical Gaze: Scientists Search for Remarkable Differences', *The Journal of Sex Research*, 27 (3) 1990, pp. 317–99.

132. Henry, George W., *Sex Variants: A Study of Homosexual Patterns*, New York: Paul B. Hoeber Inc., 1948, p. 1023.

133. Ibid., p. 700.

134. Frederick, Carlton, 'Nymphomania as a Cause of Excessive Venery', 1907, *American Journal of Obstetrics and Diseases of Women and Children*, 56 (6), pp. 742–4. Quoted in Groneman, Carol, 'Nymphomania: The Historical Construction of Female Sexuality, *Signs*, 19 (2), 1994, pp. 337–67, p. 355.

135. See Groneman, 1994, for an excellent discussion of all of these arguments in the context of the history of nymphomania.

136. See Faderman, 1991, Ch. 2, for a detailed description of this process.

137. Dr James Weir Jr., 'The Effects of Female Suffrage on Posterity', *American Naturalist*, September 1895, 24 (345), pp. 815–25. Quoted in Faderman, 1991, p. 47.

138. Quoted in Faderman, 1991, p. 49.

139. Kronemeyer, R., *Overcoming Homosexuality*, New York: Macmillan, 1980, p. 7. Quoted in Kitzinger, Celia, *The Social Construction of Lesbianism*, London: Sage, 1987, p. 40.

140. Le Vay, Simon, *The Sexual Brain*, Massachusetts: MIT Press, 1993, p. 127.

141. International Academy of Sex Research, Provincetown, September 1995.

142. There are a number of notable exceptions to this, and many recent analytic thinkers would argue that we have to theorize all sexuality. See Chodorow, Nancy J., *Femininities, Masculinities, Sexualities: Freud and Beyond*, London: Free Association Books, 1994.

143. Murphy, T. F., 'Redirecting Sexual Orientation: Techniques and Justifications', The Journal of Sex Research, 29 (4), 1992, pp. 501–23.

144. For an excellent and critical review of this literature see Pattatucci, Angela M. L. & Hamer, Dean H., 'The Genetics of Sexual Orientation: From Fruitflies to Humans,' in Abramson & Pinkerton, 1995, pp. 154–74.

145. Kallman, F. J., 'Comparative Twin Study on the Genetic Aspects of Male Homosexuality', *Journal of Nervous Mental Disorder*, 115, 1952, pp. 282–98.

146. Bailey, J. M. & Pillard, R. C., 'A Genetic Study of Male Sexual Orientation', *Archives of General Psychiatry*, 48, 1991, pp. 1089–96.

147. Bailey, J. M., Pillard, R. C., Neale, M. C. & Agyei, Y., 'Heritable Factors Influence Sexual Orientation in Women', *Archives of General Psychiatry*, 50, 1993, pp. 217–23.

148. Bailey, J. M., 'A Twin Registry Study of Sexual Orientation', paper presented at the twenty-first annual meeting of the International Academy of Sex Research, Provincetown, Massachusetts, September 1995.

149. See Garber, Marjorie, *Vice Versa: Bisexuality and the Eroticism of Everyday Life*, London: Penguin, 1995, for the development of a convincing argument that the very boundaries of 'sexual orientation' are always fluid or potentially in a state of flux.

150. Hamer, D., 'Sexual Orientation, Personality Traits, and Genes', paper presented at the twenty-first annual meeting of the International Academy of Sex Research, Provincetown, Massachusetts, September 1995.

151. Fedoroff, J. P. et al., 'A GnRH Test of Androphiles, Gynephiles, Heterosexual Pedophiles, and Homosexual Pedophiles', paper presented at the twenty-first annual meeting of the International Academy of Sex Research, Provincetown, Massachusetts, September 1995.

152. Alias, A. G., '46 XY, 5-Alpha-Reductase Deficiency: A (Contrasting) Model to Understanding the Predisposition to Male Homosexuality?' Paper presented at the twenty-first annual meeting of the International Academy of Sex Research, Provincetown, Massachusetts, September 1995.

153. *Wall Street Journal*, 12 August 1993, p. 1. Quoted in Garber, 1995, p. 271.

154. Pattatucci & Hamer, 1995, p. 155.

155. Garber, 1995, p. 115.

156. Ibid., p. 85.

157. Abramson, P. R. & Pinkerton, S. D., 'Introduction: Nature, Nurture and In-Between', in Abramson & Pinkerton, 1995, p. 11.

158. See Garber, 1995.

159. Herdt, 1987.

160. Garber, 1995, p. 149.

161. Same-sex marriage was passed as legal by the Dutch parliament in April 1996. The American state of Hawaii was also considering such legislation

at the time of writing, and Denmark, Sweden and Norway offered limited legal recognition for same-sex couples.

162. This was because he did not condemn active female sexuality or homosexuality, unlike many of his colleagues.

163. Ellis, 1946, p. 26.

164. Ibid., p. 30.

165. Ibid., p. 31.

166. Ibid., p. 15.

167. Ellis, Havelock, *Men and Women*, London: Contemporary Science Series, 1893, p. 448.

168. See Groneman, 1994.

169. Quoted in Jeffreys, S., *The Sexuality Debates*, London: Routledge & Kegan Paul, 1987.

170. Ellis, 1946, p. 263.

171. Krafft-Ebbing, 1886. Quoted in Groneman, 1994, p. 353.

172. Storer, Horatio, 'Cases of Nymphomania', *American Journal of Medical Science*, 32 (10), 1856, pp. 378–87. Quoted in Groneman, 1994, pp. 337–8.

173. Wilson, Glenn D., 'The Sociobiological Basis of Sexual Dysfunction', in *Sex Therapy in Britain*, Martin Cole & Wendy Dryden (eds.), Milton Keynes: Open University Press, 1988.

174. Masters, W. H. & Johnson, V. E., *Human Sexual Response*, Boston: Little Brown, 1966.

175. Le Vay, 1993, p. 10.

176. Wallen, Kim, 'The Evolution of Female Sexual Desire', in Abramson & Pinkerton, 1995, p. 57.

177. See Abramson & Pinkerton, 1995, for examples of this research.

178. Wilson, L. 1988, p. 50.

179. Ibid., p. 51.

180. Symons, Donald, 'Beauty is in the Adaptations of the Beholder: The Evolutionary Psychology of Human Female Sexual Attractiveness', in Abramson & Pinkerton, 1995, p. 91.

181. Wilson, 1988, p. 50.

182. Ibid., p. 51.

183. See *Social Trends*, London: Central Statistical Office, 1994.

184. Wallen, 1995, p. 57.

185. Personal communication.

186. Wilson, 1988, p. 65.

187. Wilson, 1988, p. 65.

188. Le Vay, 1993, p. 47.

189. Ibid., p. 47.

190. For a feminist critique of popularized sex manuals, see Altman, Meryl, 'Everything They Always Wanted You to Know: The Ideology of Popular Sex Literature', in *Pleasure and Danger: Exploring Female Sexuality*, Carol Vance, (ed.), London: Routledge & Kegan Paul, 1984.

191. Boyle, M., 'Gender, Science and Sexual Dysfunction', in *Constructing the Social*, T. R. Sarbin & J. I. Kitzinger (eds.), London: Sage, 1994.

192. I have discussed this issue in greater detail elsewhere. See Ussher, 1993.

193. Benton, D. & Wastell, V., 'Effects of Androstenol on Human Sexual Arousal', *Biological Psychology* 22 (2), 1986, pp. 141–7.

194. Beggs, V. E., Calhoun, K. S. & Wolchik, S. A., 'Sexual Anxiety and Female Sexual Arousal: A Comparison of Arousal during Sexual Anxiety Stimuli and Sexual Pleasure Stimuli', *Archives of Sexual Behaviour* 16 (4), 1987, pp. 311–19.

195. Alzate, H. & Londono, M. L., 'Vaginal Erotic Sensitivity', *Journal of Sex and Marital Therapy* 10 (1), 1984, pp. 49–56.

196. Hoon, P., Murphy, D. W. & Laughter, J. S., 'Infrared Vaginal Photoplethysmography: Construction, Calibration, and Sources of Artifact', *Behavioral Assessment* (6), 1984, pp. 141–52, p. 141.

197. Money, J., 'Commentary: Current Status of Sex Research', *Journal of Psychology and Human Sexuality*, (1), 1988, pp. 5–15, p. 5. Quoted in Tiefer, L., 'Commentary on the Status of Sex Research: Feminism, Sexuality and Sexology', *Journal of Psychology and Human Sexuality*, 43 (3), 1991, pp. 5–42.

198. Byrne, D., 'Introduction: The Study of Sexual Behaviour as a Multidisciplinary Venture', in *Alternative Approaches to the Study of Sexual Behaviour*, D. Byrne & K. Kelley (eds.), Hillsdale, N. J.: Erlbaum Associates, 1986, p. 2. Quoted in Tiefer, 1991, p. 5.

199. Money, 1988, p. 6. Quoted in Tiefer, 1991, p. 13.

200. For example, the International Society for Sex Research holds an annual conference which is open only to members or those sponsored by members. To become a member one must have published at least twenty papers in academic, peer-reviewed journals.

201. Masters, W. H. & Johnson, V. J., *Human Sexual Inadequacy*, Boston: Little, Brown, 1970, p. 199.

202. Masters & Johnson, 1966, p. 69.

203. Claimed by Hite in 1976 in a study of 3,000 women.

204. Reported in Garde, K. & Lunde, I., 'Female Sexual Behaviour: A Study in a Random Sample of 40-Year-Old Women', *Maturitas* 2, 1980, pp. 225–40, in a sample of 225 women.

205. All quotes are from the *DSMIII-R*.

206. Saunders, D. *The Woman's Book of Love and Sex*, London: Sage, 1985.

207. Cole, M., 'Sex Therapy for Individuals', in *Sex Therapy in Britain*, M. Cole & W. Dryden (eds.), Milton Keynes: Open University Press, p. 277. I have previously discussed this issue in Ussher, J. M. 'The Construction of Female Sexual Problems: Regulating Sex, Regulating Woman', in Ussher, J. M. & Baker, C., *Psychological Perspectives on Sexual Problems*, London: Routledge, 1993.

208. Kaplan, H. S., *The New Sex Therapy*, New York: Brunner/Mazel, 1974, p. 291.

209. Crabbe, Anthony, 'Feature-Length Sex Films', in *Perspectives on Pornography: Sexuality in Film and Literature*, Gary Day & Clive Bloom (eds.), London: Macmillan, 1988, p. 64.

210. Ibid., p. 64.

211. Cole & Dryden, 1988, p. 9.

212. See Hawton, K., *Sex Therapy: A Practical Guide*, Oxford: Oxford University Press, 1985; and Cole in Cole & Dryden, 1988.

213. See Jehu, D., 'Impairment of Sexual Behaviour in Non-Human Primates', in *The Psychology of Sexual Diversity*, Howells (ed.), Oxford: Blackwell, 1984, p. 135.

214. Pasini, W., 'Unconsummated and Partially Consummated Marriage as Sources of Procreative Failure', in *Handbook of Sexology*, J. Money & H. Musaph (eds.), Amsterdam: Elsevier/North Holland, 1977; and Catalan, J., Bradley, M., Gallawey, J. & Hawton, K., 'Sexual Dysfunction and Psychiatric Morbidity in Patients Attending a Clinic for Sexually Transmitted Diseases', *British Journal of Psychiatry*, 138, 1981, pp. 292–6.

215. Cooper, G. F., 'The Psychological Methods of Sex Therapy', in Cole, 1988, p. 137.

216. See Ussher, 1993, for a full discussion of these issues and for examples of studies suggesting these different aetiological roots for women's sexual problems.

217. See Ussher & Baker, 1993.

218. See Bancroft, J. *Human Sexuality and Its Problems*, London: Churchill Livingstone, 1983.

219. Ibid.

220. One researcher, John Money, makes a distinction between sexology and sexophosy (the latter being 'subjective', the former 'objective').

221. Altman, Meryl, 'Everything They Always Wanted You to Know: The Ideology of Popular Sex Literature', in Vance, 1984, p. 118.

222. Doyle, 1983, p. 205. Quoted in Tiefer, 'In Pursuit of the Perfect Penis', *American Behavioral Scientist*, 29, 5, 1986, pp 579–99.

223. *DSMIII-R*, p. 294.

224. Ibid., p. 295.

225. Ibid., p. 295.

226. Tiefer, 1986.

227. Melman, A., 'Development of Contemporary Surgical Management for Erectile Impotence, *Sexuality and Disability*, 1, 1978, p. 272–81.

228. Ibid.

229. See Tiefer, 1986.

230. Ibid., p. 583.

231. Kokken, S., *The Way to Married Love: A Happier Sex Life*, London: Souvenir Press, 1967, p. 93. Quoted in Jeffreys, Sheila, *Anticlimax: A Feminist Perspective on the Sexual Revolution*, London: The Women's Press, 1990, p. 140.

232. Masters, W. & Johnson, V. E., *Human Sexual Inadequacy*, Boston: Bantam Books, 1981, p. 294. Quoted in Jeffreys, 1990, p. 140.

233. The glaring absence of research on subjects such as female ejaculation was made clear with the advent of AIDS, when it was noted that there was little research information on the process of female ejaculation, let alone on the risk of transmission of AIDS through this fluid.

234. Ussher, 1989; Showalter, E., *The Female Malady*, London: Virago, 1987.

235. Maudsley, H., *Body and Mind*, London: Macmillan, 1873, p. 88.

236. Burrows, George Man, *Commentaries on Insanity*, London, 1828, p. 147.

237. Millar, J., *Hints on Insanity*, London: Henry Renshaw, 1861, p. 13.

238. Porter, Roy, 'Men's Hysteria in Corpore Hysterico?' paper presented at the Wellcome Institute symposium on the History of Medicine, History of Hysteria, 6 April 1990, London.

239. Sydenham, T., *The Works of Thomas Sydenham*, R. G. Latham (trans.), with a Life of the Author, 1848.

240. Plato, *Timaeus*. Quoted in Veith, I., *Hysteria: the History of a Disease*, Chicago: University of Chicago Press, 1965, p. 7.

241. Veith 1965:7.

242. Maddock, A., 'The Education of Women', in *On Mental and Nervous Disorders*, London: Simpkin Marshall, 1854, p. 177.

243. Ussher, 1989, p. 49.

244. Ibid.

245. See Ussher, 1989: and Ussher, Jane, *Women's Madness: Misogyny or Mental Illness*, Hemel Hempstead: Harvester Wheatsheaf, 1991, for developments of these arguments.

246. Ehrenreich, B. & English, D., *For Her Own Good: 150 Years of Experts' Advice to Women*, New York: Anchor, Doubleday, 1978.

247. See Graham, H. & Oakley, A., 'Competing Ideologies of Reproduction: Medical and Maternal Perspectives on Pregnancy', in *Women, Health and Reproduction*, H. Roberts (ed.), London: Routledge & Kegan Paul, 1981, for an analysis of the derogatory way in which medics converse with, or ignore, pregnant women.

248. Rich, Adrianne, *Of Woman Born*, London: Virago, 1986.

249. Berlin, F., 1988, p. 191.

250. Archer, John, 'Evolutionary Psychology', in *Male Violence*, J. Archer (ed.), London: Routledge, 1994, p. 265.

251. Ibid., p. 265.

252. Research on sexual attackers has shown that one third are married and having a sexual relationship with their wives at the time of the attack, and the majority are in consenting relationships. Gordon, M. T. & Riger, S. *The Female Fear*, Urbanna: University of Illinois Press, 1991.

253. Archer, 1994. p. 269.

254. Ibid., p. 269.

255. Ibid., p. 269.

256. Ibid., p. 270.

257. Ibid., p. 270.

258. Ibid., p. 270.

259. Ibid. p. 274.

260. Gallichan, W. M., *Sexual Apathy and Coldness in Women*, London: T. Werner Laurie, 1927, p. 101.

261. Chesser, E., *Love Without Fear*, London: Rich & Cowen Medical Publications, 1941, p. 66.

262. See Caputi, Jane, *The Age of Sex Crime*, London: The Women's Press, 1987, pp. 54–60, for a discussion of the hunter metaphor to describe sex killers.

263. Pavelka, M. S. & McDonald, S., 'Sexual Nature: What Can We Learn from a Cross-Species Perspective?' in Abramson & Pinkerton, 1995.

264. Smuts, B. & Smuts, R., 'Male Aggression and Sexual Coercion of the Female in Nonhuman Primates and Other Mammals: Evidence and Theoretical Implications', in *Advances in the Study of Behaviour*, P. J. B. Slater, M. Milinski, J. S. Rosenblatt & C. T. Snowdon (eds.), London: Academic Press, 1993, pp. 1–6.

265. Nadler, R. N., 'Sexual Aggression in the Great Apes', in R. A. Prentky & V. L. Quinsey (eds.), *Human Sexual Aggression: Current Perspectives*, New York: New York Academy of Sciences, 1988, pp. 154–62, p. 156.

266. Ibid., p. 156.

267. Ibid., p. 160.

268. Earls, C., 'Aberrant Sexual Arousal in Sex Offenders', in Prentky & Quinsey, 1988, p. 41.

269. Ibid., p. 41.

270. Berline, F., 'Issues in the Exploration of Biological Factors Contributing to the Etiology of the "Sex Offender" Plus some Ethical Considerations', in Prentky, 1988, pp. 188, 190.

271. Berline in Prentky, 1988, p. 191.

272. Langevin, R., Bain, J., Wortzman, G., Hucker, S., Dickey, R. & Wright, P., 'Sexual Sadism: Brain Blood and Behaviour', in Prentky & Quinsey, 1988, pp. 163–71, p. 165.

273. Langevin et al. in Prentky & Quinsey, 1988, p. 166.

274. See Archer, John, 'The Influence of Testosterone on Human Aggression', *British Journal of Clinical Psychology*, 82, pp. 1–28.

275. Ibid.

276. See Ussher, 1991.

277. See Showalter, 1987.

278. Weidegar, Paula, *Histories Mistress: A New Interpretation of a Nineteenth-Century Ethnographic Classic*, London: Penguin, 1985, p. 70.

279. Hoskins, E., 'The Hoskin Report: Genital and Sexual Mutilation of Females', *Women's International Network*, USA: Lexicon, 1979.

280. Bradford, J., 'Organic Treatment for the Male Sexual Offender', in Prentky & Quinsey, 1988.

281. Knight, Raymond, 'A Taxonomic Analysis of Child Molesters', in Prentky & Quinsey, 1988, pp. 2–20.

282. Cohen, M. L., Boucher, R. J., Seghorn, T. K. & Mehegan, J., 'The Sexual Offender against Children', presented at a meeting of the Association for the Professional Treatment of Offenders, Boston, MA, 1979.

283. Langevin et al. in Prensky & Quinsey, 1988.

284. Knight, in Prensky & Quinsey, 1988.

285. Walker, L. E., 'The Battered Woman Syndrome Study', in *The Dark Side of Families. Current Family Violence Research*, D. Finkelhor, R. J. Gellos, G. T. Hataling & M. A. Strauss (eds.), London: Sage, 1983.

286. Browne, L. *When Battered Women Kill*, London: The Free Press, 1987, p. 83.

287. Groth, A. N. & Burgess, A. W. 'Sexual Dysfunction during Rape', *New England Journal of Medicine*, 1977, pp. 764–66.

288. Halleck, S. L., *Psychiatry and Dilemmas of Crime*, LA: University of California Press, 1971.

289. Cohen, M. L., Garotrab, R., Bouscher, R., & Seghorn, T., 'The Psychology of Rapists', *Seminars in Psychiatry*, 3, 1971, pp. 307–27.

290. Revitch, E. & Schlesinger, L. B., 'Clinical Reflections on Sexual Aggression', in Prentky & Quinsey, 1988, pp. 59–61; Schultz, L. G., 'The Wife Assaulter', *Journal of Social Therapy*, 6 (2), 1960, pp. 103–12.

291. Snell, J. E., Rosenwald, R. & Robey, A., 'The Wife-Beater's Wife: A Study of Family Interaction', *Archives of General Psychiatry*, 11 (August), 1964, pp. 107–12.

292. Mendelssohn, B., 'The Origin of The Doctrine of Victimology', *Excerpta Criminologica*, vol. 3, May–June 1963, pp. 339–44.

293. Finkelhor, D. & Lewis, I. A., 'An Epidemiological Approach to the Study of Child Molestation' in Prentky & Quinsey, 1988, pp. 64–78.

294. See Frosh, Stephen, *Sexual Difference: Masculinity and Psychoanalysis*, London: Routledge, 1994, for an excellent discussion of masculinity and vulnerability.

295. Scully, D., *Understanding Sexual Violence. A Study of Convicted Rapists*, London: Unwin Hyman, 1990, p. 141.

296. Ibid, p. 104.

297. Ibid., p. 150.

298. Kelly, Liz, 'The Continuum of Sexual Violence', in Hamner, J. & Maynard, M., *Women, Violence and Social Control*, London: Macmillan, 1987, pp. 46–60.

299. For an excellent review of feminist arguments about rape, see Edwards, Anne, 'Male Violence in Feminist Theory: An Analysis of the Changing Conceptions of Sex/Gender Violence and Male Domination', in Hamner & Maynard, 1987, pp. 13–29.

300. Stiglmayer, Alexandra, 'The Rapes in Bosnia Herzegovina', in *Mass Rape: The War Against Women in Bosnia Herzegovina*, Alexandra Stiglmayer (ed.), Lincoln & London: University of Nebraska Press, 1994, p. 84.

CHAPTER FIVE

Violating the Sexual Body: Rape, Child Sexual Abuse and Sexual Murder

The law of rape stands as clear proof of the power of and force of a male rape fantasy. The male rape fantasy is a nightmare of being caught in the classic, simple rape. A man engages in sex. Perhaps he's a bit aggressive about it. The woman says no but doesn't fight very much. Finally she gives in. It's happened like this before, with other women, if not with her. But this time it's different. She charges rape. There are no witnesses. It's a context of credibility, and he is accused 'rapist'.

SUSAN ESTRICH, 1987[1]

Rape trials can be seen as a barometer of ideologies of sexual difference, of male dominance and female inferiority. Rape can be seen as a metaphor for women's rights to self determination, their right to say 'No', whether in regard to giving birth, having sex, or making other choices. An analysis of rape trials raises fundamental questions about the status of women and principles of equal rights.

SUE LEES, 1996[2]

I was petrified. It was the way he kept changing. He'd be so nice. Then all of a sudden he'd be totally different. He said 'I'm going to rape you if you like it or not.'

Statement of woman complainant in rape trial where the man was acquitted.[3]

The abstract debate on the socially constructed nature of sexual crimes, perversions or dysfunctions I have engaged in thus far may seem little more than academic navel-gazing when we turn to the material reality of sexual violence, to the subject of rape, child sexual abuse or sexual murder. To a person who is raped the fact that scientific and legal definitions of sex or of sexual crimes are both contradictory and open to change may seem an irrelevance, an issue of concern only to academics in the luxurious (or peculiar) position of being paid to think about sex. Yet the exposure of the fact that both sex and sexual crimes are socially constructed concepts that reflect hegemonic phallocentric representations of 'woman', 'man' and 'sex' is central to any understanding of the material reality of sexual violence and, in particular, the way in which both assailants and victims[4] are positioned in the machinery of the law.

In considering sexual violence, we invariably assume that it is men who are the assailants and women the victims. As I have argued, this is not always the case. Many men and boys are raped and sexually abused – although they often keep silent about such assault for fear of being told they 'wanted it really' and accruing the label 'homosexual' in a homophobic world. The law reinforces this invisibility by refusing in many contexts to categorize sexual assault against men as 'rape', as we have already seen. Conversely, women are capable of committing a sexual assault against a child, a woman, or a man – although those women who do so are in the minority, the majority of sexual assaults being committed by men. However, the focus of the discussion below is sexual violence between women and men, where man is perpetrator and woman is victim. This is because this is the most common manifestation of sexual violence, as well as the dominant representation of sexual violence within the law, and it is in representations of 'man', 'woman', and 'sex' within the law that I am interested here. Equally, as I am arguing that there is a continuity between representation and material practice in the sexual sphere and my focus is on representations of femininity framed within the boundaries of heterosexuality, I am concentrating my analysis on those practices which, arguably, represent the acting out of masculine fantasies and fears about femininity which populate art, film and pornography, examined above.

Sexual violence against women is an emotive subject, one to which many people prefer to turn a blind eye. This is understandable; it allows it to be positioned as something that happens to other people, not to us (or our mothers, sisters, friends or lovers). Yet if we look at the statistics on sexual violence it's clear that it is a subject we cannot ignore. However, 'official' statistics hardly suggest that it is a prevalent crime. Reported rates of rape in England and Wales[5] stood at 1,334 in 1983,

4,589 in 1993.[6] In the USA, according to FBI statistics, there were 109,062 attempted or completed rapes reported to the police in 1992; 106,590 in 1991; 102,560 in 1990.[7] From these statistics, it is estimated that only 1–2 per cent of women have experienced rape at some time in their lives.[8] Yet these official statistics reflect only reported crimes or offences followed by a conviction. Estimates arrived at from crime surveys or from research carried out at rape crisis centres, suggest that only 10–50 per cent of rapes are reported.[9] For example, a National Women's Study which surveyed rape in the USA in 1990 found that 13 per cent of American women had been the victim of at least one forcible rape in their lifetime and that only 26 per cent of them had ever reported the crime. This led to the estimate that one in eight, or over 21 million adult women in the USA had been raped – despite the fact that the study used a very conservative definition of rape, excluding rapes which happened to women under the age of eighteen (which constitutes six out of ten rapes). Other surveys suggest even higher rates. For example, in a random survey of women residents of San Francisco carried out in the early eighties, Diana Russell reported that 44 per cent had experienced attempted or completed rape.[10] In another study of over 3,000 women, Koss and her colleagues found that 54 per cent of women had experienced some form of sexual violence as adults, including unwanted sexual contact (14.4 per cent), sexual coercion (11.9 per cent), attempted rape (12.1 per cent) and rape (15.4 per cent).[11] These different estimates reflect the sample of women studied and the ways in which 'rape' is defined by the researchers. However, regardless of disagreements as to the actual percentage, the notion that only 1 per cent of women are the victims of rape is clearly a serious underestimate.

Focusing on men provides further confirmation of the distorted picture of sexual violence we see reflected in national statistics. In one study of known rapists and child molesters, it was reported that the sexual offences for which the men had been convicted amounted to less than half of those they had actually committed.[12] Similarly, in studies of men *not* convicted of sexual offences, a surprisingly high number of offences are admitted. In one study 2.4 per cent of men interviewed admitted to having raped.[13] More worryingly, in a study of nearly 2,000 male American college students, where men were allowed to report anonymously, Koss and Leonard found that over 40 per cent admitted to having perpetrated some form of sexual violence.[14] This included 4.3 per cent who admitted having carried out sexually assaultive behaviour, 4.9 per cent sexually abusive behaviour and 22.4 per cent sexually coercive behaviour. Other studies have reported that substantial proportions of men harbour fantasies of rape and admit that they would commit rape if they knew that they would get away with it. For example, in one study of 356 US college men 28 per cent said they would rape and use force, and 65 per cent said they would rape without force if they knew they wouldn't be caught.[15] In a further study 15 per cent of men reported that they would commit paedophilia if they could go undetected.[16]

As we have already seen adult 'rape' is just one form of sexual crime. In the 1993 statistics for England and Wales 17,350 crimes of indecent sexual assault against a woman were recorded; 268 incidences of unlawful intercourse with a girl under thirteen; 1,443 incidences of unlawful intercourse with a girl under sixteen; 484 cases of incest and 1,280 cases of gross indecency with a child (which may include boys and girls as victims). Of the twelve US states which report rape statistics in sufficient detail to distinguish juvenile from adult rape, 51 per cent of the rape victims were under the age of eighteen, and one in six under the age of twelve.[17] This has led to the estimate that, nationally, 17,000 girls under the age of twelve were raped in the US in 1992.

Arguably, these official statistics on sexual assault, and particularly childhood sexual abuse, are no more accurate than those on rape – if anything the figures are more misleading. For despite the widespread hue and cry around child sexual abuse in recent years, official statistics would suggest that less than 1 per cent of girls are sexually assaulted. Yet surveys of adult women give a very different picture, ranging from 12 per cent in a random community survey of 1,049 women carried out in Britain[18] to 54 per cent of women in a community survey of 930 in San Francisco.[19] Surveys of women attending clinics for psychological or sexual problems give even higher rates of prevalence of childhood sexual abuse – between 30 and 60 per cent.[20] Only a minority of children ever report childhood sexual abuse.[21] For example, in a study of 767 women survivors in Britain that I conducted in 1991 (see p. 380), in only 3 per cent of cases had the abuse been reported to the authorities. Only 46 per cent of women had ever disclosed the abuse to *anyone*, the majority telling husbands or boyfriends later in life if they did talk of it. So it 'officially' remains a hidden crime. As is the case with adult rape, the official statistics are merely the tip of the iceberg.

The disparity between official statistics on the recording of and convictions for sexual violence reveals much about the treatment of sexual violence in the law. Only a minority of reports eventually lead to a prosecution and an even smaller percentage to a conviction. Taking an estimate of one in ten rapes being reported, with 56 per cent of reports leading to arrest, and 36 per cent of those leading to conviction, it was estimated by Gilley in 1974 that only 0.9 per cent of rapes actually lead to conviction.[22] Today, it may be an even smaller percentage. As Sue Lees points out in *Carnal Knowledge*, her damning critique of rape law, whilst 24.4 per cent of the 1,842 recordings of rape made by the police in England in 1985 eventually led to the man's conviction, in 1994 the conviction rate was only 8.4 per cent of the 5,039 cases recorded[23] (and many of these convictions were reversed at appeal). In addition, many rape reports are 'downgraded' by the police to ABH (actual bodily harm) or indecent assault, so they never enter the rape statistics,[24] and the potential maximum penalty is reduced at the outset. This tightening of the law (or arguably the increasing inability to take the claims of women seriously) stands in stark contrast to the many press reports in both Britain and North America (and the claims of 'post-feminists' such as Katie Roiphe) that there has been an 'epidemic' of rape complaints leading to men being falsely accused and convicted.[25] It would seem from the statistics that men are *less* likely to be convicted if accused of rape today, regardless of the laudable efforts of the police to make the reporting of rape a less traumatic event for women (which may partially account for the increase in reporting).

The question is, how do we account for this? Much is explained if we look at the way in which sexual violence is positioned within the law (and by the media in their reports of rape trials). On the one hand the by now familiar phallocentric vision of 'sex' and 'woman', both reflected and reinforced by the law, serves to perpetuate myths about rape and functions to exonerate sexual crimes, which are positioned as the normal sexual behaviour of 'man' (or, paradoxically, if rape cannot be denied, as the actions of a 'mad rapist'). Arguably, it also encourages some men to carry out such crimes, because they know they can get away with it. At the same time, as Sue Lees has argued, the way in which prosecutions for rape are conducted is inherently biased against women (or men for that matter) who bring an accusation of rape. In the adversarial system used in England and the US, the complainant has no legal representation in court, no access to a lawyer before or during a trial. The state prosecuting counsel, whose role it is to be 'impartial', brings the case before the courts, yet is not allowed to meet the complainant before the case or even talk to her on the day of the trial.[26] Complainants are not allowed to see their police statement, often made a considerable time before the trial, until just before the court hearing, whilst the defence has had access to this statement for a much longer time.

In England, common-law rules on corroboration meant that, until 1995, when the Criminal Justice and Public Order Act 1994 came into force, judges had to warn juries about the dangers of relying on the uncorroborated testimony of two witnesses (it is now a discretionary warning). As Sue Lees has argued, 'The whole issue of corroboration is directly related to the question of reputation, if the woman is considered credible, then the idea is that corroboration is not necessary.'[27] Given this, it shouldn't surprise us that the whole basis of the defence in rape trials is invariably an attempt to undermine the complainant's reputation – putting her femininity, her status as 'good woman' on trial. It is here that the whole gamut of representations about 'woman' and 'sex' we have already examined comes into play, with, perhaps, the most serious material consequences. Positioning women as provocateurs, liars or simply fickle in changing their minds serves to deny or dismiss the claims of women who have been raped and to position sexual violence as simply 'sex'. This has considerable implications both for women who have been raped and for our understanding of what 'normal sex' is, as I will outline in detail below. It is understandable – and right – that men who are accused of rape should have the best defence that can be provided within the law. But when the cost is the annihilation of the woman complainant's reputation, and the reinforcement of phallo-centric myths about 'woman' and 'sex', grave questions must surely be asked about the machinery of the law.

Deconstructing 'Rape': 'It's Only a Bit of Sex, Isn't It?'

The Myth of the Reasonable Woman

The Judge

Women who say 'no' do not always mean 'no'. It is not just a question of saying 'no', it is a question of how she says it, how she shows it and makes it clear. If she doesn't want it she only has to keep her legs shut and she would not get it by force and there would be marks of force being used.[28]

The Professor of Law

Anyone who wants sex can learn to say 'yes'. No one who says 'no' should be subjected to another's sexual advances ... The transition from penetration of the mouth by the tongue to the penetration of an orifice by the penis is neither instantaneous nor unscripted. The partners will have time to object to sex acts they don't like, typically before those acts occur, and in any event immediately upon their initiation.[29]

The Doctor

A girl out of her first decade is seldom capable of being raped against her will without mark of forcible restraint or injury.[30]

I am perfectly satisfied that no man can effect a felonious purpose on a woman in possession of her senses without her consent.[31]

A fully conscious woman of normal physique should not be able to have her legs separated by one man against her will.[32]

The Rapist

At the time I didn't think it was rape. I just asked her nicely and she didn't resist. I never considered prison. I just felt like I had met a friend. (The woman was an employee of a store raped by the man as he robbed the store. He held a bayonet.)

I had intercourse with her, but I didn't hurt her at all. I didn't knock her about or anything.[33]

In essence, the law appears to reinforce the age-old view of men and women seeing the world through a different lens. Man is essentially innocent, stumbling around in the minefield of heterosexual romance, where the acts viewed as 'rape' by woman are believed to be 'sex' by a man. At the heart of the matter is the issue of consent; as many acts of consensual sex do not involve verbal discussion of willingness prior to sexual contact being initiated, the possibilities for misunderstandings or misinterpretation are always potentially present. It is assumed by the law (and, implicitly, by the man) that consent is given unless there is strong evidence to the contrary; in rape trials the prosecution counsel has to prove that the woman *didn't* consent.

In assessing evidence of consent, women are judged against the standard of how the 'reasonable woman'[34] would respond – clearly, shut her legs, say 'no', and then fight to the bitter end, according to the experts quoted above. The fact that a woman believed she was resisting, that she was saying rather than shouting 'no', is not enough; to the man this could clearly be 'normal sex'. The American case of *State* v. *Rusk*, described by Susan Estrich, is a good illustration of this.[35] Pat, the complainant, gave Rusk a lift home from a bar. No sexual intent was present – on her part. Dropping him off, he invited her up to his apartment. She said 'no', twice. Leaning over her, he took her car keys and insisted that she go inside. She did. He went to the toilet; she didn't leave. When he returned, he pulled her down on to the bed and removed her blouse. He then told her to take off her trousers, which she did. She was scared and said, 'If I do what you want, will you let me go without killing me?' She started to cry; 'he put his hands on my throat and started lightly to choke me; and I said, "If I do what you want will you let me go?" and he said "yes", and at that time, I proceeded to do what he wanted me to.'[36]

The courts did not see this as *real* rape and freed Rusk, based 'not on what Rusk did or did not do, but on how Pat responded'.[37] It was agreed that intercourse took place. It was agreed that Pat had not wanted it. But her 'resistance' was not sufficient. By being in a bar, by giving a man a lift, by entering his apartment, she was viewed as implicitly saying 'yes' to sex. So what was 'rape' to her was 'sex' to him. The court's verdict makes the situation clear:

> She may not simply say 'I was really scared' and thereby transform consent or mere unwillingness into submission by force. *These words do not transform a seducer into a rapist.* She must follow the *natural* instinct of every proud female to resist, by more than mere words, the violation of her person by a stranger or an unwelcomed friend. She must make it plain that she

regards such sexual acts as abhorrent and repugnant to her natural sense of pride. She must resist unless the defendant has *objectively manifested* his intent to use physical force to accomplish his purpose [my italics].[38]

So if *excess* force is not used the man can be positioned merely as a seducer, not a rapist. For as we are continually told, within the script of heterosexual romance, it is man's role to persist and the role of woman to resist, at least until force is *objectively manifested* (when the 'seduction' turns into assault). This highlights the phallocentric view of 'normal' heterosexual sex that underpins the treatment of sexual violence in the law: Coercion is positioned as part of the 'art' of seduction, merely an attempt to subvert the woman's initial resistance, the feigned 'no' which is part of the feminine script (the story of romantic fiction, pornography and scientific theories of sexuality). Yet women who are subjected to such threats fail to take such a benign view. To them the threat (and the rape) is 'real'.

If the legal or medical experts decide that a *reasonable* woman's will would not have been overcome in the circumstances described before the courts – because force as *men* understand it was not present – the definition of the act as 'rape' rather than 'sex' will be hard for the prosecution to prove. Central to this practice is the notion of the 'simple rape' – the representation of the rapist as a lone man and the rape as a violent encounter which a 'reasonable' woman will resist with all her power and which as a result will leave evidence of injury to validate the notion of *real* rape. Yet this is a misconception. Only 5 per cent of *convicted* rape cases involve injuries to the woman that require medical attention.[39] Most rapists do not need to batter women to gain submission; most rapists do not inflict life-threatening wounds that leave scars. Verbal threats or the fear of death are effective means of coercion. One man ensured his victim's silence by threatening her thus:

> I've raped three other women and killed them and that's what's to happen to you. Undress. If you don't hurry, I'll kill you. If you're not quiet, I'll kill you [poking knife at her nose and eyes]. Maybe I'll take off your nose too.[40]

He didn't cut off her nose. He didn't even need to beat her. No signs of 'resistance' were left for the courts to see. In these circumstances, women's fear for their lives may mean that their actions are not those of the 'reasonable' woman. The courts may believe that the 'reasonable' woman would fight, but most women would rather be raped and live, than die unviolated (they would probably be raped anyhow). It is death that is the fear at the centre of most acts of rape, a fear exploited by many rapists, as evidenced above. A woman who was raped by a cab driver described the attack:

> It was only when he got into the back of the car, pulling at the same time at his trouser belt to unbuckle it, that I realized in an instant of the purist clarity what was about to happen. I opened my mouth to scream as I edged away, but no sound came. I couldn't believe it. Surely I could *scream* at least. And then it was too late. His hand was over my mouth and I was being forced down on the floor of the car. All I could register, as the belt was pulled around my head like a noose, was that the name of the car was 'Avenger'.
>
> I shall spare you the details of what followed, mainly because I prefer to spare myself. Suffice to say that I was raped orally and anally as well as vaginally and under the continuous threat of the noose being pulled tighter I submitted, if submit is the word, because I realized I would rather be alive than dead.[41]

The contradictions in the law on this matter are illustrated by advice given to women on the ways effectively to survive a sexual assault. The dominant view given out by the police is 'Don't fight back', illustrated in a recent report on sexual offences, in which it is concluded that 'passive resistance and attempts to appeal to or reason with the assailant are probably safer and as effective as counter-attacks which may provoke more violence.'[42] As one woman raped by two men reported:

> When I started shouting he said 'Shut up or I will kill you.' He was very strong. Once I realized their intention I became very calm, almost detached from myself. I kept very still in the hope that they would do what they wanted and leave me alive.[43]

Resisting may actually result in the violence going on for longer. As a physician who treated many of the women raped during the war in Bosnia-Herzegovina commented:

> At first the women and girls were beaten black and blue, especially in the lower body region. Later on we didn't find that kind of injury on them

any more. The first ones probably told the others the best way to survive. A nineteen-year-old girl told me that she closed up tight inside. She lay down, tried to think of something else, and wasn't there; she blocked it out mentally. She said that all she felt was a foreign object penetrating her, something cold and hard that caused a ripping feeling. Then she said, 'When I could hear that he was drinking and cursing, I came to again. I stood up, and he said furiously "You're pathetic." ' The women probably figured out that that was the best way to survive and it was the least fun for the rapists. ' 'Cause if they resist, the men can take it as a challenge.'[44]

There may have been no 'marks of resistance', but there is no question that this woman was raped. Yet the paralysing effects of fear and the threat of death are denied in the law as 'reasonable' reasons for not resisting and the woman criticized for doing what many experts would advise.

The implicit assumption that 'normal sex' is violent is also evident in rape cases, where women with clear injury are not believed in their accusations of rape. In one case where the woman claimed to have been beaten and raped by two men and had extensive bruising all over her body to prove it, the defending counsel argued that this was a result of consensual sex:

Defending Counsel

There are not as many or as serious injuries as one might have expected from her account. What she does have is consistent with vigorous sexual intercourse with consent, but in rather cramped conditions . . . If she has been fighting for her honour as she says she was, there would be some sign of injury to the defendants, too. The examination shows that there wasn't – no sign of injury anywhere on them.[45]

Equally, a number of medical experts have been happy to testify that vaginal injuries are 'normal' during consensual sexual intercourse, invalidating women's claims that such injuries are evidence of rape. In the case of one woman who experienced vaginal tears which required stitching after an alleged rape, the medical witness testified:

There is not a single obstetrician who has practised over five years who hasn't seen such tears as a result of consensual intercourse in non-virgins. The dangers of inferring consent from genital injuries are commonly taught in forensic textbooks. These tears simply occur through penetration, where there is a disproportion in the size of those involved.[46]

Regardless of men's delusions of phallic grandeur, the vagina has the capacity to stretch to accommodate even the most enormous penis. No penis can match the size of a baby's head – the one thing that does 'naturally' tear the vagina during childbirth (although not in every case). Violent penetration of the vagina of a woman who is not lubricated because she is in no way sexually aroused is what results in internal tearing in women, or penetration of her vagina with an instrument that is designed to hurt. Yet, conversely, if a woman *doesn't* show internal injury, she can be positioned as having been lubricated and, by (inaccurate) implication, to have consented to sex. As one defendant commented, 'She enjoyed it. I think it got inside by itself. Or, I suppose, she was wet; she definitely wasn't dry.'[47] A similar line is sometimes taken by the defence counsel in cross-examination, as evidenced by the comments in one of the trials observed by Sue Lees:

Defence Counsel
He touched your vagina and it was lubricated.

Complainant
It was not lubricated.[48]

In the majority of rapes the vagina isn't lubricated – but even if it is, it doesn't necessarily indicate sexual arousal. Fear, alcohol and the stage of the menstrual cycle can all affect the level of lubrication, and many women have a moist vagina all the time.[49] Even if a woman *were* to respond sexually to her attack, does this mean that she is implicitly giving consent? Sexual arousal or response during the event is a not uncommon finding in both male and female victims of certain forms of sexual assault, as we have already seen.

Yet in 1975 the case of *DPP* v. *Morgan* enshrined in English law the notion that if a man *believes* that a woman consents to sex, regardless of her protestations, rape has not taken place. The case of *Morgan* v. *Morgan* concerned a husband and wife and an alleged rape by four men. Morgan and his three friends had been drinking. As they were unlucky in their quest to 'find some women', Morgan invited his three friends back to his home for sex with his wife. Whilst assured that she was compliant, if not keen, they were warned that she might struggle or feign resistance, as this was what turned her on. This, in fact was what happened during the act that was experienced by the woman as a rape. Whilst all four

men were convicted – the three friends for rape, and Morgan for aiding
and abetting – the issue discussed in the appeal to the House of Lords[50]
and subsequently in the British press was whether a man could be
convicted of rape if he believed, however foolishly, that the woman
consented. The House of Lords concluded that 'honest belief clearly
negates intent.'[51] to rape, and therefore the man could not be convicted.
Whilst the four men *were* convicted in *DPP* v. *Morgan*, as it was agreed
that no jury could have faith in the 'honest belief' of these four men
that the woman was consenting, in a later British case, using the
judgement in *DPP* v. *Morgan*, a man was acquitted of rape on the
grounds that he honestly believed in the woman's consent. The cases
were similar in that it was a man having sex with the crying wife of his
friend, the act taking place on the instigation of the husband.[52] So all
the man has to say is, 'I thought she wanted it really', and the law may
be lenient. As the representation of women enjoying rape, fantasizing
about rape and saying 'no' when they mean 'yes' is so prevalent in both
pornography and other forms of popular culture, it's not surprising to
find that so many men are exonerated.

The Triviality of 'Unwanted Sex'

Even if it can be accepted that the woman did not want to have 'sex',
the act of rape is often trivialized in the law. As one professor of law
commented in a recent debate on rape, 'Sex may be unpleasant, but it
is not the equivalent of a physical assault . . . people generally, male or
female, would rather be subjected to unwanted sex than be shot, slashed
or beaten with an iron tire.'[53] Again, the conflation of rape with sex
acts to diminish rape's importance and its effects. This can mean that
only the most severe acts (perhaps those involving an iron bar . . .) are
deemed worthy of serious punishment. Cases abound of rapists acquitted
because the act appears innocuous or because the victim *appears*
unharmed. In 1993 in Britain a fifteen-year-old boy was given a three-
year probation order for raping a fifteen-year-old girl who refused to
give him a kiss. He was told by the judge to give her £500 to go on a
holiday to 'help her get over it'. In 1986, in the 'vicarage rape case',
Jill Seward was raped by two men when a gang broke into her family
home. At the subsequent trial the judge, Mr Justice Leonard, described
her trauma as 'not so very great' (he later apologized for his comments),

and sentenced one of her assailants to five years for rape and five years for aggravated burglary, the other to three years for rape and five years for burglary and assault. Here is Jill Seward's description of her assault:

> The man is pulling down his trousers, pushing me to my knees in front of him . . . I can feel tears welling in my eyes. 'Don't you dare cry,' the man threatens. I blink back the tears and do as he demands. I am coughing and retching but how can you argue with a man who has erratic behaviour and a large knife.
>
> He orders me on to the bed, knocking Mum's neatly ironed washing to the floor. There are more instructions. Things I have never read about in textbooks. Or heard discussed at youth groups. This has nothing to do with the fulfilment of a committed relationship, special and complete. It is sordid, violent, with a total stranger who reeks of stale tobacco and beer like an old pub. I feel sick. Physically and emotionally. All I can do is pray, 'God, let me come out of this alive' . . . Man 2 launches into a fresh onslaught, this time on my own bed . . . I am being attacked from all angles, though Man 2 has an extremely limited vocabulary of four-letter words to express his demands. I switch off emotionally. This must be the kind of thing they put in pornographic movies, activities that take place in seamy studios behind darkened windows. Not in full daylight in my own room with the man's two accomplices wandering in and out at will.
>
> There is blood on the sheet. In my mouth. My blood. So much for trying to remain a virgin, saving myself for my wedding night. Who will want me now? Will I ever be able to live with myself after these depravities? I am retching again. I can't stand the sight of blood, let alone the taste, and am sickened by the acts this man seems to want me to enjoy. My body has become an object, a machine. It must stay like this if I am to survive.[54]

Jill Seward continued to be raped by two of the men, whom she says took great delight in finding out that this was her 'first time'. In meting out equal sentences for the burglary and the sexual assault, the judge considered Jill Seward's composure in court to be evidence of her recovery from the trauma. He didn't consider that she was splitting off her anguish and anger in court as she had done during the actual assault. He also took into account the young age of one of the men and his previous lack of convictions.

The view that child sexual abuse is not only innocuous, but potentially *beneficial* to the child takes the notion of rape as 'unwanted sex' one step further. Kinsey and his colleagues concluded in 1953, 'It is difficult to understand why a child, except for cultural conditioning, should be disturbed at having its genitalia touched.' Equally, in many instances, child sexual abuse is not considered as abuse if violence is not used; if the child is not otherwise physically hurt. A number of researchers have argued that any negative consequences of child sexual abuse can be attributed to reactions of parents, 'medical personnel, law enforcement and social officials, and social workers,'[55] rather than to the sexual abuse itself. As this line of reasoning goes, we would do better to leave well alone, and children would not suffer any negative consequences. These may be minority views – most people today agree that CSA is harmful to children. But some go further. Here are the confident assertions of a number of (often self-proclaimed) experts who maintain that sexual abuse has no negative effects at all, or that it can actually have positive benefits:

> [Many children] seemingly *benefited from* a sexual relationship with an adult without this preventing the development of normal sexual interests in adolescence and a sound marital adjustment in later years.[56]

> A careful review of the literature on adult-child [sexual] encounters clearly indicates that immediate negative reactions are minor or completely absent in the majority of cases, and significant long-term psychological or social impairment is rare.[57]

> In 19 years of working clinically with hundreds of adolescents and children, I cannot recall a single case of a client significantly psychologically damaged by sexual experiences. On the other hand, I can recall several tragic cases of children (and adults) psychologically devastated by stupid adult reactions to the discovery of sexual relationships.[58]

> There is little ground for saying that a paedophile experience will neces-sarily damage a child but . . . catastrophic reactions may sometimes occur in special circumstances, for instance if violence is used or if the child has some pre-existing emotional problem.[59]

In this view any negative effects of CSA are attributed to the 'meddling professionals' or to some weakness in the child, implying that pathology might have occurred anyway. Other experts may acknowledge that CSA has negative effects but dismiss their seriousness.

For example, Kinsey was quoted as saying that 'the reported fright was nearer the level that children will show when they see insects or spiders.'[60] In either case, the stark reality of statistics on the incidence and prevalence of sexual abuse can be ignored as the very notion of abuse is dismissed – it is simply 'sex'. This is a strategy effectively used by abusers as a means of keeping children silent, as the women in the survey of adult survivors of CSA I conducted confirmed when asked how they were stopped from disclosing:

> telling me we were doing nice things
> he said it was fatherly love
> by saying it was our private game
> pretending he was teaching me the facts of life
> by saying it was because he loved me[61]

Sex is not necessarily detrimental for children. As was outlined above, prior to the seventeenth century, the sexuality of children was an open and accepted part of life. Anthropologists have documented cases of societies where sexual play is not only allowed but openly encouraged between children and adolescents. Sexual games are condoned and sexual caresses to pacify children are a normal part of parenting in many societies[62] – and have no ill effects. Equally, it is undoubtedly the case that investigations in suspected cases of child sexual abuse can be damaging for the child.[63] As reported by women in rape cases, the child may experience the police questioning and the court case as a second assault and feel that they are marked as a liar if a conviction does not result. They also have to face the knowledge that they may have destroyed their family unit if the abuse is intrafamilial, or have to live with the person accused if a conviction is not brought. But this cannot be taken as evidence of the *benefits* of child–adult sexual contact or for turning a blind eye to child sexual abuse.

Any sexual activity between adult and child which occurs in the context of a power imbalance, where the sexual activity between adult and child is against the law and coercion of a verbal or physical kind has to be used as a consequence is not simply about 'sex', it is about exploitation and abuse of power. It is about physical and psychological coercion. Kinsey's seemingly innocent questioning of why children should be damaged by having their genitals touched must be seen in the context of a social order in which to touch a child sexually is taboo, forbidden and associated with serious sanctions, legal, moral and social – a social order in which child sexual abuse is seen as one of the most serious forms of deviancy. It is in this context that it is damaging to the child. When we examine in detail some of the mechanisms by which children are kept silent, it is not surprising that there are negative effects. In the aforementioned survey of 775 women survivors of CSA carried out in Britain ('n' being the actual number of women affected), the abusers maintained secrecy by the following means: saying that nothing was wrong (31.9 per cent, n =) 247), using threats/violence (28.5 per cent, n =) 221), saying it was their fault (20.5 per cent, n =) 159) and saying it would split up the family (25.4 per cent, n =) 197). Here are some of the ways in which the girls who were sexually abused were stopped from telling:

> by saying I'd be out in a home
> I belonged in a mental asylum
> it was done because I was evil
> I would be taken to hospital and Dr S. would do the same as he
> my mum and dad would be angry with me
> said no one would believe me
> by telling me he would kill me
> I'd get sent to prison
> you don't want to hurt your mother
> I'd be locked away
> saying I'd be punished
> a mad dog would get me
> he'd get my younger sister
> always telling me I was ugly
> monsters will get me
> he killed my pets

Making threats of this nature to young girls is no trivial matter – nor is the 'sex' that the threats were designed to conceal: In this study over 40 per cent had experienced sexual intercourse with their abusers; on average the abuse continued for five years; and the average age at which the abuse started was eight years of age. It was within the family that 80 per cent were abused.

Rape or child sexual abuse are distinguishable from 'sex', and have very different effects. Vast bodies of research now attest to both long-

and short-term traumatic effects of rape for a majority of women. It is commonly associated with depression, anxiety, sexual problems, eating disorders and a host of physical complaints. The same can be said of childhood sexual abuse.[64] Many women and children recover but many others are scarred for life, both psychologically and physically. Studies that ask women how it felt sexually find that no women report positive feelings or experiences. As one rape victim clearly says, 'there is no "sex" in rape. There is only pain – traumatic physical pain.'[65] Yet as Sue Lees has pointed out in her observation of rape trials, there is little or no space in the law for women to report these traumatic effects. One woman who started to explain how she felt about having been raped was silenced by the defence counsel, who said, 'This is beginning to sound like a speech.' In law, the only issue is whether 'rape' occurred, not whether it had a negative effect on the woman.

Women Enjoy Rape

The Police Surgeon

[Rape is] where a man or youth has at some time tried to take her knickers down: all the rest of the story is pure fantasy or wish fulfilment.[66]

The Lawyer

There are people [sic] who allege rape for some psychological reason. *It may be some sexual fantasy.* [my italics][67]

The Medic

It may be necessary to enquire how far lust was excited, or if she experienced any enjoyment. For without the enjoyment of pleasure in the venereal act no conception can possibly take place.[68]

The Rapist

If she told the truth she would have described me like any other girl. I try to make a girl enjoy herself as much as possible and she was no exception.[69]

One of the ways in which 'rape' is reframed as 'sex' in the law is through the myth that women enjoy rape *really*, once their initial reluctance had been overcome. One assailant who entered a woman's bedroom and then raped her as she slept claimed, 'Once she got into it, she was okay.'[70] Another, who raped a woman whom he had abducted in the street claimed, 'She told me I was a good lover and asked me where I had learned.'[71] As Diane Scully, who interviewed a series of convicted rapists, argues:

> One denier who had abducted his victim as she walked on the beach, could have been recalling a pornographic novel when he claimed: She said, 'No, I have my period. I'm a virgin.' I laughed and rubbed her back and she accepted physically. Her legs spread and she thrust up to meet me. It was telepathic. This wasn't rape. I know what rape is.[72]

A man who raped a fifteen-year-old girl on a beach at knife point echoed the view that women *have* to say 'no' because to say 'yes' would be to be positioned as 'whore':

> A man's body is like a Coke bottle, shake it up, put your thumb over the opening and feel the tension. When you take a woman out, woo her, then she says, 'No, I'm a nice girl', you have to use force. All men do this. She said 'no' but it was a societal 'no', she wanted to be coaxed. All women say 'no' when they mean 'yes' but it's a societal 'no' so they won't feel responsible later.[73]

Men may use this tactic as a means of justifying their own behaviour, during or after the sexual assault. Forcing the woman to feign pleasure or arousal can add to the man's fantasy of dominance and control. As one survivor said, 'He told me to wiggle and enjoy it. His penis was very large and he was hurting me.'[74] Others may actually believe that the woman is enjoying the assault, which explains why some rapists ask if they can see their victims again (also suggesting a very distorted view of courtship and 'sex'). As one woman who was raped commented:

> As soon as he had ejaculated he got off me, put himself straight, told me not to go to the police, because I wouldn't be believed, and he also asked me if he could phone me and take me out the next day.[75]

This is even more common in 'acquaintance rape' situations, where women are raped by men they know, or by men who have taken them on a 'date'.

The notion of a 'simple rape' – rape as an act which involves violence and is carried out by a stranger – being the norm is further discredited when we look at the statistics on 'acquaintance rape'. Over three quarters of women who are raped are violated by men that they know.[76]

This may be a friend, a 'date' or a husband. It may be another member of her family. In the majority of rape cases the woman is raped in her home, or in the home of the rapist.[77] So 'acquaintance rape' is not the exception – it is the norm. It is also the most invisible form of rape, as it has been estimated that less than 1 per cent of victims report the attack.[78] In many cases they do not believe they have a legitimate right to – they may acknowledge that they are the victims of an attack, but not _legitimate_ victims.

'Date rape'[79] – the term now coined by the media to describe all forms of acquaintance rape – has been accorded an inordinate amount of publicity by the media in recent years as a result of a number of well-reported trials in England and the United States. Three trials in England – that of the students Donnellan and Kydd, who were acquitted, and the solicitor Diggle, who was convicted[80] – as well as the trial of William Kennedy Smith in the US – were presented by the media as evidence that most accusations of 'rape' are unfounded and that the majority are the result of women changing their minds 'the morning after'. This is clearly part of a feminist backlash used to dismiss feminist arguments on rape – also seen in the inordinate amount of media publicity given to Katie Roiphe's argument that many women's accusations of date rape are spurred on by feminist propaganda which positions heterosexual sex as analogous to rape, and that women should be capable of saying 'no'. Yet this is a grossly inaccurate portrayal of cases of rape that get brought to trial – a case of what Susan Estrich has described as 'male rape fantasy' spoken through the mouth of a woman.

One of the assumptions behind the portrayal of 'date rape' is that women who put themselves in such situations deserve whatever they get, that date rape is merely casual sex, which in many circumstances a man is right to expect. Take this comment from a man who raped a woman on their second date: 'I think I was really pissed off at her because it didn't go as planned. I could have been with someone else. She led me on but wouldn't deliver . . . I have a male ego that must be fed.'[81] Another man, who abducted a woman at knife point from a party, provided a similar view; his expectations of sex, his outlay on the woman, meant that he deserved to be fulfilled:

> After I paid for a motel, she would have to have sex but I wouldn't use a weapon . . . I would have explained I spent money and if she still said

'no', I would have forced her. If it would have happened that way it would have been rape to some people, but not to my way of thinking.[82]

The law is not always sympathetic to such a view: In the Diggle case – where a woman solicitor was subjected to attempted rape by a colleague as they slept separately in the same room after a ball – the fact that the defendant claimed, 'I spent £200 on her. Why can't I do what I did to her?', when the police were called was used as evidence to indict him. However, arguably, this assumption was one of the factors which led to the acquittal of William Kennedy Smith, who was accused of raping a woman he had met in a local bar in 1991. The woman complainant had agreed to for a walk with him on a beach because, in her words, 'I was enjoying his company. He was an intelligent man. It was a nice night.' Smith wanted to swim, and took off his clothes. The woman declined:

> I turned my back. I don't think it was appropriate. I started to leave . . . I was yelling 'Good night, I'm leaving' and looking for the stair. I started up the stairs and was at the top of the steps and my leg was grabbed. It was a shock. Who could be grabbing my leg? I tried to get away. I lost my momentum and started to go down. I pushed off and started to run. I was very frightened. I couldn't figure why my leg had been grabbed. Mr Smith had been such a nice guy. If he was playing, I wanted to get away and say, 'Don't play with me.' But I never got that far.
>
> He had me on the ground and I was trying to get out from under him and I was yelling 'no' and 'stop' and I tried to arch my back but he slammed me to the ground, then he pushed up my dress and raped me . . . and I thought he was going to kill me.[83]

Smith was acquitted of rape. In his trial the judge disallowed testimony from three other women that they had been attacked in a similar way. The defence counsel argued that such an upstanding man, from a good family, could not commit rape. He had merely wanted (and had) 'sex' with a woman he had met four hours before. The case focused on proving that she was 'the sort of woman' who would do such a thing. So her underwear was revealed in court – ostensibly to demonstrate that it had not been torn, but as she had been wearing a see-through lacy bra, it served to raise questions about her morality to the court (sexy underwear signifying promiscuity). The jury believed Smith. As in all rape trials, it was merely her word against his: If the woman can be positioned as a slut, her reputation irrevocably damaged, then her word is worth next to nothing. Yet the representation of 'loose women' as 'false accusers' from whom the reputation of 'decent men' must be protected is not a recent one – it has pervaded legal considerations of rape for centuries.

'Women: The Most Decided Liars in Creation'[84]

The Lawyer

Human experience has shown that girls and women do sometimes tell an entirely false story which is very easy to fabricate but extremely difficult to refute. Such stories are fabricated for all sorts of reasons, which I need not enumerate, and sometimes for no reason at all.[85]

The Police Medical Officer

I am sure that everyone agrees that men and youths should be protected from wild accusations which can be made very easily by a woman seeking to get herself out of trouble with her husband, boyfriend or parents, out of spite or, simply, fantasy.[86]

The Rapist

I woke up being slapped around the face. I just hit out, slapped her back. She kept asking if I loved her, and I said I loved my wife. There was a row about this. She said she was going to get me for this.[87]

The positioning of 'woman' as liar is one of the oldest and most entrenched rape myths. For example, in 1865, when pontificating on the vexed subject of female accusations of rape, one eminent medical authority confidently claimed that most were in essence a 'false accusation . . . made from wilful and hysterical motives.'[88] This line of argument was used at the time to deal with a sudden increase in sexual assaults reported by women travelling alone in carriages on the newly introduced railways, the design of which ensnared the woman and her 'seducer' in a sealed compartment, isolated from the rest of the passengers on the train. These accusations of rape were viewed unsympathetically by the law, seen not as evidence of men's willingness to exploit the vulnerability of trapped women but of the fabrications of 'vile conspirators and blackmailers'. Of a hundred reported rape cases of this kind during the 1890s, one Birmingham police surgeon advised prosecution in only six. He warned that:

> The extension of railway travelling and the introduction of anaesthetics and new hypnotics, the ease with which an errant maid, when discovered, sheltered herself by making a charge of crime against her lover was then apparently made so much easier (1894, p. 226).[89]

As Susan Edwards has argued, there were two explanations for the 'false' accusations and supposed lying: Women were malevolent or, more benignly, women fantasized about seduction and thus imagined it. The increase in women's accusations of sexual assault by medics using the newly developed anaesthetics in the late nineteenth century were not examined seriously for evidence of abuse of power – or abuse of the woman's chemically induced vulnerability – but dismissed as the wanderings of the errant female mind. This comment is echoed almost a century later by a medico-legal expert, showing the continuity of the belief in female fantasy, either from innocence or ill will:

> There is particular risk in medicine and dentistry of unfounded allegations of indecent assault, either through malice or through confusion following anaesthetics for dental or minor operations. The allegations of a woman when recovering from the effects of gas and oxygen or intravenous barbiturates are not always malicious, the effects of the narcosis sometimes leaving genuine belief in a woman's mind that she suffered sexual interference.[90]

We might question whether it is to protect women from sexual violation or to protect men from false accusations that a female nurse or assistant now has to be present when any anaesthetics are used.

The more malevolent view of women making supposedly 'false' accusations of rape is that women of loose morals change their minds, absolving themselves of all responsibility for sex by simply saying 'no' after the event. Historically, these women have been doubly guilty – not only have they lied, casting an unpardonable slur on a man's good will and character, they have also been sexual outside the controls of matrimony and so are at risk of being positioned as 'whore'. In asserting that 'it must be remembered that every alleged act of rape is not necessarily one', Gaister advised the legal profession of 1925 that:

there were many adult females of loose morals who, though consenting parties to sexual connection at the time, later [became] conscious-stricken, and to alter the complexion of their act after it (had) been committed, (laid) a charge of rape against the partner of their illicit romance.[91]

Another interpretation of a woman's 'lie' is that she is confused, she just does not know her own mind. As one nineteenth-century expert sagely commented, 'sometimes really she does believe subsequently that she did not consent to intercourse at the time.'[92] Or as a defendant in a recent rape trial commented, 'I'm saying she wanted it. Her body wanted it, but her mind was somewhere else.'[93] The corollary to this view of the fickle or forgetful woman is that in reality she has a deep pathology which motivates a woman to fabricate a rape charge. As an authoritative text of 1940 declares:

Modern psychiatrists have amply studied the behaviour of errant young girls and women coming before the courts in all sorts of cases. Their psychic complexes are multifarious, distilled partly by inherent defects, partly by diseased derangements or abnormal instincts, partly by bad social environment, partly by temporary physiological or emotional conditions. One form taken by these complexes is that of contrary false charges of sexual offences by men. The unchaste . . . mentality finds incidental but direct expression in the narration of imaginary sex-incidents of which the narrator is the heroine or the victim.[94]

Here the whole gamut of accusations levied against 'woman' are exposed. She has 'inherent defects' – the natural weakness reminiscent of Darwin's view that women were closer to nature, more like animals and children than men. She is afflicted by 'diseased derangements or abnormal instincts' – echoes of the myth of female malady, woman's instinctive proneness to madness or lability, which litters psychiatric treatises from the nineteenth century to present day.[95] She is afflicted by 'physiological or emotional conditions' – perhaps her raging hormones or her fluctuating irrational moods? This sustains the myth that 'woman' is victim of her emotions, driven by changing whims and moods, but unreliable and open to influence. The allusion to 'bad social environment', to the 'unchaste mentality', rounds off the picture. Woman is not only mad, she is potentially bad. Whatever the interpretation, her word is not to be trusted. And this is not a historical anachronism. In a recent trial the defence counsel argued, 'I am not suggesting that she is barking mad, but she may have underlying problems that have brought her to lie this way.'[96] In another trial, where a man was accused (and acquitted) of raping his daughter, his barrister declared: 'These are allegations made by a mental patient against a man of good character. The notes [her medical notes] show gross disturbances. The notes reveal that she is prone to fantasize about such matters.'[97]

The fact that the law accepts these misrepresentations of 'woman' means that one of the most common defences used by men in rape cases is that women change their minds, that they seek revenge on a man, or simply that they want sympathy and attention. Yet what woman would go through the horror and degradation of a rape trial for such motives? This again reflects *men's* fears rather than women's – the fear that an innocuous action will be misunderstood, that a simple flirtation will result in a cry of rape, that *they* could be standing in the dock, accused by a confused or malevolent woman. This is undoubtedly one of the reasons why the press greeted the acquittal of student Austin Donnellan (who was accused of raping a fellow undergraduate at King's College London) with glee.[98] In being presented as a wrongly accused man fighting for his rights and his reputation he stood for the fears of many men.

Yet not all acts of sexual violence can be deconstructed in this way – recategorized as 'sex' and therefore as enjoyable or acceptable or dismissed as the fantasies of a hysterical lying woman. In many cases the rape is too violent or too abhorrent, the child or woman clearly abused. Yet the reputation of the woman is still not immune from attack in such cases; rape and sexual abuse can still be denied, and the man excused and exonerated, through the myth of female precipitation.

Man Can't Resist Her

The Seductive Woman
Pretty girls cannot go on to beaches and not expect to have advances made towards them. But they should not be violent or threatening advances.[99]

The Seductive Child

A certain amount of coy seductiveness among small girls tends to be encouraged as natural and charming, provided that the sexual element is not too overt, but some girls will actively solicit and seem to enjoy the sexual attentions of adults.[100]

The Vulnerable Man

We are all liable to fall, gentlemen; we must be lenient.
(Judge sentencing man for a sexual assault on a seven-year-old girl.)

I am satisfied we have an unusually sexually promiscuous young lady. And he [the defendant] did not know enough to refuse. No way do I believe [the defendant] initiated sexual contact.[101]
(Judge sentencing a man to ninety days' work for sexually assaulting five-year-old daughter of his lover.)

The most pervasive rape myth is that sexual violence is woman's fault. Through being seductive or desirable, or being in the wrong place at the wrong time, she incites man to rape. So men have been exonerated from rape because the woman was hitchhiking, drinking or because she accompanied a man out of a bar:[102] Her alleged assailant acted as men naturally do in such situations – he 'seduced' her. This reflects and reinforces the myth of uncontrollable male sexuality – once roused, necessarily expressed. There is also an implication that if a woman is seductive or if she makes herself attractive, she is marking herself out as willing, because she must know the effect she has on man. This justifies the display of women's underwear in rape cases (the man's is never shown) and the discussion of her general clothing or appearance. This positions rape as a response to desire, a 'normal' man's reaction to an attractive woman. As the judge asked the defendant in a rape trial, 'Did you find her attractive as a woman, a girl?' Answered in the affirmative, he continued, 'When you went into the bedroom you must have thought it was Christmas and Easter put together when you found her naked in your bed.'[103] This view of rape as response to an attractive woman was evident in a report of a recent British Home Office survey on sexual violence,[104] in which women's appearance is clearly deemed paramount (or if she is *not* attractive, some other explanation is needed):

[The fact that half the rape victims were women aged between thirteen and seventeen] probably reflects the *ages of maximum attractiveness* and availability to offenders (my italics).[105]

It has also been noted that victims can be of singularly plain and unprovocative appearance. This might be particularly understandable where the motive is not primarily sexual. Moreover, it may be that some rapists, especially those with sexual inhibitions, are put off by girls who look aggressively sexual.[106]

A classic double bind: Women are at risk if they are attractive but also if they are *un*attractive – sackcloths and ashes are clearly no protection. The irony here is that women are positioned as 'asking' for rape if they follow the traditional feminine masquerade – if they wear make-up, high heels and 'sexy' clothes – if they 'do girl' as they are told that they should. This is an interesting reversal of the more ubiquitous notion that femininity is 'natural'; here it is implicitly positioned as something about which women have a choice. In rape law, it appears that in choosing to wear feminine (or in any way sexy) clothes, women are seen to be choosing to look like a 'tart' or a 'slag' and thereby putting themselves at risk. This is used to imply that she actually *is* a tart and thus to exonerate the man accused of rape (because for woman positioned as whore, rape is deemed impossible). As one rapist who abducted a woman at knife point commented, 'to be honest we knew she was a damn whore and whether she screwed one or fifty guys didn't matter.'[107] The law manipulates this prejudice against women: In a recent study interviewing defence lawyers, the majority admitted they attempted to create a 'smokescreen of immorality around the girl'.

In Britain, the first legal admission of moral character as evidence against the woman raped was the case of *R v. Hodgson* (1811–12).[108] This set the precedent of putting the reputation of the woman on trial, meaning that any woman deemed 'whore', any woman who is sexually available or solicitous, is at risk of being denied the protection of the law. One rapist said in his own defence, 'She wanted it. She wanted it all ways, so I done it up her arse. She's a slag. She needs sorting out.'[109] This is analogous to the excuses put forward by three men who raped a woman they met in a pub: She was just a whore, 'sex' was what she wanted, so 'sex' (in their minds) was what she got:

First Defendant
A girl came in [the pub] and she had a row with her boyfriend. She was buying drinks. She was putting herself about, just a slag. It was 'Hello, darling, you in the red shirt, I fancy you.'

Second Defendant
She was drunk when she came in. She got herself a gin. She was joined by her boyfriend and bought a pint. She was over everybody. She smelt like an old fishpond. She pulled someone to her knee, she was dancing about.

Third Defendant
The way she behaved, I thought she was a bit of an old bag.[110]

In this case the sexual availability of the woman ('just a slag'; 'over everybody') was compounded by her being 'drunk', foul mouthed and having 'a row with her boyfriend' – all emphasizing her lack of femininity. Her supposed smell – 'like an old fishpond' – further stressed her difference from the good 'feminine' woman, who is always fragrant and pure.[111] Yet it isn't just what a woman does *now* which puts her at risk of being designated 'whore', it is anything she has ever done in the past. Few women are immune from castigation.

Before the previous sexual history of a woman was deemed inadmissible evidence in rape trials,[112] it was very likely to be used as a mainstay of the defence if a woman brought an accusation of rape. However, in her study of rape cases at the Old Bailey in London, Zsuzsanna Adler found that in over 60 per cent of rape cases where the identity of the man was unquestioned, an application was made to introduce evidence of the prior sexual history of the woman complainant.[113] If a woman steps outside the narrow boundaries of the feminine script – as so many women do – it can be used to discredit her testimony and dismiss her allegation of rape.

Such was the case in three trials where the female victims were aged between fourteen and seventeen – an age at which 'good' girls should be innocent of all experience of sex. The young women were not virgins, which was used as grounds for application under s.2 of the 1976 act that is, the man believed the woman consented.[114] The implication was clear: If she has had sex once, she will easily do so again. Or the rape is merely 'sex'. As one defence lawyer proclaimed:

> The defence [for the man accused of rape] is consent, and this is relevant to establish consent: the fact that this was not the complainant's first experience of sexual intercourse. If it were, it would be heavily against the defendant. The matter ought to be before the jury, or, in view of her age, they might draw inaccurate conclusions about her virginity.[115]

In another case, the defence for a 'coloured' man who raped a white woman was based on the same line of argument, as the defence counsel argued:

> I want to show that the complainant was not averse to having sexual intercourse with coloured men. The jury should have no presumption of lack of consent because of the colour of the people involved here. Her sexual experience was almost entirely with coloured men.[116]

This woman was 'guilty' of sex outside her racial group; in a racist society a white woman having sex with a black man may be deemed perverse and be likely to be condemned. Saying 'yes' to one 'coloured' man is constituted to imply she would say 'yes' to all – so, by definition, 'rape' cannot have occurred. In another case, the fact that the woman had had sex with a man prior to being raped was brought forward as a mitigating circumstance in the attack. The defence counsel argued: 'The defendant wore a contraceptive and there should not have been any semen in the complainant when in fact there was. The only explanation is that she had intercourse with another man that evening.'[117] By implication, a woman who has recently had consensual sex is incapable of being raped, or, she was sexually active and therefore rape (seen as 'unwanted sex') was less traumatic than if she had been a virgin. Unsurprisingly, for women working as prostitutes, a rape allegation is even more difficult to prove.

Technically, the law in Britain did recognize that a prostitute could be a victim of rape as long ago as 1841, in the case of *R* v. *Hallett*;[118] yet the fact of a woman being a prostitute continues to be used in a court of law as a means of dismissing a charge of rape to this day. Even in the case of *R* v. *Hallett*, the eight men who raped a woman who was known to be a prostitute were convicted of assault, not rape. The jury who passed such a verdict were undoubtedly influenced by the comments of the presiding Judge Coleridge, who declared:

> It is well worthy of your consideration whether, although she at first

objected, she might afterwards (on finding that the prisoners were determined) have yielded to them, and in some degree consented; and this
question is more deserving of your attention when you consider what
sort of person she was, what sort of house she lodged in, and that she
herself told them that she would make no objection if they came one at
a time.[119]

As Susan Edwards has argued, throughout the late nineteenth and
twentieth centuries, lawyers repeatedly used the allegations of prostitution as a defence for rape. In *R* v. *Clay* in 1951, the testimony of a
policeman that he had seen the woman working as a prostitute twenty
years before was allowed.[120] In *R* v. *Greenberg* in 1923 the presiding
judge seemingly dismissed the possibility of rape of a woman working
as a prostitute, commenting that 'people do not always ask for what
they expect';[121] and in *R* v. *Bashir & Manzur* in 1969 Mr Justice Veale
allowed the defence counsel to introduce evidence that the complainant
was a prostitute, saying that whilst in any other case he might not allow
such evidence, with rape 'special rules apply'.[122]

Attacking Man's Property

Rape is often positioned not as an attack on women, but as a violation
of the property of man, as this tract on rape in a Yale law journal of
1952 makes clear:

> The consent of a woman to sexual intercourse awards the man a privilege
> of bodily access, a personal 'prize' whose value is enhanced by sole
> ownership . . . the man's condemnation of rape may be found in the
> threat to his status from a decrease in the value of his sexual possession
> which would result from forcible violation.[123]

A raped wife is clearly a soiled wife. This is arguably why the rape
of an 'honest', married woman, or the rape of a virgin is deemed much
more serious in the eyes of the law. Her worth has been lowered within
the boundaries of the heterosexual script. So prior to the Matrimonial
Causes Act of 1857, s.59, a British husband cuckolded through seduction,
rape or adultery could bring an action for damages against the man who
had violated his property – his wife[124] – even if they were already
separated. And whilst women murdered by their husbands make up

over three quarters of all matrimonial murders,[125] men who are suspected or known to be involved with a man's wife are often killed as part of retribution or revenge. The law does not officially condone but, again, is sympathetic in such cases.

This implicit positioning of woman as property is also recognized by many rapists; they know that to rape a woman is to attack a man. The motive for rape can spring from a realization of this fact – an attack on man through the violation of his woman. As one rapist recounted:

> I grabbed her and started beating the hell out of her. Then I committed the act. I knew what I was doing. I was mad. I could have stopped but I didn't. I did it to get even with her and her husband.[126]

Rape within war can be interpreted similarly. Woman as the spoils of war – symbolic desecration of the enemy through the possession of woman. In the mass rapes of Bosnian women reported in the war in the former Yugoslavia and the civil war in Rwanda, the women were doubly victims – raped by the enemy soldiers and subsequently rejected by their own communities, particularly their men. It is arguable that this systematic abuse of women, only recognized as a crime against humanity in 1992, in a United Nations Security Council statement, is one of the most effective means of attacking men – damaging and degrading their possessions, their women, and ensuring a complete breakdown of all social order. Families are riven apart by these women being rejected, a situation which adds to the trauma of the women who have been raped and results in many of the rapes going unreported.

Many men react to the rape of 'their' woman with revulsion and blame, often feeling great anger about the fact that their woman has 'allowed herself' to become 'damaged merchandise', 'unclean' or 'tainted'. One man reported feeling physically disgusted when he went near his wife after her rape.[127] This can add to women's shame, guilt and sense of complete violation, as well as the feelings of self blame. These are the comments of one woman, Sedeta, talking about the rape of herself and her friend during the Bosnian war:

> She was much worse off than me. She said that she and her mother and two sisters had been at home when the Chetniks came. One of them asked who was still a virgin. She told them she was, 'cause you could see she was anyway. He told her to go with him so she could pick out a man.

They tortured her and beat her. Luckily, she survived. And she didn't get pregnant either.

Maybe that's their way of hurting Muslim women and Croatian women, and the whole female race. It's a lot more fun to torture us, especially if they get a woman pregnant. They want to humiliate us . . . and they've done it too. Not just in my case, either, all the women and girls feel humiliated, defiled, dirty in some way for the rest of their lives . . . I feel dirty myself somehow. And I feel as though everybody can see it when they pass me in the street. Even though it isn't true, no one could know about it. But the humiliation is there.[128]

All this blaming of the victim of sexual violence – for being seductive, foolish or beneath contempt – serves to focus on woman as provocateur rather than on man as rapist. Public circulation of these myths acts to keep women in check and ensure that they don't stray too far from the confines of femininity, because they know what their punishment could be. It's not surprising that women blame themselves for rape.

I kept wondering if I had done something different when I first saw him that it wouldn't have happened – neither he nor I would be in trouble. Maybe it was my fault . . . My father always said whatever a man did to a woman, she provoked it.[129]

I felt guilty. I felt it was my fault because I had been drinking. I felt angry at myself for not having fought or screamed louder.[130]

Yet the notion that the rapist targets only loose or seductive women or that women are to blame is patently untrue. In her study of men who rape, Diane Scully provides chilling evidence for the random nature of the majority of the sexual attacks, particularly where the victim is not known by her attacker. Many women were raped because they just happened to be there – nothing special about them caught the rapist's eye. In one case a pregnant woman in a supermarket car park became the rapist's victim because she was the first person to come along: 'She was an easy target.' He threatened her with a knife and raped her, saying afterwards, 'I wasn't thinking about sex. But when she said she would do anything not to get hurt, probably because she was pregnant, I thought "Why not?" '[131]

Like many women raped, this woman's 'mistake' was to be in the wrong place at the wrong time. But many defence lawyers will still look (and find) reason to condemn the woman, given the narrow boundaries of 'respectable' femininity women are judged against in the law. Men who rape are clearly aware of this and may view the law – as well as women's fear of reporting rape – as giving them a license to abuse. Here are the comments of two convicted rapists interviewed by Diane Scully:

> At the time I didn't think of it as rape, just fucking, but I knew I was doing wrong. But I also knew most women don't report rape and I didn't think she would either.

> I knew what I was doing. I just said, the hell with the consequences. I told myself what I was going to do was rape . . . but I didn't think I would go to prison. I thought I had gotten away with it.[132]

This is chilling in the light of the research cited earlier that shows that a high percentage of men would rape if they too thought they could get away with it.

Gang Rape – 'Running a Train'

In gang rape many of the misogynistic assumptions underlying both the execution and representation of sexual violence can be seen at their clearest. Documentation of gang rape comes mainly from North America, where campus rapes of women by male college students have been reported to be alarmingly common.[133] This is perhaps the most extreme and brutal version of 'date rape', often involving serious injury to the victim. In most cases the rape is deliberate and planned. The formula is simple. One member of a gang asks a woman out on a date. Unbeknown to her, the other members of the gang are waiting in a predetermined spot, usually an isolated and deserted place where the woman is taken. The whole gang then rapes her.

Diane Scully interviewed a number of men who reported taking part in over thirty of such 'gang date rapes'.[134] One man reported that he and his friends had gone as far as to rent a house for the purposes of such 'recreation'. They excused their behaviour by the familiar tactics of claiming that the woman enjoyed it or that she was a whore, or that she provoked it (by the crime of wearing lacy clothing in one case, no bra in another). When all else fails, she was positioned as having only reported it because the men left her after the 'sex'. In one case, a woman had been abducted on the street after having left a library. As Diane Scully, who interviewed one of the men, describes:

> The victim was blindfolded and driven to the mountains, where, though it was winter, she was forced to remove her clothing. Lying on the snow, she was raped by each of the men several times before being abandoned near a farm house.

One of the men – who described gang rape as 'the ultimate thing I ever did'[135] – argued that the woman reported it only because the gang who abducted her subsequently abandoned her, not doing the 'gentlemanly thing' and spending the night with her. In a case of four football team-mates from Glenn Ridge, New Jersey, accused of sexually assaulting a 'mentally incapacitated' woman with a broom handle, a baseball bat and a stick, as well as forcing her to perform fellatio and masturbation, the defendants claimed that the woman consented to the acts in order to gain affection, friendship, and a date.[136] In court, the woman was said to be 'sex obsessed'; her injuries were dismissed by the defence on the grounds that she was a 'full-breasted, full-bodied' woman, who was on the Pill[137] (and, by implication, ready for sex). Both of these cases represent the most extreme distortion of the view that women desire male attention and affection and will put up with extreme violation to obtain it, or that women want the 'beast'.

As women rarely report gang rape, arguably, men are supported in their fantasy that the victim wanted the 'sex' really. Yet it is not surprising women don't report it. They are often known to the men involved and have agreed to go out on a date (allowing the men to claim that the woman knew what she was letting herself in for). What woman would want to relive the ordeal of a trial when she had publicly to expose this ultimate violation, often by men she thought of as 'friends', who would all back each other up in their own defence? She has no hope.

Perpetrators of gang rapes in American colleges have been almost impossible to prosecute. In one study of twenty-four cases, of which nineteen were reported to the police, only one conviction resulted.[138] It appears that the courts, the college authorities and the relatives of the 'respectable men' who stand accused cannot believe that such acts of violence can be carried out by decent men. The myth of the monstrous man as rapist works to support their defence. The men can argue that gang 'sex' took place not rape, that the men were merely 'running a train' on the woman.[139] It is interesting that group sex with a distressed and subsequently injured woman is considered normal sexual practice for these 'good upstanding men'.

This also assumes that some women are amenable to participation in group 'sex' (with in many cases up to twenty men), that being the object of 'running a train' is erotic and arousing. What woman would agree, except perhaps in the pages of pornographic fiction? In the case of the gang rape of a seventeen-year-old woman by seven college students at Michigan State University in 1984 the 'fact' that the woman was a whore who wanted group sex was the main argument of the defence. The high moral standing and middle-class status of the seven men were contrasted with the low status of the female victim, who was depicted as a 'streetwise ghetto kid.'[140] On the same lines, one young college man interviewed on the subject of rape talked of how a woman was selected weeks in advance for 'running a train' because she was promiscuous and therefore supposedly wouldn't mind.[141] Her 'promiscuous' nature merely acted to excuse their vicious abuse. Other gang rapists position the woman as invisible, as a non-person, and similarly exonerate their own action. One rapist commented, 'We felt powerful, we were in control. I wanted sex and there was peer pressure. She wasn't like a person, no personality, just domination on my part. Just to show I could do it – you know, macho.'[142]

Many of these college gang rapes take place in fraternities, often by athletes, in particular football- or basketball-team members.[143] They are also very common in war. Being part of a masculine 'gang' appears to encourage abuse of a woman. As was the case with the group viewing of porn, gang rape can serve the function of maintaining group solidarity. The normal inhibitions regarding sexual violence held by individual men are lifted in the group pressure of the rape situation and allow men to act out a violent fantasy. Men can demonstrate that they are 'man'; they are heterosexual, potent and able to be in control of 'woman'. They can ward off anxieties about impotence, about homosexuality (despite gang rape being a potentially homoerotic act), and about being vulnerable, needy or romantic – all despised 'feminine' traits. Being 'man' they can publicly fuck without needing to have thoughts or feelings about the object of their desires. Men who refuse to engage in gang rape may be at risk of being seen to fail as 'man'. One woman raped in Bosnia reported:

> Drago [the commandant] brought different gangs who were supposed to rape me . . . Some men didn't want to go along with it. He hit them and asked, 'You mean, you really don't want her?' and then they did rape me after all.[144]

Research on gang rape has shown that it is characterized by a greater degree of denigration and violation of the woman's body. Sue Lees comments that it is twice as likely that gang rape will involve 'insult, forced fellatio, pulling, biting and burning the breasts, urinating on the victim, and putting semen on her body'.[145] We could interpret this as an acting-out of a pornographic script – where these are common depictions of 'sex'. Or we could say that both the representation and the practice of this denigration of 'woman' reflect the deep-seated dread and disgust which pervades the psyches of many men. One woman, Marija, described her rape in Bosnia in 1991:

> He knocked on the window. 'Open up, I'm bringing you guys a real lioness.' When he led me into the house he said, 'Here she is, I've done my job.' They stripped me naked right away and forced me to kiss and lick their penises. Seven of them raped me and I had to satisfy them orally. I had the blindfold on the whole time. They raped me, one after the other. They held knives to my breasts and other parts of my body. When one of them pressed a knife to me again, I heard one of them call out, 'Obrad, we didn't agree to that!' For me the worse part was that I had to swallow their semen and urine. The whole time someone kept swearing, 'Fuck the Ustasha mother, where's the gold your son stole?' He grabbed my breasts several times and punched me in the belly. When I couldn't swallow anything any more they threw me out on to a cement floor. Later they brought me back in again. The whole thing lasted two hours.[146]

Can this ever be conceived of as 'sex'? It is the humiliation, degradation and desecration of woman through *her* sexuality; it is a violent act of assault through which men assert their phallic power and their contempt and disdain for woman as object. When she is treated thus, she is not fearful, she does not challenge their authority or control; she is meant to be used and abused. In some instances – such as the use of 'comfort women' by the Japanese army during the war – this is legally considered to be 'sex', not rape; another example of the law protecting man's right to the body of woman, regardless of her will or desire.

Legalizing access to women

Marriage: A Licence for Violence

> But the husband cannot be guilty of a rape committed by himself on his lawful wife, for by their mutual matrimonial consent and contract the wife hath given herself in this kind unto the husband which she cannot retract.   CHIEF JUSTICE OF ENGLAND, 1736

> If you can't rape your wife, who can you rape?
>   CALIFORNIA STATE SENATOR, 1980

The 'marital exemption' to rape, first outlined in the sixteenth century, is perhaps the most ubiquitous form of legalized violence against 'woman'. Until 1991 rape within marriage was not recognized in English law. Its introduction in the statute-books did not result in a flood of accusations of rape – (the fear of many men). Only two cases were brought in between 1991 and 1993, both from women no longer living with their husband. In North America, in 1990, rape within marriage was still not legally recognized in seven states unless the couple were living apart, legally separated or had filed for divorce.[147] In seventeen states wife-rape is a crime regardless of whether the couple are living together or apart, and in a further twenty-six there are limited exemptions, for example, the fact that, in California, the wife must report the rape within ninety days.[148] Yet rape in marriage is not an infrequent crime: one survey reported that one in seven married women has experienced rape by their husbands.[149] Few, if any, report it. Ironically, in this context the wife is in a worse position than the prostitute, whose violation is at least legally acknowledged, even if rarely acted upon.

Marital rape is not a case of women engaging in sex when they'd rather be reading a romantic novel or having a cup of tea – it's not 'altruistic sex'. Rape within marriage is commonly associated with some degree of violence. It is typically combined with battering, occurring as a part of general marital abuse.[150] One woman, Susan Dyas, made a complaint of rape after her husband raped her in every room in the house. She dropped the charges because the police told her, 'I know you're telling the truth but I can't see you standing up to him in court.' The first rape happened on her wedding night – a violent and angry attack. She had had four miscarriages as a result of her husband's attacks, on the last occasion being tied to a radiator, raped and sexually assaulted with a broom handle. She commented, 'Can you imagine what it's like having an abortion when you're awake?'[151]

Diana Russell has claimed that 'the continuum of violence and the continuum of sex merge in the act of wife rape.'[152] As rape is ignored or denied within marriage, or seen to be legitimate, so, historically, was domestic violence. Official dictates from the Roman era through to the twentieth century are littered with examples of legally sanctioned wife-battering.[153] One Roman husband who beat his wife to death because she drank some wine was considered to have meted out 'exemplary punishment' because 'any woman who drinks wine immoderately closes her heart to every virtue and opens it to every vice.'[154] In the nineteenth century, in Britain, a movement to outlaw wife-battering gained publicity with the publication of the watershed book *The Subjugation of Women*, by John Stuart Mill. He argued in 1869 that 'Marriage is the only actual bondage known to our law. There remain no legal slaves except the mistress of every house.'[155] In 1878 Francis Power Cobbe produced a document entitled 'Wife Torture in England', which estimated that, based on judicial statistics, 6,000 women had been 'brutally assaulted' in the previous three years. Cobbe concluded that the positioning of the wife as object was a major factor in this abuse: 'The notion that a man's wife is his property, in the sense in which a horse is his property . . . is the fatal root of incalculable evil and misery.'[156] Parliamentary changes in England in 1878 allowed women to cite cruelty as grounds for divorce for the first time. Yet the long-held belief in the right of the man to beat (and rape) his wife was too ingrained for an immediate reversal of public opinion. The advice of a magistrate in 1915 that a man could legitimately beat his wife, 'provided that the stick used was no wider than a man's thumb,'[157] makes this clear. Giving her whole self over to her husband in marriage, the best a woman could hope for was that he treat her gently.

These are not merely historical horror stories. Domestic violence is still prevalent, even if it is *officially* condemned by the law. In one survey covering 2,000 homes of married couples, researchers reported that 28 per cent had experienced at least one incident of physical assault, and

16 per cent had experienced violence in the year prior to study.[158] In a Harris poll carried out in 1980, 21 per cent of married couples reported that they suffered physical violence. In North America, it is estimated that 3−4 million women each year are battered by their male partners. In Britain, the figure is estimated to be 530,000.[159] This, again, is an invisible crime, as it has been estimated that only one out of 270 incidents of wife abuse are reported to the authorities.[160] When the police are informed, incidents may be dismissed as a 'domestic' and the woman expected to drop charges. Women often do, which reinforces police apathy and inaction. One woman, Pat Hayes, whose husband raped her on her return from hospital after the birth of her first child, before her post-natal stitches had healed, didn't bring charges because 'the police still treated it as a domestic.' She said she felt 'ashamed and dirty'.[161] This is a common response. Any visible scars woman bears signify *her* criminality, her deviance, not that of the man. As one battered woman commented, 'I have learned that the doctors, the police, the clergy and my friends will excuse my husband for distorting my face, but won't forgive me for looking bruised and broken.'[162]

Wife Murder: 'If I Can't Have You . . .'

> I swear if you ever leave me, I'll follow you to the ends of the earth and
> kill you.   *People* v. *Wood*[163]

Arguably, marriage is far more than a raping licence − in the law, it can be a licence to kill (at least if woman is not 'good'). I'll start with some statistics lest there be a protest that I am taking an extreme case and setting it out as the norm. Of 231 women killed in Britain in 1993, 40 per cent were killed by a spouse or lover. The comparable figure for women killing their male partners was 6 per cent in the same year (out of 375 men killed). These figures are in line with statistics collected in North America, which report that 41 per cent of women are murdered by a husband or lover (compared to 10 per cent of men murdered by their wives).[164]

In many countries the figures are much higher. A report issued by the Russian government stated that in 1993, 14,500 Russian women were murdered by their husbands and another 56,400 were disabled or seriously injured.[165] In India between 1981 and 1982 official figures record that 637 women were burned to death 'accidentally', in what are widely acknowledged to be cases of 'dowry murder', a woman being killed by her husband and his family because her dowry is inadequate. It is estimated that thousands of women have been burned to death in this way, the majority of the crimes going unpunished because the deaths are recorded as 'suicide'.[166]

Most legal systems do not condone a husband taking the life of his wife; most culprits will be given custodial sentences. But the law does view his case with sympathy, at least in cases where he claims he was provoked. In England, for example, the law of provocation enshrined in the 1957 Homicide Act has resulted in scores of men literally getting away with murder. Provocation is defined as:

> some act or series of acts done by the deceased which would cause in any reasonable person, and did cause in the accused, a sudden and temporary loss of self control, rendering him so subject to passion as to make him not for the moment the master of his mind. The sufficiency of the provocation shall be left to the determination of the jury, which shall take into account everything both said and done according to the effect which, in their opinion, it would have on a *reasonable man*.

Adultery – whether real or imagined – is one of the major factors deemed justifiable grounds for provocation. Romanticized as a 'crime of passion', the murder of adulterous wives has a long history. Henry VIII had two of his six wives (Anne Boleyn and Katherine Howard) beheaded for this crime. In the case of Anne Boleyn, sullied for centuries as whore, harlot, witch and temptress, there was little evidence for the supposed adultery and many recent historians have attested to her innocence.[167] Yet even the *accusation* of female adultery has long been sufficient evidence for a sentence of marital death. The husband, driven mad – like Othello by Desdemona – and wild in a jealous frenzy, is excused and understood. It is still the case today in the state of Texas and, until recently, in Italy and France,[168] that a 'crime of passion' can lead to an almost automatic acquittal.

In court men put forward sexual jealousy as justification for the anger and outrage that turns into killing. This Canadian man shot his estranged wife:

> I know she was fuckin' around. I had been waiting for approximately

five minutes and seen her pull up in a taxi and I drove over and pulled up behind the car. I said, 'Did you enjoy your weekend?' She said, 'You're fucking right I did. I will have a lot more of them too.' I said, 'Oh no, you won't. You have been bullshitting me long enough. I can take no more.' I kept asking her whether she would come back to me. She told me to get out of her life. I said 'No way. If I get out of this it's going to be both of us.'

Separation from her husband is no protection for an errant woman. This man stabbed to death his twenty-year-old common-law wife after they had been separated for six months:

She said that since she came back in April she had fucked this other man about ten times. I told her how can you talk love and marriage and you been fucking with this other man. I was really mad. I went to the kitchen and got the knife. I went back to our room and said were you serious when you told me that. She said yes. We fought on the bed, I was stabbing her and her grandfather came up and tried to take the knife out of my hand. I told him to call the cops for me. I don't know why I killed the woman. I loved her.[169]

Imagined infidelity fares no better. In one study of wife murders carried out in Dayton, Ohio, between 1974 and 1979, in which the researchers found that jealousy accounted for 64 per cent of all such killings, one man killed his wife because he returned home to find her talking to someone on the phone whom he assumed was her boyfriend. The police confirmed that she had simply been talking to a relative and that there was no evidence for her having a boyfriend.[170] Yet sexual provocation is not the only 'feminine' wile which is seen to drive men to murder. Three of the Dayton murders were for insurrection: women refusing sexual advances, refusing to get the man more wine and refusing to give him her money – punishment of women stepping outside the narrow confines of the feminine script?

So *is* marriage a licence to kill? It's not surprising that many men think so, as the law often concurs. In 1985 Nicolas Boyce was sentenced to five years only for killing his wife. His defence that she 'nagged' him was treated with great sympathy by the judge, who implicitly condoned the murder in his summing up by saying, 'You were provoked, you lost self control, and . . . a man of reasonable self control might have done what you did.' His defence counsel argued, 'She constantly bullied him and remorselessly ground him down until he finally snapped and strangled her with an electric flex. What he wanted, all he ever wanted was some peace and time to spend with his children.' The defamation of Christabel Boyce's character went unchecked. The fact that she had wanted to leave him, had been frightened for her life and had told friends that he had recently been violent was not mentioned during the trial.[171] Neither was the fact he had been reading up on criminal law.

The defamation of a woman's character is not unusual. In 1981 Peter Wood clubbed his lover Mary Bristow to death with a meat tenderizer whilst she slept. The provocation accepted by judge and jury was the fact that she refused to enter into a monogamous relationship with him, preferring to keep her independence.[172] In his summing up the judge drew attention to the dangers of such 'unorthodox' behaviour, seeming to suggest that female intelligence, independence and sexual freedom together posed such a great threat to man that he could not fail to rise to the bait. He went on to draw a clear distinction between 'a villain shooting a policeman, and a husband killing his wife or lover at a stage when they can no longer cope'. Wood was sentenced for manslaughter not murder and consequently served a four-year prison sentence. The British tabloid press dubbed the case the 'Savage Killing of a Women's Lib Lover' (the *Sun*), implicitly suggesting that any man would be exasperated by such female independence. As laws of defamation do not hold for the dead, any slurs on a woman's character can be made by the defence counsel during a murder trial. Peter Wood's claims that he and his lover engaged in 'kinky sex' were used as part of the general calumny – positioning her as 'whore', and implicitly suggesting that she courted her violent fate. This was reiterated in the tabloid press under the banner heading 'Mary's Sex Games Turned Jealous Lover into Killer' (the *Star*). Under English law (as it then stood) witnesses could not be called to challenge evidence brought by the defence which defames the character of a murder victim, so a web of lies can easily be spun.[173]

This case is not an exception, dragged out of the archives. The depressing fact is that a whole litany of such cases can be recited. Here are a few British cases where provocation has been accepted as mitigating circumstances:

Gordon Asher, 1981, strangled his wife and buried her naked body in a chalk pit. Sentence: six months, suspended.

Peter Hogg, 1985, strangled his wife and buried her body in the Lake District. Provocation: alleged infidelity and promiscuity. Sentence: three years; served: fifteen months.

Nicolas Boyce, 1985, murdered his wife, dismembered her body in the bath and cooked parts of her in order to conceal that they were human flesh. He dumped the body in plastic bags all over London. Provocation: nagging and insubordination (including refusing sex). Sentence: six years; served: three years.

Leslie Taylor, 1987, knifed his wife to death. Provocation: seeing her kissing another man at a wedding and alleged infidelity. Sentence: six years.

Stephen Midlane, 1989, strangled and cut up his wife's body, depositing it on a rubbish tip. Provocation: alleged infidelity. Sentence: five years; served: three.[174]

In 1994 in Britain Alan Hunt was given an eighteen-month suspended sentence for strangling his wife during an argument over an affair he was having with another woman. Hunt claimed that he and his wife were having an argument in the car, when his wife had tried to get out and had started kicking him. Trying to restrain her, he killed her. Judge Kenneth Taylor was sympathetic, commenting during the sentencing that he was 'quite satisfied you were outrageously provoked'.[175] In the same month, across the Atlantic, Kenneth Peacock received a similarly light sentence of eighteen months for shooting his wife in the head with a hunting rifle after coming home to find her in bed with another man. Judge Robert Cahill apologized for having to send him to prison at all, but said that he had to impose the sentence 'to make the system honest'. Apparently condoning the violent murder, he commented, 'How many men would have the strength to walk away without inflicting some corporal punishment?'[176]

Few women kill their husbands. But the law is harsh on women who attempt to use claims of provocation as mitigating circumstances. The law clearly operates a double standard – the law of provocation applies to 'a reasonable *man*'. Self-defence is more frequently put forward as a defence plea by women in such circumstances. However, there are many renowned cases where the law is harsh, sentencing women to life for murder even when they have been repeatedly beaten and sexually abused for years – such as the case of Sara Thornton, who was jailed for life in Britain in 1990 after stabbing her violent and alcoholic husband to death. (She was released on appeal in 1995.) However, it is still the case that systematic abuse and violence by a man is not viewed as seriously as female adultery or insurrection.

Sexual Murder: The Lust to Kill?

This examination of the sexualized violation of the body of 'woman' cannot ignore the most extreme violation – that of sexual murder. Murders involving a clear sexual component are not solely confined to women victims, there being many cases involving boys or men. However, with one or two notable exceptions,[177] sexual murderers are men. In the way these murders are positioned by the media, by the courts and by the men who commit such crimes we see the most malevolent material consequences of the cornucopia of misogynistic misrepresentations of 'woman', 'man' and 'sex'.

Sexual murders include women killed during or following the act of rape; cases where orgasm or sexual pleasure are experienced by the murderer only during or following the killing (which sometimes involves necrophilia); murders where the woman's body is attacked or dismembered in a sexual way after her death; and murders where the motive for killing is explicitly of a sexual nature. Many cases involve all of these elements combined.

These cases appear to incite a morbid fascination which can seem to glorify the crime. For example, Michael Newton, author of an encyclopaedia of serial killers, has been quoted as saying, 'my all-time favourite was Ed Gein. He used to make suits out of women's skin – breasts, vagina and all. When they went into his home they found a belt made of nipples, and nine vaginas in a shoebox.'[178] This case was glorified more publicly in providing the basis for the character Hannibal Lecter in the film *Silence of the Lambs* – sexual murderer elevated to the status of anti-hero, voyeuristically celebrated by millions. Outlined below are a number of notable cases[179] – not to elicit voyeurism or to shock, but to provide clear evidence of the reality and the pervasive nature of this crime and to illustrate the depths to which sexual violation and the desire to desecrate can sink:[180]

> 'Jack the Ripper', the Whitechapel murderer, London, England. Killed six prostitutes in 1888. Sexually assaulted the victims and mutilated their bodies.

> David Berkowitz, the 'Son of Sam', shot six people dead in the late seventies. He claimed to target 'pretty women'.

> John Christie, killer of seven women in London during the forties and fifties. Women were made to inhale carbon monoxide, strangled, and raped after death.

> Edward Cole, executed in 1985, brutally murdered fourteen women, most of them married women whom he had had sex with. He claimed that as a boy his mother had taken him on her adulterous excursions and made him dress up as a girl.

> Norman Collins, killed seven women in Michigan, USA, in the late sixties. They were tied up, raped and sexually abused, beaten, stabbed and mutilated.

> Ted Bundy, North American serial killer of over thirty-six women between 1974 and 1976. The women were bitten, beaten, raped and strangled.

> Albert De Salvo, the 'Boston Strangler', killed thirteen women and raped or sexually assaulted thousands more in the sixties. He left the women with their legs spread wide, often with objects such as broom handles stuffed into their vaginas.

> 'Hillside strangler', strangled, raped and sexually tortured ten women in the late seventies in Los Angeles.

> Joseph Kallinger, North American killer who stabbed a woman to death for refusing to chew off the penis of a man being held at gunpoint. He committed many other sexual assaults and fantasized about mutilated women's bodies.

> Edmund Kemper, killed at least six students in California in the early seventies, sexually violating and decapitating the women after killing

them. He also killed, raped and decapitated his mother and confessed to cannibalism.

Henry Lee Lucas, North American serial killer who claimed up to 360 victims, mostly women travelling alone, in the late seventies and early eighties. He strangled the first girl he had sex with when he was fourteen and claimed that he had murdered by every method other than poison, having shot, stabbed, burned, beaten, strangled, hanged and crucified his victims, and that some had been filleted like fish.

Peter Sutcliffe, the 'Yorkshire Ripper', killed thirteen women between 1975 and 1981. He stabbed the bodies repeatedly in the breast and abdomen and raped one dying victim. His main targets were prostitutes.

Frederick West, killed twelve young women in Gloucester during the seventies and eighties. Many were sexually assaulted, including his first wife and two of his daughters. The women were buried in the garden of his home.

When caught, these men *are* legally condemned: In the US states that still enforce the death penalty, they are thought to deserve it. In all other cases they are given life imprisonment – or more (Joseph Kallinger was sentenced to eighty years in prison). Their time in prison is not easy, many being kept in solitary confinement for their own protection, as violence and assaults directed at sexual criminals are rife in the prison system. Many are murdered – for example, Albert De Salvo, the Boston strangler, convicted in 1967, was killed by a prison inmate in 1973. Yet the media still appear to glory in the mythology of the sexual murderer.

Take the nicknames – Jack the Ripper, the Yorkshire Ripper, the Boston Strangler – which somehow position these men as folk heroes. These men, and their actions, are normalized through such representation, and our initial shocked reaction to this extreme of sexualized violence dims as we become inured to it. This violence becomes an aspect of urban life that is almost taken for granted. The focus on the mythology of sexual murderers also diverts attention away from the reality of these crimes and the underlying implications of their becoming increasingly common.

The gory fascination with sex murders is demonstrated by the number of bestselling books published on the subject (the novels of Patricia D.

Cornwell; Stephen King's *The Dead Zone*; scores of books on actual cases), films (*Psycho*; *Halloween*; *Pieces*), and by the continued popularity of sex-murder museums (the London Dungeon, or the Ripper tableau at Madame Tussaud's in London) which provide 'entertainment' analogous to the implicit celebration of the witch trials in the museums at Salem – Sex murder as Saturday entertainment, terror as titillation.

Newspapers lavishly describe every gory detail in cases of sexual murder – particularly if the victims are women. As Jane Caputi has argued in *The Age of Sex Crime*, it is notable that in the cases of murders that involve men or boys as victims, the crimes are not so graphically described. Perhaps the media have less voyeuristic interest in descriptions of male rape, castration and dismemberment. Yet, as we have already seen (pp. 129–34), they have no such qualms with women. Here, the sex murderer is represented almost as the epitome of virile male sexuality – both deviant and aberrant, but at the same time motivated by the drives somehow dwelling within all men. As one male commentator eulogizes at the beginning of a fictional account:

> Jack the Ripper is with us now. He prowls the nights, shunning the sun in a search for the blazing incandescence of an inner reality . . . let the Ripper rip into you an awareness of the urges and forces most of us will neither admit to nor submit to.[181]

A whole industry has developed in reverence to the serial sex killer, an underground American system of killer literature including trading cards, comics, poetry, memorabilia and 'killer art' – paintings by the serial killers themselves. Salaciously sensationalized, the sexual murderer is given the status of cultural icon, enjoying far more than his proverbial fifteen minutes of fame. For example, one disciple, Michael Newton, glories in their acts as he records them in his data bank of 1,263 serial slayers, commenting:

> [There is] an aspect of those guys which is the ultimate outlaw. These guys are in the twilight zone, doing whatever comes to mind. Jesse James was robbing banks, these people are eating human hearts. In the sixties, the FBI had two serial killers a year. By the Seventies it was 18 a year. Since the Eighties I've been finding one every 10 days.[182]

Newton presents us with a narrative of romance, grossly parodied: 'Man' as ultimate hero, 'having' the woman who lies helpless in his power – except that in these cases she really is dead. Given this celebration of the sexual murderer, is it surprising that there are so many 'copy-cat' crimes when the police release details of ongoing cases?[183] The fact that many men identify with sex killers is evidenced by the thousands of crank letters the police receive which claim to be from the killer himself when such crimes are still unsolved – in the case of 'Jack the Ripper' only three out of the many thousands are now thought to be genuine, and even that is in doubt. In their analysis of sex murders, Deborah Cameron and Liz Frazer present this description of one of the killings of Jack the Ripper for the *Pall Mall Gazette* on 10 November 1888, in order to remind us of the horror of sex killings. That men would want to copy such a crime is almost beyond belief.

> The woman lay on her bed, entirely naked. Her throat was cut from ear to ear, right down the spinal column. The ears and nose had been cut clean off. The breasts had also been cleanly cut off and placed on a table that was beside the bed. The stomach and abdomen had been ripped open while the face was all slashed about, so that the features of the poor creature were beyond all recognition. The kidneys and heart had also been removed from the body and placed on the table by the side of the breasts. The liver had likewise been removed and laid on the right thigh . . . the thighs had been cut.[184]

The obsessive detail in which crimes of sexual murder are recorded and recounted arguably acts to remind all women of their potential fate. Judith Walkowitz, amongst others, has deemed the Ripper a 'modern myth of male violence against women' who reminds us of the potential for female genocide. As with rape, this is particularly the case if we stray from the feminine masquerade. For when the victims of sexual murders are women of 'loose morals' the press and police have treated them as less of a serious concern, a fact which murderers frequently use in attempts to exonerate themselves from their crimes:

> I am down on whores and I shan't quit ripping them until I do get buckled.   JACK THE RIPPER, 1888, letter to the police

> Stacey was a whore . . . I'd kill her again. I'd kill them all again.
>   DAVID BERKOWITZ, the 'Son of Sam'

> The women I killed were filth, bastard prostitutes who were just standing
> round littering the streets. I was just cleaning the place up a bit.
>
> PETER SUTCLIFFE, the 'Yorkshire Ripper'[185]

Apparent police apathy over the murder of prostitutes has been noted again and again. For example, there was a distinct absence of police attention on the 'south side killer' in a small area of Boston, where at least seventeen women were murdered in the early eighties. All the women were described as prostitutes, runaways or drug addicts, by implication 'deserving to die'.[186] To compound this, they were also predominantly black. Racism abounds in sex crimes – in a number of cases where the women have been black the police reaction time has been said to be much slower, the crime apparently thought less serious. This stands in contrast to the outrage greeting the murders of men such as Ted Bundy, who attacked 'America's daughters', nice middle-class white girls, who hadn't stepped out of line.

A similar picture can be painted of the reactions to the crimes of Peter Sutcliffe, the 'Yorkshire Ripper'. It was only when he turned his attention from prostitutes to 'ordinary' young women that public outrage crescendoed. That the police shared this bigoted attitude is encapsulated most clearly in the comment from Police Chief Constable Jim Hobson as he appealed to the then uncaptured killer:

> He has made it clear that he hates prostitutes. Many people do . . . But
> the Ripper is now killing innocent girls. This indicates your mental state
> and that you are in urgent need of medical attention. You have made
> your point. Give yourself up before another innocent woman dies.

George Oldfield, who led the police investigation, reiterated this belief at a press conference called after the murder of Josephine Whittaker, who was stabbed twenty five times, three times in her vagina. She was not a prostitute. Oldfield commented, 'This girl is perfectly respectable' and that 'the next woman could be anyone's wife, daughter, or girlfriend.'[187] This is again a parallel to the comments of judges that 'good girls' are more traumatized by rape.

In this view, as prostitutes are not 'innocent', dying in a horrific manner is deemed to be a risk of the job (as is rape). Killing them is seen not as a sign of madness, but as perfectly understandable. This is hatred of female sexuality, of the woman who steps outside man's control, at its most blatant. This is killing the object of hate, annihilating that part of 'woman' which signifies 'sex'. It's not a coincidence that sex murderers attack the vagina – that object of disgust, anger and fear, which we see attacked (or negated) in art, film, literature and pornography. These are men acting out the fantasy. The 'vagina denta' is literally desecrated and despoiled.

Sexual science provides us with individualistic theories which explain sexual violence as the pathology of an individual man, drawing attention away from the roots of violence in 'normal' masculinity. The law, in contrast, appears to position men accused of rape as 'normal men', just doing what men do – seducing and having sex with women. It is an interesting contradiction. The process of blaming women for provoking sexual assault, dismissing rape as 'sex' or implicitly positioning certain women as unworthy of legal protection (or incapable of being 'raped') draws our attention to the inherent power imbalance and the potential for violence in 'normal' heterosexual sex. Whilst the law ostensibly stands as a protector of 'the family', with laws being constructed and applied to suit the interests of man, in its treatment of rape, the law focuses sharp attention on the widespread acceptance of men's denigration and violation of women. It reveals the misogynistic fears and fantasies about 'woman' and 'sex' in the most obvious and materially consequential manner. For the law implicitly acknowledges that most men accused of rape are no different from any other man. They merely stand at the extreme end of a continuum where sexual power over women is deemed a male prerogative and where masculine pursuit and feminine resistance is central to the script of 'normal' sex. This is a phallocentric fantasy fictionalized in the mass media, art, film and pornography. Through being enshrined in the law on sexual violence, it provides legitimation for the material enactment of misogynistic control of the sexual bodies of individual women. Castigating the few men convicted of 'real rape' may allow the law-makers to complacently assume that they are championing the rights of the sexually violated and abused. But the fact that so few sexual crimes are ever prosecuted, and even fewer proceed to conviction, demonstrates that the law acts to protect and reinforce phallocentric power over women.

Science and the Law: Framing Woman, Framing Sex

The last two chapters may seem a depressing litany of sins associated with science and the law. Both act in unison to define what is acceptable (or not) in the realm of the sexual; both reflect and reinforce phallocentric myths about 'woman', 'man' and 'sex'; both reify monogamous hetero-sexuality and reproductive sex as natural and right, defining as deviant or dysfunctional anything which falls outside this sphere. These stances and the material consequences that derive from them allow the condemn-nation of 'woman' as wicked temptress who seduces and then accuses the unknowing innocent man, positioning women who contravene the narrow boundaries of femininity as 'whores' who ask for and deserve everything they get. This is a familiar story by now – we have seen it played out in mass media imagery, in art, film and pornography. Yet here there are direct material effects, arising from the medico-legal practices which literally contain and control the bodies of women and men and police the boundaries of acceptable sex.

We have seen that the categories of sexual crime or illness which have been unconditionally accepted within science and the law can be deconstructed: the notion of the 'homosexual' or 'heterosexual'; of 'paraphilias'; of sexual crimes; of vaginal penetration as 'sex' (and failure in this sphere as 'dysfunction'); of disinterest in sex or premenstrual distress as an 'illness'. Arguments highlighting the assumptions under-lying the current construction of these categories in many ways parallel the arguments made in the seventies about the need to deconstruct categories of mental illness – the danger in labelling someone as 'schizo-phrenic' or 'depressed' and assuming that these are 'real' illnesses which are just waiting to be found, rather than being social categorizations placed on sets of symptoms or behaviours which deviate from the 'healthy norm'; and the pathologizing of those who threaten the status quo and the peace or power of dominant social groups.

Yet there is a downside to this deconstruction. When we question the validity of social categories and the ideological intent behind them, we can be left with a scenario where nothing is 'real', where everything is just a social label, an invention of those in power. We find ourselves in a situation where there is no such thing as a sexual problem, a sexual crime, no such thing as perversion, as a 'homosexual' or a 'heterosexual'. This may discount the experiences of many women and men. Women who suffer anxiety and stress associated with sexuality, who experience changes in mood across the menstrual cycle, are not happy to be told that these are merely 'social constructions', not valid problems. Men who cannot achieve an erection, or who can only do so when dressed in particular clothes may feel similarly. Equally, telling a gay man or lesbian that 'homosexuality' as an identity was an invention of the sexologists will invariably be met with derision. The positive adoption of a gay or lesbian identity has been one of the ways in which many men and women have celebrated and made positive their position as sexual outsiders. The difference between heterosexuals and homosexuals is often emphasized rather than ignored.

This type of deconstruction has also been used by those who would prop up phallocentric privilege. We have seen how 'rape' is often reframed as 'seduction' within the law, implicitly positioning sexual violence enacted by men towards women as 'normal sex', blaming the woman for her unlucky (or unwise) fate,[188] and providing a script of exoneration used effectively by men who rape. In a similar vein, social-constructionist arguments concerning the age of consent – the idea that there is no absolute age when it is *natural* first to have sex, so the definition of sex with minors as 'abuse' is arbitrary – have been used to support the sexual activities of paedophiles. At a recent conference on sexuality, the veteran sex researcher John Money deconstructed the notion of paedophilia by ironically drawing attention to the number of men suffering from 'twentyphilia' or 'thirtyphilia' – attraction to women in their twenties or thirties. Implying that there was no distinction to be made between those who are specifically attracted to women of a certain age (or women of a certain body type) and those who were specifically attracted to children, he went on to argue that many men who became sexually engaged with children were positive and loving in their relationships with them. In a social context in which sex with children was normal, and children had a free choice in whether to engage in it or not, his arguments may have some validity (although whether there can ever be a free 'choice' when there is so great a power imbalance is always questionable, and is one of the reasons for laws on age of consent). However, when adult–child sexual activity is against the law, and where the majority of adults who engage in such acts use threats or coercion, often leaving the child in a state of shame and self blame, such libertarian deconstructions simply do not wash. The motivations of those apologists for paedophilia must be seriously questioned.

So what is the answer? Firstly, we must be critical of the supposed rational objectivity of social institutions such as science and law on the subject of sex and sexuality. These are literally man-made rules and regulations which act to support phallocentric privilege and power. We must look beyond the rhetoric, beyond the technical or professional language, to the fears and fantasies which underlie the practices of science and law – the fear and hatred directed towards the female, towards that which threatens heterosexual hegemony, towards the sexual outsider; or the fear associated with homoerotic desire. It is these fears which lead to desperate attempts to maintain a narrow notion of what is 'normal sex', following the traditions of the theological prelates, where notions of 'naturalness' are espoused as a means of defence.

This is not to dismiss the existence of sexual identity, sexual problems or sexual crime. It is not to say that there aren't a range of expressions of sexuality, some of which may be problematic because they cause distress to the individuals who experience them (often because of the way behaviour is categorized or judged in a particular social context). To understand these aspects of sexuality we need to move beyond a monolithic and unidimensional theory, to stop looking for a simple biological or psychosocial *cause* for our sexual feelings and behaviour and acknowledge the complex interaction of social, psychological and biological factors in our sexual lives. Take the case of sexual desire. It is not devoid of a biological component – changes in hormones, our genetic make-up and the configuration of the brain can all play a role in sexual desire. But so do social and psychological factors. That which is sexually desirable changes across cultures and across history; it is affected by sexual laws and moral mandates. The expression of desire is influenced by what we learn and what we see around us. The rituals of courtly love enacted by the medieval knights and the macho man strutting in a modern bar differ enormously, but they are both enactments of desire shaped by the cultural context. How an individual person reacts to this, whether they accept or reject it, is related to their own unconscious fantasies and desires. Some women desire macho men, others deride them. The tenor of the response will depend on many interacting factors – one cannot predict how 'woman' will respond.

Similarly, take the case of 'sexual orientation'. There seems to be some evidence from the sexual scientists that there is a biological component, at least for male homosexuality. This fits in with the intuitions of many gay men and lesbians, who say they have always 'known' that they were different. As one woman I interviewed said:

> 'Those who say being gay is a choice obviously haven't been there themselves. I knew I was gay before I even knew such a thing existed. I was always attracted to women. I've never fancied a man. From when I was a teenager I knew I wasn't the same as everyone else.'

Yet we cannot simply say that homosexuality or heterosexuality are biological givens. Many other gay men and lesbians go through 'normal' heterosexual adolescence, only to 'discover' their sexual attraction to the same sex later in life. They certainly experienced desire for those of the opposite sex at some point in their lives. Their experiences would seem to contradict the notion of a simple homosexual gene. And as I have argued above, the notion of a homogeneous category of homosexuality which explains the experiences of everyone who is categorized as such is nonsensical. There is no *simple* biological or social root cause for 'sexual orientation'. Again, many social and psychological factors interact with biology to result in the complicated thing which is sexual attraction and love for the same or opposite sex. To be 'homosexual', 'heterosexual' or 'bisexual' is not the same experience for everyone – to imply that it could be so is naïve. We must move away from these monolithic theories and allow for the complexity of individual experience. But at the same time we must bear in mind the meaning of these categorizations in different social contexts. Being 'homosexual' will have a very different meaning in a context where it is illegal than in a context where it is normal or allowed. It may be a positive statement of pride in one context, a cause of criminal indictment in another. The context will clearly affect the experience of individual women and men and the meaning behind the categorizations of the sexuality they choose (or are given). For many people it is not even an issue about 'sex'. As one woman who identified as lesbian commented, 'It's more about love, about who I like, and who I get on with the best. It's about commitment. The fact that I have sex with a woman is only a small part of my being a lesbian.'

Similarly sexual problems may have a physical manifestation – anorgasmia, vaginismus or erectile dysfunction do not simply exist in the mind of the beholder but have 'real' effects on the physical body – but they cannot be reduced to a physical response. The actual 'problem' itself can result from a complex interaction of physical, psychological and social factors. The fact that the inability of the body to function as it 'should' is seen as such an important issue has to be viewed as a social issue. In a cultural milieu in which penetration of the vagina by the penis is not pre-eminent the inability of the penis to become erect might not be seen as such a 'problem'. We might also ask why inability to talk about sex or refusal to explore a wide avenue of sexual experiences is not seen as a 'problem' whereas the inability to fuck *is*. Many people obtain sexual pleasure outside this narrow sphere, and subscribe to a very different notion of what 'sex' is. We cannot deny that heterosexual intercourse is an essential part of human reproduction (IVF aside), and for that reason alone it might be given priority over other expressions of pleasure and desire by many people. But most people don't have sex to reproduce, so the fact that heterosexual intercourse is elevated to the status of being the only 'normal' form of sexual expression has nothing to do with 'natural' factors – it is to do with our living in a phallocentric sphere in which 'man' proves himself through the actions of penis as phallus and woman's rightful place is as enthusiastic receptacle, propping up both his ego and his phallic power.

Applying these arguments to sexual violence is a more sensitive issue. We could look to Pauline Bart's argument that there is a continuum of rape ranging from consensual sex to altruistic sex (going along with it because you feel sorry for the man or would feel guilty about saying 'no') to compliant sex (going along with it because the consequences of saying 'no' are worse than giving in) to rape. The majority of women have engaged in both altruistic and compliant sex sometimes in their lives – indeed so had the majority of men I interviewed. Both men and women talked of having sex when they were too tired, but wanted to avoid an argument; having spent an evening with someone, not really fancying them, but going along with sex because it had started to happen; not wanting to get the last bus home, so staying with someone who had a crush on them, then agreeing to sex because it would make the other person happy; having sex when they'd rather have a cup of tea/watch televison/go to sleep. Defence lawyers may attempt to suggest the opposite, but women who got to court with accusations of rape do not fit into the above categories – they can distinguish between compliant sex and 'rape', and few (if any) would put themselves through the exposure and trauma of a rape trial if they had not experienced the act as a sexual assault. I am not arguing that women (or men) *should* have altruistic or compliant sex, and if they say 'no' it should certainly cease, but it is a dangerous move to try to position all rape as the result of women crying 'rape' when the man thinks he is engaging in 'sex'.

At the same time, it is important to acknowledge that rape, child sexual abuse and sexual murder are not simply about sex, regardless of what the perpetrators of such acts profess. They are about anger, hatred, control and power – enacted by men, primarily on the bodies of women,[189] a desecration of the object of his desire and disgust. These acts are 'sexual' in that the hatred is directed at the sexual body – it is the *woman's* sexuality that is violated. They are also 'sexual' in that the penis is often used as a weapon, an instrument of power and control, or because the enactment of such violence often parodies that of a non-abusive sexual encounter. In every other way these are acts of violence, degradation and defilement – as far from a consensual sexual experience as most women could ever possibly contemplate. Yet the fact that the law, and many men who rape, position these acts as 'sex' tells us everything we need to know about the distorted, if not perverse, view of 'normal' sexuality that dominates in so many spheres. 'Sex' means 'man' as active, controlling, coercive if necessary – but ultimately always able to perform.

This is not 'sex' from the perspective of 'woman' but 'sex' in a phallocentric masculine gaze. In judging men on their sexual performance or their penis size – as many women do – women are feeding into the view of 'sex' and sexuality. It may provide short-term pleasure (at least for women who like to fuck), but ultimately it reinforces the inordinate pressure on men to live up to the myth of the phallic hero, leading to anxiety, dread and fear of failure which is projected outwards on to the bodies of women in sexual violence, or results in men completely splitting off and avoiding the intimacy and merger which many women actually want. We need to completely re-evaluate the whole meaning of 'sex' and the positions of 'woman' and 'man' in relation to each other if we are really to deal with sexual violence, sexual problems and issues of discrimination around sexual identity and practice. Only when sexual science and the law take on this task, developing more pluralistic definitions of 'sex' which don't simply reinforce the power and authority of the heterosexual man will any progress actually be made.

NOTES

1. Estrich, Susan, *Real Rape*, Cambridge, MA: Harvard University Press, 1987, p. 5.
2. Quoted by Lees, Sue, *Carnal Knowledge: Rape on Trial*, London: Penguin, 1996, p. xxvi.
3. Ibid., p. 230.
4. I use the word 'victim' advisedly here – to refer to the fact that the person is positioned as victim both by their attacker and by the law. Later I will talk of survivors, the term preferred by many who have experienced sexual violence.
5. These statistics don't include Scotland, which has a different legal system. See *Criminal Statistics in England and Wales*, London: HMSO, 1993.
6. In the government report which accompanies publication of these statistics the increase is dismissed with the statement, 'the number of recorded sexual offences has risen at a slower rate than crime in general: about 4 per cent a year – reassuring us that in an apparently increasingly violent society, sexual violence is increasing at a relatively slower rate.' Ibid., p. 32.
7. These statistics don't reflect the number of 'unfounded' complaints, as the FBI remove any accusations found to be 'false' from their official figures. The rate of 'unfounded' complaints is relatively high (in 1991 8 per cent of rape allegations were unfounded, compared to 2 per cent of any other serious crime). *Fordham Law Review*, vol. 63, October 1994, p. 135.
8. Stanko, Elizabeth A., *Intimate Intrusions. Women's Experience of Sexual Violence*, London: Routledge & Kegan Paul, 1985.
9. See Parrot, Andrea & Bechhofer, Laurie, *Acquaintance Rape: The Hidden Crime*, New York: Wiley, 1991.
10. Russell, D. E. H., *Rape in Marriage*, New York: Macmillan, 1982.
11. Koss, M. P., Gidycz, C. A. & Wisniewski, N., 'The Scope of Rape: Incidence and Prevalence of Sexual Aggression and Victimization in a National Sample of Higher Education Students', *Journal of Consulting and Clinical Psychology*, 55, pp. 162–70.

12. Groth, A. N. & Burgess, A. W., 'Rape: A Sexual Deviation', in *Male Rape: A Casebook of Sexual Aggression*, A. M. Scacco Jr (ed.), New York: AMS Press, 1982, pp. 231–40.

13. Koss, M. P. & Oros, C. J., 'Sexual Experiences Survey: A Research Instrument Investigating Sexual Aggression and Victimization', *Journal of Consulting and Clinical Psychology*, 50, 1982, pp. 455–7.

14. Koss, M. P. & Leonard, K. E., 'Sexually Aggressive Men: Empirical Findings and Theoretical Implications', in *Pornography and Sexual Aggression*, N. Malamuth & E. Donnerstein (eds.), New York: Academic Press, 1984, pp. 213–32.

15. Briere, J. & Malamuth, N., 'Self-Reported Likelihood of Sexually Aggressive Behaviour: Attitudinal versus Sexual Explanations', *Journal of Research in Personality*, 17, 1983, pp. 315–23. In a second study, of 172 US men 37 per cent said they would rape if they knew they wouldn't be caught.

16. Tieger, T., 'Self-Rated Likelihood of Raping and Social Perception of Rape', *Journal of Research in Personality*, 15, 1981, pp. 147–58.

17. Bureau of Justice Statistics survey of rape, 1992, Patrick A. Langan & Caroline W. Harlow, Crime Data Brief, June 1994, NCJ 147001; distributed on the internet.

18. Baker, A. W. & Duncan, S. P., 'Child Sexual Abuse: A Study of Prevalence in Great Britain', *Child Abuse and Neglect*, 9, 1985, pp. 457–67.

19. Russell, D. E. H., *The Secret Trauma: Incest in the Lives of Girls and Women*, New York: Basic Books, 1986.

20. For reference to these studies, see Ussher, J. M. & Dewberry, C., 'The Nature and Long-term Effects of Childhood Sexual Abuse: A Survey of Adult Women Survivors in Britain', *British Journal of Clinical Psychology*, 34, 1994, pp. 177–92.

21. There are many reasons for this under-reporting. Some women repress memories of sexual abuse experienced as children, and either split them off from their other experiences of themselves as 'woman', thereby allowing themselves to experience a positive sexual identity as adults, or simply 'forget' them altogether. This is a form of psychological defence mechanism which isn't peculiar to sexual abuse. We can 'forget' many difficult or disturbing experiences that happen to us as children – or as adults – repressing the memories of these events in order to be able to survive the psychic pain which they precipitate. Some women never 'remember' sexual abuse that occurred to them as children. In a recent

study of 129 women with previously documented histories of sexual abuse in children, 38 per cent as adults had no recollection at all of the event. Those women who had been abused by someone they knew or who were younger at the time of the abuse were more likely to have no recall of the events. (Williams, Linda Meyer, 'Recall of Childhood Trauma: A Prospective Study of Women's Memories of Child Sexual Abuse', *Journal of Consulting and Clinical Psychology*, 62 (6), 1994, pp. 1167–76).

22. Gilley, J., 'How to Help the Raped', *New Society*, vol. 612, 27 June, 1974, p. 28.

23. A distinction needs to be made between reporting of rape and police recording of rape for, as Sue Lees points out, in many cases the police will record the crime as sexual assault – a lesser crime in the eyes of the law.

24. Lees, 1996, p. xi.

25. See Lees for a discussion of the misrepresentation of rape in the media and the inaccurate portrayal of the reality of rape in Roiphe's work. See Lees, 1996, pp. 74–7, for a discussion of the changes in media reporting over the last twenty-five years.

26. Ibid., p. 106.

27. Ibid., p. 110.

28. Judge Wild, Cambridge Crown Court, 1982, reported in the *Sunday Times*, 12 December, 1982. Quoted in Adler, Zsuzsanna, *Rape on Trial*, London: Routledge & Kegan Paul, 1987, p. 9.

29. Donald Dripps, Professor of Law, Illinois College of Law, *Fordham Law Review*, 1994, pp. 141, 146.

30. Simpson, K., *A Doctor's Guide to Court*, London: Butterworths, 1962.

31. Tait, R. L., *Diseases of Women and Abdominal Surgery*, Leicester: Richardson, 1989, p. 56.

32. Camps, F. E., 'The Medical Aspects of the Investigation of Sexual Offences', *The Practitioner*, 189, 1129, 1962, pp. 31–5. Camps was a forensic pathologist.

33. Quoted by Scully, D., *Understanding Sexual Violence. A Study of Convicted Rapists*, London: Unwin Hyman, 1990, p. 104.

34. Estrich, Susan, *Real Rape*, Cambridge, MA: Harvard University Press, 1987, p. 71: 'Under the force standard courts still judge the woman, not the man . . . as she compares (poorly) to the court's vision of the reasonable woman.'

35. *State* v. *Rusk*, 289, Md 230, 424, A.2d, 720, 733 (1981). See Estrich, 1987, pp. 95–6.

36. *Rusk* v. *Stafel*, 43 Md App. 476, 478–479. Estrich, 1987, pp. 62–5.

37. Estrich, 1987, p. 64.

38. *Rusk* v. *State*, 43 Md App. 476, 478–479. Quoted in Estrich, 1987, pp. 62–5.

39. Wright, R. & West, D. J., 'Rape: A Comparison of Group Offences and Lone Offences', *Medicine, Science and the Law*, 21, 1981, pp. 25–30. This study was of rape cases in six counties in Britain over a five-year period.

40. Holmstrom, L. L. & Burgess, A.W., 'Rapists Talk Linguistic Strategies to Control the Victim', *Deviant Behaviour*, 1979, 1, 105–6. Quoted in Stanko, 1985, p. 45.

41. Quoted in Stanko, 1985, p. 41.

42. 'Howard League Working Party Report', *Unlawful Sex: Offences, Victims and Offenders in the Criminal Justice System of England and Wales*, London: Waterlow, 1984, Section 2:15, p. 11.

43. Quoted in Lees, 1996, p. 53.

44. Quoted in Stiglmayer, Alexandra, *Mass Rape: The War against Women in Bosnia Herzegovina*, Lincoln and London: University of Nebraska Press, 1994, p. 90.

45. Adler, 1987, p. 115. This case was observed by Adler at the Old Bailey.

46. Quoted in Estrich, 1987, pp. 93–4.

47. Quoted in Lees, 1996, p. 117.

48. Lees, 1996, p. 118.

49. Ibid., p. 118.

50. The House of Lords is the highest British court.

51. Lord Hailsham (quoted in Estrich, 1987, p. 93).

52. See Estrich, 1987, pp. 93–4.

53. Dripps, *Fordham Law Review*, 1994, p. 141.

54. Seward, Jill with Green, Wendy, *Rape: My Story*, London: Bloomsbury, 1990, pp. 29–31.

55. Walters, D. R., *Physical and Sexual Abuse of Children*, Bloomington: Indiana University Press, 1975, p. 113.

56. Wilson, M., *The Man They Called a Monster*, North Ryde, Australia: Cassell, 1981.

57. Constantine L. L., 'The Sexual Rights of Children: Implications of a Radical Perspective', in *Love and Attraction: An International Conference*, M. Cook & G. Wilson (eds.), Oxford: Pergamon, 1979, p. 505. Quoted in

Howitt, D., *Child Abuse Errors*, Hemel Hempstead: Harvester Wheatsheaf, 1992, p. 66.

58. Ryder, R., 'Child Abuse', *The Bulletin of the British Psychological Society*, 2 (8), 1989, p. 333. Quoted in Howitt, 1992, p. 68.

59. 'Howard League Working Party Report,' 1984, p. 22, referring to the conclusions of Powell, G. E. & Chalkey, 'The Effects of Paedophile Attention on the Child', London: Batsford, 1981, in *Perspectives on Paedophilia*, B. Taylor (ed.), London: John Churchill, 1981.

60. Kinsey, A. C., Pomeroy, W. B., Martin C. E. & Gebhard, P. H., *Sexual Behaviour in the Human Female*, Philadelphia & London: Saunders, 1953, p. 121.

61. Ussher & Dewberry, 1994.

62. 'Howard League Working Party Report', 1984, p. 20.

63. See Howitt, D., *Child Abuse Errors*, Hemel Hempstead: Harvester Wheatsheaf, 1992.

64. Recognition of the deleterious long-term effects of CSA initially arose from the identification of high proportions of CSA in female psychiatric populations: For example, rates of 33 per cent, 30 per cent and 64 per cent were reported by Rosenfeld, Q., Nadelson, C., Krieger, M. & Backman, J., 'Incest and Sexual Abuse of Children', *Journal of the American Academy of Child Psychiatry*, 16, 1979, pp. 327–39; Spencer, J., 'Father–Daughter Incest: A Clinical View for the Correction Field', *Child Welfare*, 57, 1978, pp. 581–90; and Surrey, J., Swett, C., Michaels, A. & Levin, S., 'Reported History of Physical and Sexual Abuse and Severity of Symptomatology in Women Psychiatric Outpatients', *American Journal of Orthopsychiatry*, 60, 1990, pp. 412–17, respectively. Comparisons of adult women who have experienced CSA with control groups (e.g. Bagley, C. & Ramsey, R., 'Sexual Abuse in Childhood: Psychologic Outcomes and Implications for Social Work Practice', *Journal of Social Work and Human Sexuality*, 1986, pp. 33–47; Fromuth, M. E., *The Long-Term Psychological Impact of Childhood Sexual Abuse*, unpublished doctoral dissertation, Auburn University, 1983; Russell, 1986, suggests significantly higher rates of problems for those who have experienced CSA. The most commonly reported long-term effects include depression, anxiety, fear of men, sexual problems, self-destructive behaviour, substance abuse, low self-esteem and a tendency towards later victimization (see Cahill, C., Llewelyn, S. P. & Pearson, C., 'Long-Term Effects of Sexual Abuse which Occurred in Childhood: A Review', *British Journal of Clinical*

Psychology, 30, 1991, pp. 117–30; Browne, A. & Finkelhor, D., 'Impact of Child Sexual Abuse: A Review of the Research', *Psychological Bulletin*, 99 (1), 1986, pp. 66–77, for reviews of the literature). Whilst there are disagreements over the magnitude and extent of effects, the major dispute arises over the question of which factors associated with CSA are more likely to lead to later problems.

65. Extract from a letter to *Village Voice*, 22 October 1979, reprinted in Stanko, 1985, pp. 34–5.

66. Blair, L. M., 'The Problem of Rape', *Police Surgeon*, Spring 1977, p. 16. Quoted in Edwards, S., *Female Sexuality and the Law*, Oxford: Martin Robeson, 1981, p. 169.

67. Defence counsel in a rape trial. Quoted in Adler, 1987, p. 74.

68. Farr, S., *Elements of Medical Jurisprudence* (trans. and abridged from *Elementa Medicinae Forensis* by J. Faselius), 1815, p. 46. Quoted in Edwards, 1981, p. 123.

69. Comment from a rapist who had broken into his victim's home. Quoted in Scully, 1990, p. 13.

70. Ibid., p. 106.

71. Ibid., p. 113.

72. Ibid., p. 114.

73. Ibid., p. 104.

74. Lees, 1996, p. 226.

75. Ibid., p. 233, for examples of this.

76. See Russell, D. E. H., 'The Prevalence and Incidence of Rape and Attempted Rape of Females', *Victimology*, 7, 1982, pp. 81–93, in Koss, Gidycz & Wisniewski, 1987.

77. Parrot, A. & Link, R., *Acquaintance Rape in a College Population*, paper presented at the eastern regional meeting of the Society for the Scientific Study of Sex, Philadelphia, PA, 1983.

78. Parrot & Bechhofer, 1991, p. 11.

79. The term was first coined by the US feminist rape researcher Mary Koss to describe a specific form of rape, but has been criticized as a misnomer more recently, as it has been used by the media to describe all forms of acquaintance rape. See Lees, 1996, pp. 77–8.

80. See Lees, 1996, Ch. 3, for a discussion of these cases and the media reporting that resulted from them.

81. Scully, 1990, p. 144.

82. Ibid., p. 110.

83. *Independent*, 15 December 1991, p. 15.
84. Routh, address to the British Gynaecological Society, 1886. Whilst describing women as 'the most decided liars in creation', Routh cautioned that gynaecologists were particularly at risk from unwarranted accusations of assault as a result of fantasies fuelled by a 'perverted sexual instinct'.
85. *R* v. *Henry and Manning* (2968) 53 Cr. App. R. at 153. Quoted in Adler, 1987, p. 15.
86. Blair, L. M., 'The Problem of Rape', *Police Surgeon*, Spring 1977, p. 16. Comment by a police medical officer of the Greater Manchester Police.
87. Rapist who argued that the woman fabricated the accusation of rape out of spite. Quoted in Adler, 1987, p. 93.
88. Taylor, A. S., 'The Principles and Practice of Medical Jurisprudence', London: John Churchill, 1865, p. 989. Quoted in Edwards, 1981, p. 126.
89. Quoted in Edwards, 1981, p. 128.
90. Comments of barrister at law Bernard Knight. In Knight, B., *Legal Aspects of Medical Practice*, London: Churchill Livingstone, 1972, p. 167.
91. Glaister, J., 'Legal Medicine for Members of the Legal Profession and Police Forces', Glasgow, 1925, p. 146. Quoted in Edwards, 1981, p. 131.
92. Arnold, 'Psychology Applied to Legal Evidence', London: G. F. Arnold, 1906. Quoted in Edwards, 1981, p. 131.
93. Quoted in Lees, 1996, p. 118.
94. Wigmore, J. H., *A Treatise on the Anglo-American System of Evidence in Trials at Common Law*, (3rd edition) vol. 3, pp. 459–60. Boston: Little Brown, 1940.
95. See Ussher, Jane, *Women's Madness: Misogyny or Mental Illness*, Hemel Hempstead: Harvester Wheatsheaf, 1991; Showalter, E., *The Female Malady*, London: Virago, 1987.
96. Quoted in Lees, 1996, p. 126.
97. Reported in *Guardian*, 29 March 1995.
98. See Lees, 1996, p. 79.
99. Comments made by the judge in the trial of a man convicted of making indecent, disgusting advances to women on a beach. *London Evening Standard*, 16 June 1993.
100. Mohr, J. W., Turner, R. E. & Jerry, N. B., *Paedophilia and Exhibitionism*, Toronto: Toronto University Press, 1964.
101. Quoted in Stanko, 1985, p. 95.
102. Ibid., p. 94, for a discussion of these cases.

103. Quoted in Lees, 1996, p. 142.

104. Howard League, 1985.

105. Ibid., 1985, p. 39.

106. Ibid., 1985, p. 39.

107. Rapist who abducted his victim at knife point from the street, quoted in Scully, 1990, p. 108.

108. *R* v. *Hodgson* [1811–12] E.R. 168 at 765. Cited by Edwards, 1981, p. 63.

109. Lees, 1996, p. 108.

110. Quoted in Adler, 1987, p. 99.

111. See the comments of the judge in the case of the author and former politician Jeffrey Archer, who was accused of consorting with a prostitute and brought a case of libel against a number of British newspapers. In his summing up of the cases, emphasizing the ludicrous nature of the accusation, the judge commented on the 'fragrant' nature of Archer's wife Mary – a woman held up as the epitome of femininity.

112. In England this occurred in 1976. Until the late eighties men's sexual history was also deemed inadmissible.

113. Adler, Z., 'The Reality of Rape Trials', *New Society*, 2 February 1982, pp. 90–1.

114. See Adler, 1981, p. 76.

115. Defence counsel in a rape trial. Quoted in Adler, 1987, p. 78.

116. Quoted in Adler, 1987, p. 79.

117. Adler, 1987, p. 76.

118. *R* v. *Hallett*, 1841. E.R. 173, at 1038. Cited by Edwards, 1987, p. 61.

119. *R* v. *Hallett*, 1841. E.R. 173, at 1038. Cited by Edwards, 1987, p. 61.

120. *R* v. *Clay*, 1851, 5 Cox CC at 146.

121. *R* v. *Greenberg*, 1923, 17 Crim. App. Rep. at 106. Cited by Edwards, 1987, p. 62.

122. *R* v. *Bashir & Manzur*, 1969. 3 All E.R. at 692. Cited by Edwards, 1987, p. 64.

123. Griffin, Susan, 'Rape: The All-American Crime', *Ramparts*, September 1971, p. 30. Quoted in Tong, Rosemarie, *Women, Sex and the Law*, New Jersey: Rowman & Allanheld, 1987, p. 90.

124. Edwards, 1987, p. 31.

125. See Wilson, M. & Daly, M., 'Till Death Us Do Part', in *Femicide: The Politics of Women Killing*, Buckingham: Open University Press, 1992.

126. Scully, 1990, p. 139.

127. Silverman, D. & McCombie, S., 'Counselling the Mates and Families of

Rape Victims', in *The Rape Crisis Intervention Handbook*, S. McCombie (ed.), New York: Plenum Press, 1980.

128. Stiglmayer, 1994, p. 96.
129. Raped woman quoted by Burgess, A. & Holmstrom, L. L., 'Rape Trauma Syndrome', *American Journal of Psychiatry*, 131, 1974, pp. 981–6, p. 983. Quoted in Stanko, 1985, p. 42.
130. Raped woman quoted by Hanmer, J. & Saunders, S., 'Blowing the Cover of the Protective Male: A Community Study of Violence to Women', in Garmanikow, E., Morgan, D., Purvis, J. & Taylorson, D., *The Public and the Private*, London: Heinemann, 1983. Quoted in Stanko, 1985, p. 43.
131. Scully, 1990, p. 142.
132. Both extracts from Scully, 1990, p. 159.
133. See O'Sullivan, Chris, 'Acquaintance Rape on Campus', in Parrot & Bechhofer, 1991, pp. 140–56, for a good review of this issue.
134. Scully, 1990, pp. 155–8.
135. Scully, 1990, p. 157.
136. In re. B.G., 589 A.2.d 637, 640–41 (NJ Super. Ct. App. Div. 1991) *Fordham Law Review*, p. 129.
137. *Newsday*, 17 October 1992, p. 17.
138. O'Sullivan in Parrot & Bechhofer, 1991, p. 151.
139. Pierson, D. K., 'Mixed Bag of Reactions Following Rape Trial Verdict', *Lansing State Journal*, 1 April 1984, 1B–2B, reporting the case of seven college students accused of raping a seventeen-year-old woman in a college dorm at Michigan State University.
140. O'Sullivan in Parrot & Bechhofer, 1991, p. 144.
141. Ibid., p. 150.
142. Scully, 1990, p. 156.
143. See Garrett-Gooding, J. & Senter, R., 'Attitudes and Acts of Sexual Aggression on a University Campus', *Sociological Enquiry*, 59, 1987, pp. 348–71, who reported that fraternity men were more likely to have engaged in coercive sex (35 per cent) than men not affiliated with any organization (11 per cent). Hoffman, R., 'Rape and the College Athlete: Part One', *Philadelphia Daily News*, 17 March 1986, p. 104, reported an FBI study in which football and basketball players were reported to the police for assault 38 per cent more often than the average male on campus.
144. Stiglmayer, 1994, p. 133.
145. Lees, 1996, p. 39.
146. Stiglmayer, 1994, p. 147.

147. Russell, D. E. H., 'Wife Rape', in Parrot & Bechhofer, 1991, pp. 129–39. The seven states are Kentucky, Missouri, New Mexico, North Carolina, Oklahoma, South Carolina and Utah.

148. See Russell, 1991. Another example of an exemption remaining in certain US states is to allow rape if the wife is unable to give consent because of a mental or physical disorder.

149. Russell, 1982, in Koss, Gidycz & Wisniewski, 1987.

150. Frieze, I. H., 'Investigating the Causes and Consequences of Marital Rape', Signs, 8 (3) 1983, pp. 532–53.

151. *Independent*, 24 October 1991, p. 3.

152. Russell, 1982, in Koss, Godycz & Wisniewski, 1987, p. 357.

153. See Dobash, R. E. & Dobash, R., *Violence against Wives. A Case against the Patriarchy*, London: Open Books, 1979, Ch. 4, for an excellent description of this history.

154. J. O'Faolain & L. Martin (eds.), *Not in God's Image: Women in History*, London: Virago, 1974, p. 55.

155. Mill, John Stuart, *The Subjugation of Women*, London: Debt, first published, 1869, 1955, p. 296.

156. Cobbe, Francis Power, 'Wife Torture in England', *Contemporary Review*, April 1878, pp. 55–87, p. 63.

157. Young, J., *Wife Beating in Britain: A Socio-Historical Analysis 1850–1914*, paper presented to the American Sociological Association, August 1976, New York City, p. 9.

158. Straus, M. A., Gelles, R. J. & Steinmetz, S., *Behind Closed Doors: Violence in the American Family*, New York: Doubleday, 1980, survey.

159. British Crime Survey, 1994.

160. Steinmetz, S., *The Cycle of Violence*, New York: Praeger Publishers, 1977.

161. *Independent*, 24 October 1991, p. 3.

162. Quoted in Stanko, 1985, p. 48.

163. *People* v. *Wood*, 391 N.E. 2d 206.

164. For example, see Wilbanks, W., 'Criminal Homicide Offenders in the US: *Black* v. *White*', in *Homicide among Black Americans*, D. F. Hawkins (ed.), New York: University Press of America, 1986, pp. 43–55.

165. Report in the *Guardian*, June 22 1995, p. 2.

166. Kelkar, G., 'Women and Structural Violence in India', *Women's Studies Quarterly*, 13, 3–4, 1985, pp. 16–18.

167. See Fraser, Antonia. *The Six Wives of Henry the Eighth*, London: Mandarin, 1992, for a fascinating account of all of these much maligned women.

Fraser claims that Anne Boleyn was guilty only of having fallen out of favour with her lord and master, as he had fallen in love with someone else – Jane Seymour, his next wife. The only evidence for Boleyn's adultery came from a manservant who was tortured.

168. Dell, S., *Murder into Manslaughter*, Oxford: Oxford University Press, 1984.
169. Both interviews are part of Catherine Carlson's study interviewing spousal homicides investigated by the Ontario police. Carlson, C., *Intrafamilial Homicide*, unpublished B.Sc. thesis, McMaster University, 1984. Quoted in Wilson, Margo & Daly, Martin, 'Till Death Us Do Part' in *Femicide: The Politics of Woman Killing*, Jill Radford & Diana H. Russell (ed.), Buckingham: Open University Press, 1992.
170. Campbell, J., 'If I Can't Have You No One Can. Power and Control in Homicide of Female Partners', in Radford & Russell, 1992, pp. 99–113.
171. See Lees, Sue, 'Naggers, Whores and Libbers: Provoking Men to Kill', in Radford & Russell, 1992, pp. 267–88, p. 278.
172. See Radford, Jill, 'Retrospect on a Trial', in Radford & Russell, 1992, pp. 277–323, for an account of the case.
173. Lees, in Radford & Russell, 1992, p. 283. In other countries, such as Australia, Canada and the United States, the prosecution can insist that evidence in rebuttal should be brought.
174. All four cases described by Lees in Radford & Russell, 1992, p. 275.
175. Reported in the *Guardian*, 29 October 1994, p. 1.
176. Reported in the *Guardian*, 27 October 1994, p. 14.
177. For example, Myra Hindley, the British 'Moors murderer', who with her partner Ian Brady sexually assaulted and murdered a number of children in the early sixties. See Cameron, L. D. & Frazer, L., *The Lust to Kill*, London: Polity Press, 1989. Rosemary West, convicted of the murder and sexual assault of twelve women in 1995, is another example.
178. Ed Vulliamy, *Observer*, 24 April 1994, p. 18.
179. A number of these cases are outlined by Deborah Cameron and Liz Frazer in their critique of sex killings, *A Lust to Kill*. Others appear in Jane Caputi's *The Age of Sex Crime*, London: The Women's Press, 1987.
180. See Master, R. E. L. and Lea, E., *Sex Crimes in History: Evolving Concepts of Sadism, Lust Murder and Necrophilia From Ancient to Modern Times*, New York: Julian Press, 1963, for an analysis of such crimes across history.
181. Robert Bloch, introducing 'The Prowler in the City at the Edge of the World', a story by Harlan Ellison, in *Dangerous Visions*, H. Ellison (ed.), p. 130. Quoted in Caputi, 1987, p. 17.

182. *Guardian*, 24 April 1994, p. 18.

183. One of the reasons we will never know the exact number of murders which can be correctly attributed to 'Jack the Ripper' is that there were clearly a number of imitators. This wasn't difficult, given the detailed descriptions of the murderer's actions given in the nineteenth-century press, a practice avoided by current police forces in order to ascertain whether they have caught the 'real' murderer when they question suspects (as well as to reduce the actual copy-cat crimes).

184. Cameron & Frazer, 1989, p. 123.

185. All three were cited by Jane Caputi, 1987, p. 33.

186. Caputi, 1987, p. 46.

187. *Daily Mirror*, 7 April 1979.

188. Unwise in the sense that they made themselves vulnerable by their behaviour – one of the dominant rape myths.

189. Men and boys are subjected to sexual violence, and it is not unknown for women to perpetrate such acts (although very infrequent). See pp. 276–8 for a discussion of this.

CHAPTER SIX

Reframing Femininity: Reframing the Boundaries of Sex

Fantasies of Femininity Framed in a Masculine Gaze

I started with fairy stories and have ended with sexual violence and sexual murder. A thread of fictions and fantasies about 'woman' and 'sex' runs between them. I have addressed the questions: Why have representations of 'woman' come to be synonymous with 'sex'? In whose interests are these sexual visions created? Whose concerns do they reflect? What is their influence on the lived experience of women, and of men? Are they a reflection of what women really are or a fantasy about what 'woman' could (or should) be? Why are the boundaries of 'sex' so narrowly defined? After journeying through the various genres of representation and examining their influence on individual women and men, we can now proffer a number of answers to these questions.

We have seen how representations of femininity and masculinity play a central role in the formation of the subjectivity and sexuality of women and men.[1] We understand ourselves as 'woman' or 'man' in relation to the social representations of what it means to be so, in relation to historically and culturally specific definitions and constructions of femininity and masculinity. Our knowledge about these constructions is not inborn or inbuilt. We continuously learn and rehearse what it is to be a 'woman' or 'man' in a process of negotiating these symbolic representations of femininity, masculinity and sexuality.

As we have seen, representations of 'woman' are framed primarily within a masculine gaze and thus reflect the fantasies, fears and desires of man. Sex is central to these fantasies of femininity, because it is in the arena of sex and sexuality that the differences between the genders, which are so central to the maintenance of order and power in a phallocentric social sphere, are constructed and defined. As heterosexuality is hegemonic, the scripts of masculinity and femininity which circulate at any point in time are irrevocably tied to the boundaries of heterosexual sex. As the boundaries of 'sex' shift and change across cultural contexts and across time, so do the scripts of what is acceptable for 'woman' and 'man'.

Sex is also central to masculine fantasies of femininity because it is the primary arena in which men prove themselves to be 'man'. Sex stands as a site of power and pleasure, but also of fear and dread. It affords intimacy and, simultaneously, vulnerability. It may produce ecstatic joy, or feelings of failure and despair. As long as heterosexual 'sex' is defined as vaginal intercourse, with man's phallic performance central to successful accomplishment of the sexual act, anxiety will never be absent. If a man (or rather his penis) cannot perform, 'sex' (so defined) cannot occur. His very status as 'man' is placed in doubt. Given the fragile nature of the organ, it isn't surprising that fears of failure and anxiety underlie the apparent sexual bravado of man or that woman is the primary site of projected anger, anxiety and despair.[2]

We see evidence of this projection in the images of 'woman' framed within the masculine gaze. In art, film and pornography we have seen how representations of the sexuality of 'woman' are juxtaposed with those of the phallic mastery of 'man': the avenging prince whose sword pierces the 'vagina denta'; the slave master with his naked harem; the female nude exposed to the all-penetrating gaze; the whore who is raped; the saint who is tortured; the porn star who is fucked. We have also seen the adoration and aggrandizement of the idealized, almost *a*sexual woman: the Madonna with child at breast; the good wife; the angel in the house; the luminously beautiful cinema star. The objectification of 'woman' that underlies these sexual visions, whether enacted through denigration or adoration, acts to alleviate her threat – the threat that she will laugh, that she will reject or that her fecund sexuality will never be satiated. These images are not reflections of what women *are*, or of how women should be; they are fantasies of what and how many men would *like* women to be – in their imaginations at least. If woman is put on a pedestal – or, conversely, crushed by the mythical all-mighty phallus – man has no need to feel either envy or fear. Instead he can worship and adore – or conquer, destroy and maintain the illusion of invincible masculine power. Envy is replaced by aggression, anxiety by (temporary) satisfaction.

This, to me, was one of the most surprising aspects of the interviews I carried out with men – their anxiety, vulnerability and insecurity in the face of the sexuality of women. It stood in stark contrast to the images of powerful, vengeful phallic men that populate the pages of both patriarchal treatises and many radical feminist texts. These interviews caused me drastically to rethink my own original thesis, in which man was positioned as exerting a machiavellian or malevolent control on female sexuality – the more usual feminist tale. Faced with repeated stories of vulnerability, fear and dread, the picture looks very different.

However, whilst men fear women because they might laugh at them, women fear men because they might rape or kill them. Which is worse?

As we have seen, it is not only in the imagination, or the world of symbolic representation that these sexualized fantasies and fears are played out – many men deal with their dread of 'woman' by diminishing or degrading the women who are objects of their desire or by seeing sex simply as an arena for the enactment of phallic power and control. We see evidence of this enacted in the denigration of women as sex objects and in the debasing and defiling of woman positioned as 'whore' – men systematically seducing and then rejecting women for being 'slags' of easy virtue or men acting out their sexual fantasies with women working as prostitutes. No fear of rejection here. No need to invest undue anxiety in the performance of penis as phallus. No fear of failure with these (non)women.

We can also see these fears and fantasies played out in the whole gamut of ideologies and practices associated with sexual crimes, sexual problems and, in particular, with sexual violence. We are presented with models of sexuality which narrowly define heterosexual intercourse as 'normal sex'. At the same time, anything which is a threat to the hegemony of heterosexual man is pathologized or condemned, homosexuality being the prime example. We are also presented with a model of 'normal' heterosexuality which legitimates or normalizes masculine power and control, feminine passivity and resistance. The most extreme example of the enactment of this phallocentric fantasy of omnipotence can be seen in serial sexual murder, but it is also evident in rape and child sexual abuse. The combination of misogyny and male insecurity underlying this systematic violation of women is concealed by the legal and medical professions. They act to divert attention from the nature of phallocentric masculinity and the pervasive nature of these abusive practices by focusing on female precipitation (the law) or on the biology and pathology of individual men (science).

This is not just a story about sex. As Michel Foucault argued, the control and regulation of sex is central to the regulation of the whole social sphere. Sexual practice is not arbitrary or coincidental, a negotiation in the privacy of the bedroom (or wherever else we care to practise our pleasures). How we express our sexuality, how we define what is permitted and what is forbidden, who is the taker and who is the taken, all reflect and construct the whole of our social order. Sex laws and sexual mores underpin social hierarchies and structures of power, reifying the legitimacy of those in positions of authority, whilst concealing this very process by positioning the practice of 'sex' in the realm of the private – even in these days of mass exposure of sex few people would consider their sexual lives to be anything other than a private matter, an expression of personal desire, a matter of free choice. We may resist the notion that we are reproducing deep-seated power relations through our sexual activities and through our definition of ourselves in various sexual roles (wife, girlfriend, mistress, heterosexual, bisexual, lesbian . . .), claiming it to be a personal preference, or perhaps a 'natural' state we take for granted. We would be wrong. The maintenance of the boundaries of sex and sexuality are central to the maintenance of phallocentric order and power, and central to this process is the symbolic meaning of dominant constructions of the sexuality of 'woman'.

The ways in which female sexuality is contained or allowed to be expressed both symbolize and reinforce power relations between women and men. Lévi-Strauss has argued that the literal exchange of women in kinship systems, in particular in marriage, symbolizes and maintains a patriarchal social order. When the father passes his daughter to her husband on her wedding day, when the father pays a dowry, or a 'bride price', this is not merely a quaint custom or an arbitrary ceremony. It is imbued with meanings whereby the woman's position within the social order, her worth and/or powerlessness – in contrast to man's power – are communicated. In the act of marriage the exchange of a woman from one man to another symbolizes phallocentric power and the 'correct' hierarchy of sexual relationships which underpin patriarchal culture – woman as object to be owned and exchanged, man as arbiter of that exchange. Equally, the rules of heterosexual romance that dictate that women should wait and men should actively pursue act to position women as passive objects to be chosen (or rejected) and men as agentic subjects with a right to dictate whether sexual relationships succeed or fail.

Yet to talk of phallocentric power and the limitations it places on the lives of individual women is not to point the finger at every living breathing man. Many men deserve such criticism, as analyses of the detrimental effects on women of the social dominance of heterosexual masculinity illustrate, in particular, in the arena of sexual violence and abuse. But many others do not. Equally, the story of the material regulation of female sexuality which has unfolded in this book cannot be the story of all women, any more than the phallocentric fantasies and fears which underpin it is the story of all men. It is naïve to imagine that we can develop an argument which will encompass the experience of the sexuality of women as a homogeneous group – there are as many differences between women of different ages, race, class and culture as there are similarities. I have not focused on these differences; they have been fully explored elsewhere. I have focused on the symbolic construction of 'woman' in what is still a phallocentric sphere and on the implications this has for the lived experience of many women, the construction of our sexual identities, the expression of our sexuality and the maintenance of the power of men.

The separation of the symbolic construction of 'woman' or 'man' from the examination of the experience of women and men as living and breathing subjects[3] moves us away from the pernicious situation in which individual women (or groups of women) can undermine or attempt to undermine carefully and meticulously constructed feminist critiques[4] with the following comments: 'I have never experienced abuse or sexual violence'; 'In my experience women are treated as equal to men'; 'Men are not sexist; feminists are paranoid'. These are the sentiments engendered by the feminist backlash[5] being uttered through the mouths of indignant women, their voices as 'woman' giving legitimacy to misogynistic or blinkered views and acting as insidious ammunition against feminist resistance to phallocentric control. Ironically, many younger women who enjoy the benefits of feminist critiques and campaigns (education, equal-pay legislation, control over reproduction . . .) seem to be ever-ready to reject or condemn the label 'feminist',

'I'm not a feminist, but . . .' being a common retort.[6] They may be guilty merely of taking for granted gains that were hard won, but they may also be buying into and giving voice to masculine fears about independent, questioning women, symbolized by the connotations of aggressiveness, ugliness and 'ball-breaking' that 'feminism' continues to have in many men's eyes. Their own desirability and allegiance to men is signified by their rejection of 'humourless' feminist women and the denial that objectification or sexual violence could ever happen to them.

At one level what they say may be true – not all women experience physical sexual oppression; not every woman is a victim. And perhaps most importantly, at least for those women who are attempting to make a success of a heterosexual relationship, denigration and degradation of women is not the favourite practice of every individual man. Relationships with men can be fulfilling at both an emotional and a sexual level. Many men have reframed and remoulded phallocentric masculinity, allowing them to have relationships with women which are egalitarian and devoid of objectification. These men may not identify so readily with the fantasies of femininity which have been explored in this book. The story of fear, anxiety and dread may not resonate in them, or may be effectively repressed. But for many others, it is a story which is all too true.

The analysis of sexual violence I have carried out illustrates without a doubt that many individual women are abused. Many women experience rape, sexual harassment and, as children, sexual abuse.[7] Many women are defined by their sexuality, in a way that positions them as second-rate, the eternal second sex. Many women lead desperately unhappy lives attempting to live up to impossible standards of feminine perfection, believing that it is they who have failed if life doesn't live up to the romantic dream. Equally, many women suffer extensive damage, both physically and psychologically, as a result of pervasive denigration and abuse. Those who escape this to lead happy, healthy, fulfilling lives may be superwomen, token women or simply women deluding themselves. They may be exceptions or simply lucky (or privileged). They may have forged an effective resistance. But their very existence does not allow us to turn a blind eye to all those women who cannot or have not escaped and to the perpetual sexualization of 'woman' which pervades all our lives.

Equally, we must not forget that the way in which science and the law define and treat sexual deviance, sexual problems, sexual violence and, by implication, 'normal sex' is simply one example of phallocentric fantasies and fears being translated into the material regulation of women's lives. We can see analogous practices in psychiatry and psychology, where femininity and female sexuality are seen as signs of madness; in the regulation and restriction of women's reproductive bodies; in sexual surgery; and in what has been termed 'sexual slavery'. We must also not forget the many political and economic controls of women's lives – in employment legislation and opportunities, educational inequalities and social policy.

So, whilst it is important to distinguish between analyses of the symbolic representation of 'woman' or 'man' and the lived experience of women and men, the two levels of analysis are irrevocably linked. This suggests that, whilst this book is not a catalogue of man-hating or man-blaming, with women as innocent victims who are misogynistically maligned, individual men are not to be let off the hook completely. Whilst we may in part focus on the realm of representation and the fantasies which circulate in the imaginary or symbolic domain, it is important to keep hold of the grounded nature of sexuality and its role in the maintenance of a phallocentric social sphere which supports the interests of many individual men and negates the interests of many women.

Denying or Defending against Misogyny

Karen Horney first wrote of man's dread and denigration of woman in the thirties. Her words are still percipient today, yet many women wish to ignore or deny these facts. Why? Man fears woman, yet will not (or cannot) acknowledge that fear. It is essential to his illusion of mastery that he is positioned as strong, that he represses his dread. Many women are successfully fooled into believing men to be invincible and deem them inadequate failures if they are not, thereby adding to the pressure on men to live up to being 'man'. It is one of the great ironies of heterosexual relationships: Man has convinced woman that she wants what he wishes himself to be. It is something he can achieve only at great cost, through continual adherence to the masquerade of phallocentric masculinity. The price of such deceit, of such difficult disguise, is passed on to and paid by women.

This is something to which many women turn a blind eye. Like the repression of memories of childhood abuse, the most effective defence is not to see at all. This is not surprising, for if women allow themselves *really* to see the charade which masculinity is and acknowledge the misogynistic machinations which have such deleterious consequences for women, how can they continue to coexist quietly and compliantly in their relations with men? For heterosexual women this problem is arguably most acute. How can they reconcile their own sexual practices and preferences with the realization of what it means to be 'man'? Some women deal with this by idealizing one individual man – 'My man is different'; 'I'm lucky to have found the perfect man.' They can thus hold the critical analysis of gender relationships that is taken for granted by today's 'post-feminist' women whilst continuing to remain in sexual relationships with men.[8] Along with this, many women position their own man as vulnerable, in need of sensitive care, inoculating themselves against any criticism of women's role in relation to men. In contrast, other women continually complain about the treatment meted out to them by men; it is one of the points of commonality or solidarity in conversations between heterosexual women. Yet, because all agree that 'This is what men are like,' these women remain in a state of permanent frustration or complaint.

These are ultimately dysfunctional defences, for they merely perpetuate the existing hierarchy of phallocentric power. Idealizing, or protecting the vulnerability of an individual man may prevent women from facing the horror of masculine abuse and allow them to accrue the protection afforded to individual women in the surface safety of the heterosexual domain, but it also opens women to the restrictions and abuses that exist in that sphere – the narrow constraints of the feminine script and sexual and marital violence. The idealization or protection of man also renders any effective resistance almost impossible. What is there to resist? Equally, complaining about men yet seeing little possibility for improvement or change leaves women powerless and impotent, reinforcing the view that misery is a woman's rightful fate. This also acts to focus attention and blame for injustice or feelings of inadequacy on the woman herself; if women refuse to face up to the magnitude of the continuum of violence and the disparagement systematically dealt out to women as a sex, the ultimate recourse is to blame themselves or to believe it is true when they are told that they are to blame. Man's flight from his fear of woman is aided by many women's modes of denial or defence.

We shouldn't be surprised to find that so many women have taken this tack. Historically, the systematic undermining of the self-respect of women has worked effectively to render many women impotent and overly dependent on the attentions and esteem of a man; they could not live without his praise, convinced that they were lucky, or privileged, to receive it. Their sense of self came from a relationship with a man. The circulation of narrow, sexualized representations of 'woman' – the fantasies of femininity found in the images of 'woman' aimed at and consumed by women and girls in fairy stories, romantic fiction, teenage magazines, soap opera and advertising imagery – acted constantly to remind women that they were worthless without a man. In this fantasy of femininity it is 'man' who is powerful and controlling and woman who is passive and resistant; 'nice girls' still wait to be asked (and invariably say 'no') and sexual girls are 'slags'; man stands as sexual conqueror whilst woman lies down and is 'seduced'; women are encouraged to transform themselves into the object of masculine desire and given detailed instructions how to achieve this goal – how to change themselves into creatures of beauty and charm, shedding or concealing their natural faults. The lesson is how to *be* and what to *do*. Woman may put up with all manner of ills, as it is better to have *any* man than no man at all. As women are continuously reminded that 'a good man is hard to find' and even more difficult to catch and to keep, is it surprising that so many women stay with what they've got rather than risk isolation and the associated stigma of 'spinsterhood'? Far better to have a man to moan about, than no man at all.

However, this isn't the only story to be told. I am not ending this journey with a wringing of hands or a cacophany of cursing about the sorry state of heterosexual masculinity or indeed the misogynistic motives of many individual men. As has already been made clear, women are not passive dupes. They do not simply lie down and accept the narrow scripts of femininity which are currently on offer. Equally, it is certainly not the inevitable fate of women to end up as victims of objectification or abuse. As we have seen, women are fully able to negotiate the fantasies of femininity which currently dominate the world of symbolic representation and, in the process, act to reframe the very meaning of what it is to be 'woman' or 'man'. The reaction to the pervasive regulation of women's sexuality in this case is resistance rather than resignation. I have identified three levels at which women actively resist – through deconstructing or reframing masculine fantasies of femininity; through active resistance to material control; and through negotiating a script of femininity which acts to reframe the boundaries of sex. To illustrate the complexity of these strategies of negotiation, I will examine each in turn.

Women Negotiating Fantasies of Femininity

Reframing Femininity through the Female Gaze

At a theoretical level, feminist critics have deconstructed and resisted the sexualized representations of 'woman' that circulate in the symbolic sphere – in art, film, literature, pornography and the mass media. In exposing the unconscious fantasies, fears and desires that underpin the masculine gaze, the foundations for an effective re-reading of the meaning of 'woman' and for new forms of representation framed within a female gaze have been laid, as we have seen.

Deconstructing phallocentric images of 'woman' exposes as much of the creators and consumers of these fantasy forms as it does about the construction of 'woman' – whilst these sexual images may initially appear to be about women, in reality they are about what it is to be 'man'. Heterosexual masculinity is defined by difference from 'woman' and all that feminine sexuality connotes, so men define themselves as 'man' through their difference from the sexualized representations of 'woman' in the media. However, as we have seen in the analysis of mass media imagery aimed at women, or in feminist art and film, representations of women within a female gaze[9] tell a different, more complex, story of what it is to be 'woman'. They have taken the form of a critique of what it is to 'do girl', in which visual representations of archetypal femininity are parodied and exposed for the sexualized fictions they are. They have also explored the tensions involved in reconciling aspects of female experience that might traditionally have been restrictive – such as beauty, sexuality or mothering – with women's desire to be an autonomous agentic subject. This demonstrates that women do not have to throw the baby out with the bath water, rejecting everything deemed 'feminine' in their quest to be something other than the 'second sex'. Reclaiming or reframing the body, sexuality or the relationship between mother and child can provide a very different interpretation of what it means to be 'woman' than that represented in archetypal representations of the Madonna or whore. But the female gaze can also be subversive and troubling, as we have seen in the case of lesbian pornography, re-visions of masculinity and representations of 'woman' taking up what is the traditional position of 'man' – the powerful, autonomous sexual subject or the independent active agent who is subjugated by no one. And, unlike in film noir, where the strong sexual woman is ultimately destroyed, these women survive. We also see evidence of this resistance in representations of 'woman' outside a sexualized gaze, women not defined by their bodies, by beauty or by their relationships with men.

Today, we can see that *women's* fantasies and desires are also reflected in the different genres of representation they consume – fantasies of power and feminine pleasure, as well as of masochism and pain. Teenage magazines now depict girls who are in control, even if only covertly so. Sex is no longer forbidden – even the heroines of romantic fiction now indulge. We also see images of women in positions of authority and control, refusing to bow down to any man, often juxtaposed with images of woman seduced, humiliated or literally possessed. These are all representations of 'woman' that are complex and contradictory and often the antithesis of what the romantic hero has traditionally come to expect.

Women Resisting Material Control

As the regulation of 'woman' and feminine sexuality is not simply a case of ephemeral representations without material consequences, so is women's resistance far wider than that which takes place in the symbolic sphere. I have examined the ways in which phallocentric myths about 'woman' and 'sex' are used to justify the material control of women's bodies and lives. All these practices have been resisted and negotiated at the levels of theory and practice – in the refusal of individual women to accede to regulation of their bodies and lives; in political lobbying or activism; and in academic critiques – of law, science, medicine, education – which have had a direct impact on the way in which the institutions of the state are able to regulate sexuality and what it means to be 'woman'. In North America and much of Europe great changes have been brought about by these organized bodies of resistance: Women have the vote; the right to education and paid employment; legal rights of redress for rape or domestic violence; access to contraception and abortion; rights of custody over their children; rights of property ownership; and the right legally to live autonomously as independent citizens – which increasing numbers are choosing to do. However, the gains hard won by a century of feminist campaigning are not universal; in other cultural contexts women are still legally categorized as second-class citizens and have few rights over their own bodies or their own lives. Sexual slavery is not a thing of the past; millions of women are each year forced into prostitution or arranged marriages; are subjected to clitoridectomy; and are legally the property of man, whether he be husband or father. We should not forget that it was only a hundred years ago that a woman in England or North America could not vote, did not have access to the same education or employment as men and could legally be beaten by her husband. Only sixty years ago women were locked up in mental institutions and castigated by 'respectable' society for becoming pregnant out of wedlock. Thirty years ago abortion was illegal. We should not take for granted the gains that have been won (and which in the backlash against feminism may still now be lost) and should recognize that it is a relatively recent luxury for women's negotiation of what it is to be 'woman' to be allowed to take place at all.

Women Negotiating Femininity

However, it isn't just overt objectification and abuse that is negotiated and resisted by women, it is also the very meaning of what it means to be 'woman'. At an individual level, women and girls negotiate the scripts of femininity in order to take up or resist the position of 'woman'. Becoming 'woman' is something women *do* rather than something women *are*; it is always at least in part a charade or a masquerade. In order to 'do girl' women have to negotiate the scripts of femininity which are currently in play and then reconcile the contradictions and inconsistencies, if they want to get it 'right' (or reject and subvert the scripts if they choose deliberately to get it 'wrong'). Women have to find a fit between what they want (Freud's now infamous question) and what they are supposed to be. Whilst the meaning of what it is to be 'woman' is always situated in a particular cultural milieu, with representations of femininity providing the boundaries of normality and acceptable performance, personal development, the impact of previous experiences and a changing social or familial context can precipitate a move to a different identificatory site. This will be influenced by conscious and unconscious psychological factors, by a woman's age and stage of life, by her relationships with other women and men and the reactions of others to the scripts she adopts.

In order to illustrate the pluralistic and fluid nature of this process, of what it is to be (or do) 'woman', I will outline below four different positions which women take up in their negotiation of femininity taken from the many interviews I have conducted: being, doing, rejecting or subverting 'girl', 'girl' being that archetypal fantasy of perfect femininity we see framed within the boundaries of heterosexual sexuality and romance. These are not four different personality typologies, or fixed positions which can be rigidly differentiated. These are *performances*, not a new taxonomy of what women inevitably *are*. Women will slide or shift between these different positions at different points in time, and often neither the woman herself nor those who would wish to interpret her particular interpretation of the masquerade will be able to pinpoint her exactly. Few performances are perfect. As Judith Butler has commented, 'to the extent that gender is an assignment, it is an assignment which is never quite carried out according to expectation, whose addressee never quite inhabits the ideal s/he is compelled to approximate.'[10] How we interpret the performance of any individual woman will depend as much on her intentions as on the assumptions we bring to our reading of her performance. But as intentions are not always conscious and our assumptions will be influenced by the gendered position we adopt ourselves this is a complicated affair.

Being Girl

I will start with the most familiar – the archetypal position of 'woman', the position taken up when a woman wants to *be* rather than merely *do* femininity, when she wants to live out the role of the romantic heroine in the fairy stories of childhood. Beauty, goodness and the ability to attract the admiration of men are the key attributes of being girl. This is the script of femininity found in romantic fiction and fifties

Hollywood films, the script every good girl ought to follow. In order to be girl, the body must be worked on, moulded and skilfully transformed from base matter into beauty (magazines and cosmetic companies tell us how). Any imperfections must be eradicated or disguised. If all goes to plan and a man is attracted and kept, life is 'happy ever after'. If not, misery may result. As one woman I interviewed said, 'Men have so many expectations about a woman's body and performance and that – I'm frightened I couldn't live up to that.' However, as *being* girl is about optimism not cynicism, feelings of inadequacy are invariably followed by renewed attention to the artifice of feminine charm and the rigours of cosmetic disguise.

In order to take up the position of being girl, there has to be complete suspension of disbelief in the rituals of heterosexual romance, complete acceptance of the notion that differences between women and men are natural or right. Being girl positions woman as the mirror to man, the 'living doll', the myth of the mother/Madonna made flesh (although in the late-twentieth-century version, in the privacy of the marital bedroom she may also act out the fantasy of the whore). Being girl means acceptance of the 'law of the father', never challenging or threatening masculine authority, power or control, accepting the phallocentric boundaries of 'sex'. As one woman told me, 'My boyfriend makes me feel wanted, and protected, and I would do anything to make him happy.' Or another, 'I've never wanted a career, I enjoy being a wife and mother. A mother's place is with her children.' To classify being girl as the myth of the fairy-tale princess come true is not to say that this is inevitably a position of weakness or vulnerability. Being girl in the late twentieth century is not about masochism or being a victim (although for some women, masochism can be the only explanation why they remain in this role). Thirty years ago, women may have had little choice in whether they wanted to be girl or not – only the foolhardy, the brave or the rich were able to step out of this archetypal position. Today, due to the impact of feminism and the availability of many other scripts of femininity women who want to be girl (either some or all of the time) invariably construe themselves as powerful and strong, as *choosing* femininity, as being the one who is *really* in control (as do the heroines of romantic fiction who manipulate men into fulfilling their romantic dreams).

Today, being girl doesn't necessitate being the 'little wife' at home;

women with career aspirations can take up this position as easily as those who do not. What being girl is associated with is an acceptance of the myth that one day the prince *will* come and, if he does, a woman should observe the rigid rules of heterosexual romance to the letter – courtship, marriage, monogamy and a maintenance of respectable appearance and demeanour. There is little risk of the woman who masters this performance being designated 'whore'. She is the 'reasonable woman' that rape law sets out to defend and protect, the one on whom all the privileges of heterosexuality are bestowed. *Other* women, who step outside the boundaries of femininity (or who contravene the rules of heterosexual romance) – the 'slag', the adulteress, the single mother, the lesbian, the career woman – are the ones who are condemned. In refusing to be 'good girls', they deserve all they get. Being girl invariably involves castigating and criticizing other women; the competitiveness between women we are taught in fairy stories and romantic fiction is made reality in the material world.

Being girl can mean motherhood; it invariably involves marriage. Motherhood will be joyous and fulfilling (or at least presented as such); marriage will be monogamous and lasting, based on devotion, mutual fidelity and 'love'. If man plays out his role as prince and is protective and faithful (or at the very least discreet), being girl can be a position of satisfaction and freedom from strife. The glowing mother/Madonna, the satisfied wife, the devoted girlfriend do exist outside the pages of romantic fiction and Hollywood films. The question is – for how long? The fairy tale often has an unhappy ending. The cracks are not always easy to paper over. What if a girl cannot find her romantic hero? If she can, what if he leaves her, refuses to love her or his fidelity fades? What if he beats her, rapes her or merely treats her like dirt? What if another woman steals him away? What if her beauty fades? If she gets fat? What happens when she gets old? What if motherhood is difficult, depressing and not the answer to a woman's dreams? Being girl is a potentially precarious position, a site of potential disappointment, failure and despair. Outside fairy tales few women manage to remain in the position of being girl for life. It can be nice while it lasts, for the few moments, days or sometimes years when a woman can maintain the mask of perfect femininity, when youth, beauty, the power of sexual attraction or the fulfilment of early motherhood are on a woman's side. If and when the mirror cracks and being girl is revealed as a fragile masquerade

– and all the more damagingly if the revelation is not acknowledged – misery and despair may ensue.

Mental health statistics tell us that it is women who try to be 'good wives and mothers' within the traditional script of femininity who are most at risk of depression and anxiety, women attempting to be girl full time. We should not be surprised. The role of the princess – self-sacrificing, subordinate to man, looking to her romantic prince or to idyllic motherhood for fulfilment – is a recipe for masochistic misery. The fairy-tale ending is something few women manage to make 'real', or to sustain. Joy and delight are only responses to domesticity and subjugation in fantasy and in fairy tales; depression, dejection and a sense of alienation are the responses of any sane woman to the annihilation of self which is central to this traditional position of 'woman'. Staying in a violent or dissatisfying relationship in the hope that a man can be reformed or will change or that underneath his harsh exterior burns a heart of gold is something which brings rewards only in romantic fiction or in fairy stories such as 'Beauty and the Beast'. In 'real life' it merely results in the steady decline of a woman's sense of self-worth. Equally, believing the beauty myth and trying to be perfection made flesh is a recipe for continual disappointment, not for fulfilment. Blaming the body for unhappiness and the failure of the romantic dream, as so many women do, can only make matters worse. Only by numbing herself to ambivalence and despair (Valium has now been overtaken by Prozac) or by hoping that someday things will change will women be able permanently to sustain the position of being girl. It is a position which requires the annihilation of self, of autonomy, of active desire.

Many women who have tried to live out the fairy-tale script and have repressed their desire for a secret life shift out of the position of being girl as they grow older. Maturity, experience and the eventual realization that the romantic dream is a myth results in a change in priorities and expectations. One interviewee, Helen, felt that her priorities changed after she had children. Sex, romantic love and the pressure to be beautiful no longer seemed of such central importance in her life. The anxieties of her teenage years – looking right, getting a boy, having a perfect body – seemed now to be trivialities:

'I now worry about the right school for my child, and whether I will be able to juggle work and home, and still find a moment for myself. The love I feel for my child surpasses anything I have ever felt before . . . and it puts all of the ridiculous games I used to think I had to play into perspective. I do have a good relationship with my partner, but it's based on commitment to a shared enterprise, not on him fulfilling my dreams. I now know that nobody else can do that for me. I wish I'd known it at seventeen – I'd have spent less time worrying about clothes and make-up, and wondering what I should do to be attractive and desirable, and more time thinking about what's going on in the world.'

It's an interesting irony. In many ways motherhood is central to the very definition of what being 'woman' is – the glowing Madonna idealized by artists and poets, fulfilling what the sociobiologists might see as her biological destiny. But for many women it throws the illusory nature of the romantic myth – and the myth of the Madonna – into sharp relief and can result in a greater self-assurance and sense of autonomy and power (or in depression if women believe that it is *they* who have failed). Motherhood changes priorities. Sex no longer seems so important, nor the attention of a man so essential. For women who find men who can make this shift with them, who can embark upon a more egalitarian relationship, who can enjoy a sexual and romantic life alongside other aims and goals in life, motherhood can comfortably exist within the traditional confines of heterosexual monogamy. For many women, however, this is another impossible dream. As divorce statistics and the growing number of 'single' mothers indicates women are increasingly choosing to leave the bounds of marriage that for previous generations of women, restrained by social and economic factors, were indissoluble ties. They are giving up being girl and the romantic myth that goes with this role in order to embark upon a more autonomous and agentic – as well as risky, in terms of phallocentric fantasies of femininity – life.

Other women stop attempting to be girl when they realize that moving outside the archetypal position of 'woman', resisting male dominance and power or developing an autonomous identity can lead to greater happiness and more positive mental health, or when the unconscious desires and fears that underpin this subservient role have somehow been resolved. However, for many women, there was never any question about their *being* girl; femininity has always been something that they *do*.

Doing Girl

In taking up the position of doing girl a woman will perform the feminine masquerade and, to all intents and purposes, may appear to be the 'good girl' incarnate. But she knows the fragility of the façade of femininity and the fact that doing girl is about playing a part. As one interviewee commented, 'I put on my face in the morning, and I feel as if I can do anything I want to. It's the most effective currency a woman has. But it isn't really me.' There is no attempt to be the fairy-tale princess here. Doing girl is arguably femininity harnessed for the pleasure and empowerment of the woman who enacts the display. However, it is a careful balancing act entailing manipulation and deceit, which results in the common refrain, 'Being a woman is great – we have the best of both worlds these days. I don't let on to men, though. They like to think they're in control.' This is not a position of compromise. There is no bending to the 'law of the father' here; playing at being a 'nice girl' will only last as long as it suits the woman who does it. Women who are doing girl may allow a man to believe himself to be in control – let him make the first move, let him believe that he has chosen her – but at the same time she positions herself as in control of her sexuality and, arguably, of his. One woman told me:

> 'Men are so easy. You just waft around in front of them in tight clothes and they're salivating. My mates and I have a laugh and see how many we can pull in a night. We always tell them we don't normally do this and they always believe it.'

This aspect of doing girl may not be so easy for women who fall outside the traditional boundaries of feminine attractiveness; they can't guarantee the male response that confirms a successful performance. It is always a fragile and, arguably, time-limited masquerade.

Women who are doing girl will openly acknowledge that many men are threatened or frightened by women and need to be cajoled, protected or treated carefully so that they do not bruise or become frightened and 'turn' violent or run away. They may massage the male ego by feigning devotion, desire and orgasmic response. One woman said, 'You never tell a man he isn't good in bed. He'd die of shame – and never get it up again. So you always tell him he's the best.' A woman who is doing girl will 'have sex' if she wants to, if she enjoys it, or even because she is 'in love' – but if sex (or the man) does not live up to expectations (and standards these days are high) the woman who is doing girl doesn't stay. She knows that 'Mr Right' is nothing but a myth, so she won't sacrifice herself in the hope that someday her chosen man might transform himself into a handsome prince (or a sexual athlete). Resignation is not part of this particular script. This inevitably means that the women who are doing girl spend time on their own (few men can live up to the myth of phallic masculinity we are sold in the modern versions of the fairy-tale script), but they are always on the look-out for a suitable romantic partner, whom they will expect to do masculinity as well as they do girl.

It might seem to be a contradiction that when women do girl they often claim to want a 'real' man (handsome, protective, strong, sexually potent . . .) – after all, there is a strong element of feminist critique in this apparently knowing and cynical stance. However, if gender is a performance and a woman is going to go to the trouble of doing girl well, why shouldn't she expect a man to play his part? Then she can reap the rewards (and not just bear the restrictions) of following the feminine script; she can receive the 'fiery brand' and all the other benefits of harnessing phallic power. Interestingly, this is also a dominant fantasy for gay men who do girl – epitomized by the character played by Terence Stamp in the film *Priscilla Queen of the Desert* – the fantasy of the 'strong, dark hero' who will make everything right and complete.

For many women taking up the position of doing girl there can be genuine delight in everything associated with the performance of femininity, in taking up what appears to the unknowing observer to be the traditional position of 'woman'. There can be a delight in beauty, make-up, clothes, in the company and conspiracy of women. Tongues may be firmly in cheeks, but doing girl is an activity that can be fun. Shopping, talking, swapping beauty tips, sexual secrets, details of the foibles (and penis size) of men is all part of the game; this is a performance which partly exists for the purpose of knowing display. The ability to shift between appearing to be girl and ridiculing the very performance of femininity and the rituals of romance is part of the pleasure. In doing girl a woman may work at her body and the masquerade of beauty and justly expect to achieve her rewards: 'I deserve adoration with all the effort I put in.' Women doing girl are likely to espouse feminist critiques of the 'beauty myth' – criticizing advertisers, women's magazines and regimes of fashion – but they still follow and claim to enjoy these beauty rituals. However, if they can't pull off the performance of feminine perfection because of aging or perceived inadequacies in themselves they are as likely to feel as devastated and despondent as the woman who wants to be girl, even if in doing girl the façade of femininity is acknowledged to be just that.

For many women doing girl it is *women* who are deemed to deserve respect (in contrast to those women who are being girl, for whom other women are always a threat). With women friends the 'real' woman can come out – the bawdy, needy, funny, frustrated, angry, intelligent sides of herself which, if exposed, risk destabilizing her position as 'woman'. One woman said, 'I can really be myself with my mates . . . whether I'm feeling miserable or pissed off, or whether I feel like having a good time. You just don't have to pretend the way you do with men.' On the other hand, for some women who do girl, there appears to be a contempt for femininity – the masquerade is a mask for a deeper ambivalence towards everything associated with being 'woman'. There is a stronger identification with men, who are positioned as gullible dupes fooled by skilfully executed feminine wiles but are still deemed more worthy of regard than that much derided group, *other* women. Like Snow White's wicked stepmother, who would stop at nothing to ensure that she was the most beautiful of all or the woman with the 'queen bee syndrome' who uses her femininity to keep other women down (and out) at work, these women might masquerade as girl, but they would like nothing more than to have all the power and advantage of being 'man'. As one woman I interviewed commented, 'I'm a woman from the neck down.' She used her body, her sexuality and her ability to play the doe-eyed 'girl' to skilful advantage to achieve power, as well as the admiration and attention of men, whilst she annihilated other women (her competitors) along the way. As the Marquise de Merteuil tells the Viconte de Valmont in the film *Dangerous Liaisons*:[11]

V: I often wondered how you managed to invent yourself.

M: Well, I had no choice, did I, I'm a woman. Women are obliged to be far more skilful than men. You can ruin our reputation and our life with a few well-chosen words, so of course I had to invent not only myself but ways of escape no one's ever thought of before. And I've succeeded because I've always known I was born to dominate your sex and avenge my own.

V: Yes, but what I asked was how.

M: When I came out into society I was fifteen. I already knew that the role I was condemned to, namely to keep quiet and do what I was told, gave me the perfect opportunity to listen and observe. Not to whatever people told me, which naturally was of no interest, but to whatever it was that they were trying to hide. I practised detachment. I learnt how to look cheerful while under the table I stuck a fork into the back of my hand. I became a virtuoso of deceit. It wasn't pleasure I was after, it was knowledge. I consulted the strictest moralist to learn how to appear, philosophers to find out what to think, and novelists to see what I could get away with. And in the end I distilled everything to one wonderfully simple principle – win or die.

V: So you're infallible, are you?

M: If I want a man I have him. If he wants to tell, he finds out that he can't. That's the whole story.

Perhaps the biggest risk to the woman doing girl is that her duplicity will be exposed. She will then be punished for not really *being* girl. She has wandered towards the edges of the boundaries of acceptable femininity, by mocking or only mimicking the feminine ideal. The fact that she might sometimes be sexual outside the confines of heterosexual monogamy, that she may reject, deride or dismiss the attentions of men, that she is ultimately concerned with herself, that she wants power, or merely that she refuses to subjugate herself to the phallocentric ideal, to *be* the fantasy creature who inhabits the imaginations of men, puts her in a position of great vulnerability. This is why concealment – at least in the company of men – is always central to this performance. If a woman is exposed her reputation may be ruined (and to women doing girl reputation is all). She may be designated 'slag' or 'whore'. She may be subjected to sexual violence – and if she complains of it to the authorities, her (assumed) duplicity and sexuality will position her as provocateur and be used to exonerate the man (who is merely enacting the rage of all men in his assault). She has knowingly stepped outside the protection of the patriarchal 'family unit' and as a result is thought to deserve all that she may get.

This is the phallocentric punishment for the mockery, rejection and masquerade of those who do girl – depicted so clearly in pornography, in depictions of rape in mainstream film and in the ruin of the Marquise de Merteuil in *Dangerous Liaisons*. Duplicitous femininity rarely remains unchallenged or unchecked. Perhaps the only exception is the woman born into the upper social classes, who can 'sleep around' as a teenager and be positioned as a 'wild child', while her working-class counterpart will be called a 'slag'; and can commit adultery with impunity as an adult, while other women are castigated for the same. Yet even these women are not safe from scandal and scorn – to which the British media treatment of Sarah Ferguson stands as evidence. For straying from the role of 'good wife and mother' (as well as for being too fat), she was condemned. Perhaps her real sin was an absence of shame – she was not only adulterous, but was clearly enjoying herself too much.

Most of the young women I interviewed could be positioned as doing girl rather than being girl. Few claimed that they believed in the traditional script of femininity, but they said that they were willing to enact the rituals of romance in order to 'get a man', for the shared pleasure of the display or to gain power. But they also wanted autonomy, freedom and the right to choose their own destiny at the same time. The divide between autonomous desire and the restrictions imposed by the boundaries of sexuality acceptable in a phallocentric sphere sets up inherently impossible contradictions which girls and women have to reconcile or negotiate. This divide can produce a fragmentation of self, with feelings of disconnection from the role a woman feels compelled to perform and discontentment with the limitations of the traditional feminine script. It can involve a splitting of different aspects of desire, in order that inherently oppositional needs can be met or inherently oppositional roles followed. This can lead to a compartmentalizing of different aspects of life, with women appearing to take up very different positions in different contexts: cynicism with friends, acquiescent femininity with a man, condemnation of the myth of romance, juxtaposed with a deep desire to be 'in love'; a desire to be independent, alongside a desire to be looked after and protected.

Arguably, inherent contradictions are central to both masculinity and femininity today. Men, too, are faced with contradictory scripts of masculinity, which are difficult, if not impossible, to reconcile. However, women's negotiation of femininity takes place in a context where 'woman' is still positioned as dangerous or deviant if she appears outside the traditional boundaries of femininity. Heterosexual men who take on masculinity as a knowing masquerade (such as the 'new man' who is laddish with his mates) are not subject to condemnation or criticism to the same degree (in contrast, gay men *are*); it is women who are invariably punished or derided if they are seen to be attempting anything other than being girl, as we have seen. Given this, and the difficulties in reconciling desires for agency and autonomy within the confines of the archetypal feminine script, it's not surprising to find that many women are increasingly rejecting the notion of being or even doing 'girl' altogether.

Resisting Girl

When women take up the position of resisting girl, that which is traditionally signified by 'femininity' is invariably ignored or denied (often derided) – the necessity for body discipline, the inevitability of the adoption of the mask of beauty and the adoption of coquettish feminine wiles. Yet this doesn't necessarily mean a rejection of all that is associated with what it is to be 'woman' – attention to appearance, motherhood or sex with men (although it can). It is the rigid rules which are laid out within the phallocentric scripts of femininity and heterosexual romance which are resisted. Women who resist girl have little interest in massaging the egos of men. But it isn't about a reversed sexism or a desire to do to men what over the centuries has been done to women. It is about stepping outside the traditional boundaries of sex and romance, within which 'woman' is passive, responsive and stands as a mirror for the narcissistic desires of men. This is the position of 'woman' not defined by 'sex' or by femininity. But this doesn't mean that it is woman either trying to be man or having to reject man. Many women who resist girl have positive, fulfilling relationships with men. They are not passive, waiting victims, or even pretending to be so, but want to be treated the same as, or at least as equal to, men.

Heterosexual women who take up the position of resisting girl are able openly to show their desire for men. They can make the first move, ask for what they want, say 'goodbye' (or 'I'll see you again') if that's what they feel. There is no need for shame. There is no need to adopt traditional feminine wiles: 'If I fancy a bloke I ask him out. No one has ever said "no". I can't be bothered with games. It's an insult to my intelligence.' Many women who resist girl are able to enjoy their own sexual pleasure and freedom with no need to disguise or conceal the adoption of a sexual role normally seen to be the prerogative of man. There may be a series of lovers, one committed relationship, or no lovers at all. There is no apology either way. This is not 'woman' defined by her position in relation to man or by the narrow rules of an outmoded sexual script.

Many women who resist girl are deliberately disinterested in the artifice of beauty, in the attempts to change, conceal or disguise who they are and how they appear. This is not the adoption of the 'natural' look that takes hours (and a fortune in cosmetics) to produce. It is the position of woman whose sense of herself as 'woman' doesn't simply come from her appearance, the shape of her body or her ability to attract a man: 'I don't care about being thin at all. I eat what I want, what I enjoy'; 'I can't be bothered with make-up and all that stuff. What's the point? I can't stand girly things.' In signifying her resistance to all that is deemed 'girly' and ensuring that she is not positioned as a sexual object in relation to men, a woman may adopt an androgynous 'look' – short hair, no cosmetics, clothes which defy the regimes of fashion; she may shave her head; she may pierce her nose, eyebrows or lips, or have tattoos. She may merely adopt a garb identical to that of her male friends – the 'grunge' look, skinhead girls, punks, goths, riot grrls, 'feminists' in dungarees and 'hippies' are all archetypal examples (although the very categorization into any one of these 'types' may be met with derision). Other women deliberately put on weight or make themselves look 'plain'. As one interviewee commented, 'Men don't look at me when I dress down. It makes me invisible. I'm not a sex object, I'm a person. I prefer it that way.' In contrast, many women who resist girl take pleasure in their appearance and are fully able to engage in many of the rituals of feminine beauty. But it is never the centre of their lives and their sense of self does not come from being able to manipulate or beguile. Women who resist girl are as likely to reject the artifice of beauty on any given day as they are to adopt it. This is not about pleasing a man, it is about a woman pleasing herself.

This isn't a position which is easy for a woman to adopt. We are bombarded with representations that tell us that women are defined by their beauty, by their bodies or by the judgements and reactions of men. So resisting girl continuously can be a struggle or an act of defiance and always comes with the risk of condemnation, both from other women and from men. 'I overheard some colleagues of mine talking about how I'd let myself go,' one woman told me. 'I tried to laugh it off, but it hurt. Sometimes I think it would be easier if I just dolled myself up, like them. But I'd just feel as if I was selling out to men, so I don't.' Women who resist girl clearly run the risk of falling into the fate feared by all fairy-tale princesses – not getting a man. Resisting femininity even as a masquerade can appear to make woman the Medusa incarnate – the threatening, sexually voracious creature which, as we have seen, appears to feature very largely in the fantasies and fears of men. Clearly some men are happy – if not enthusiastic – to engage in relationships with women who do not play out the archetypal feminine game. Their own masculinity is not predicated on dominating or disempowering women. But this experience, which was described by one of my interviewees, is possibly more common:

> 'I had just ended my marriage because I was dissatisfied with the relation-ship, and I was happy to spend some time alone. One of my male friends made me feel really depressed when he announced one day that I'd never meet another man, because I am so independent and strong. He said I'd only attract someone who was a masochist, or wanted to be mothered. Some friend.'

For women who resist girl and have nothing to do with men at all this is less of a problem. Identifying as lesbians (or as dykes, or queer), they refuse to take up the position of sexual other to man, rejecting everything associated with 'compulsory heterosexuality' and with the binary positions of 'woman' and 'man'. 'I only sleep with women. I never want to be underneath a man – literally or metaphorically,' one woman commented. Lesbian theorists such as Monique Wittig have taken this a step further, arguing that lesbians are not women, as 'woman' is constructed within a heterosexual matrix and always defined in relation to 'man'. In this view, if we take 'man' out of the picture, 'woman' does not exist. To be 'lesbian' and 'woman' is thus viewed as a contradiction in terms. However, in contrast, whilst many lesbians may resist all that is signified by femininity, rejecting the positions of being or doing girl they simultaneously take up a positive sexual subject position as women, reframing the very meaning of what it is to be 'woman': 'In the lesbian community you can be a woman who is a really hot fuck which you know you can't . . . with men.' There can also be a strong identification with other women – heterosexual or lesbian – and a strong identification *as* women, but alongside a rejection of the hegemonic (within a phallocentric symbolic sphere) of 'woman' as other, always seen in relation to man, defined by appearance, by her ability to attract and keep a man and her skills in the performance of the script of heterosexual romance. As one interviewee commented: 'I'm all woman. I'm also a dyke. I'm proud of being both.'

Many lesbians who resist girl – epitomized by the lesbian feminist movement of the seventies and eighties – condemn masculinity as vociferously as they deride being or doing girl, so this is not about taking up positions of phallocentric sexuality, but about reframing what it is to be 'woman'. Vanilla sex replaces fucking; loving sisterhood replaces eroticized power differences. However, for many lesbians (as well as for an increasing number of heterosexual women) resisting 'girl' *can* mean embracing the sexual 'other' – playing with masculinity, with phallocentric power. These women are arguably acting to subvert the script of heterosexual sex and romance.

Subverting Femininity

When women subvert femininity they knowingly play with gender as a performance, twisting, imitating and parodying traditional scripts of femininity (or indeed masculinity) in a very public, polished display. Polly, who adorns the cover of this book, attributes her own (much copied) subversion of the archetypal feminine 'look' to personal pleasure and empowerment:

> For me style has always been a matter of presence – of having the confidence and skill to present yourself in a way that truly reflects your inner personality. When I was thirteen or fourteen I discovered the joys of make-up and hair dyes. So while my school friends were busy adoring pop stars from afar, I was happily experimenting with many different hairstyles, make-up styles and ways of altering my natural appearance . . . I first got my body pierced in 1991 because I love any type of body adornment and thought it would be fabulous to wake up every morning wearing my jewelry.[12]

This is a woman subverting the rules of feminine beauty for her own interest and pleasure. The fact that she may also provoke attention or condemnation is undoubtedly part of the game.

For other women subverting femininity is about playing with sexual power, an act of 'gender trouble',[13] which in its perverse parody and play, serves to draw attention to the charade of the phallocentric 'original':

'It's about freedom . . . why should the man hold the power . . . I'm usually a top with men and a bottom with women.'

'It's in yer face perversion . . . like at gay pride walking around in full bondage . . . I love the looks you get especially off some other dykes . . . I suppose I like outraging people . . . upsetting the balance, you know, girls are supposed to be like this, or sex is supposed to be like that.'[14]

These are gendered positions celebrated within 'queer theory' – and a knowing academic analysis often influences the choice of masquerade and display. As one interviewee, a drag king whose performance involved wearing male garb, facial hair and 'packing', commented, 'I think it's brilliant . . . taking on the phallus.'[15] But this isn't just about strap-ons: The lesbian who is openly 'femme' (the 'lipstick lesbian' so fêted by the media in the apparently 'queer-friendly' early nineties), who rejects the script of heterosexual romance but seemingly follows the masquerade of femininity in her adoption of the mask of 'beauty', subverts femininity: 'I love going out looking like a girl, and then showing how hard I am underneath. I'm a femme top that no one gets the better of.' In subverting the 'natural' end of the fairy-tale romance, whilst at the same time *apparently* taking up the position of 'beautiful princess', the lie that exists at the very centre of the script of heterosexuality is exposed. It challenges so many assumptions about 'woman' and 'sex'. As one interviewee said, 'The comment men make when they find out I'm a dyke is, "But you're gorgeous." Even if they don't say it, I know they think it. I love it, it's so undermining of the whole hety game.'

The counterpart of the 'femme' is the 'butch', the lesbian who takes up much of that which is associated with the position of 'man' (a rare creature in reality, but one whose image fills the fantasies of many fearful men). The 'stone butches' of the fifties were for many years the most skilled performers of this particular brand of subversion. In recent years, there has been a revival of the 'butch femme' masquerade and of 'butch femme' sexual play. We see this in the case of the lesbian and the phallus – the woman who wears a strap-on dildo and fucks women – normally a position which is the prerogative of 'man'. The heterosexual woman who fucks her male partner is enacting a similar charade. Neither wants to *be* a man; they don't necessarily envy men; but they want to have the power to take up the role of sexual predator or performer – and enjoy the knowledge that they will never lose their sexual power: 'I like to fuck women. I know that I'm a good shag.' In wearing the strap-on as a fetish woman parodies both 'man' and 'sex'. Equally, the 'drag king' – the lesbian who dresses as 'man' but is in no way transsexual – subverts both masculinity and femininity. She can adopt masculinity as a masquerade, yet at the same time be recognized (by the cognoscenti at least) as 'woman'. Unlike the woman who is merely doing girl, in subverting femininity there is no attempt to conceal the duplicity of the performance. Those who read it as 'real' are not the target audience; indeed, the very fact that 'outsiders' are fooled undoubtedly heightens the pleasure in the play. As one interviewee commented, 'I sometimes get told I'm in the wrong place, when I go in the women's toilets. I love the look on their faces when I say I'm a girl. When one woman wouldn't believe me, I showed her my tits.'

Subverting femininity isn't the sole prerogative of lesbians. Male drag queens do girl in a way which often makes them indistinguishable from the 'original'. In adopting a perfect masquerade (often more 'perfect', in terms of 'supermodel' beauty criteria, than the 'real thing', as they have the bodies of boys – the slim thighs and tight buttocks many women would 'die for') they demonstrate how 'authentic' femininity is nothing but a masquerade. Equally, straight women, such as Madonna, can openly play with and subvert the feminine masquerade – at one moment doing girl, at another openly taking up the position of 'whore', harlot, vamp, temptress, or of 'lipstick lesbian'. Madonna's extended photo-essay *Sex* was a celebration of subversion, in all its myriad forms. As she plays with her own desires, she plays with the desires of her readers, and demonstrates that desire and the positions we take up are never 'natural', always constructed, always a performance, which is open to resistance, modification and change.

One of the problems with this line of resistance is that it could be seen to be reinforcing or reifying the feminine or heterosexual original it sets out to subvert. This has been one of the major criticisms of lesbian sado–masochistic practice or phallic masquerade – that it does not subvert, but mirrors masculine hegemonic power. Equally, we have to ask whether complex readings of the subtleties of subversive performance are made by anyone other than the well-informed. We have seen this argument made as a critique of the photographs of Cindy Sherman – that whilst she knowingly parodies femininity, the unknowing reader may read her work as a simple celebration of being girl. The woman who subverts femininity or heterosexuality in her manner or garb may also be subjected to such criticism, her performance interpreted as her wanting to *be* woman (in the case of the exaggerated femme), or wanting to *be* 'man' (in the case of the woman who takes on traditional masculine signifiers of phallic power). The other major problem with subverting (or rejecting) femininity is that it potentially places the individual woman herself at great risk, as stepping outside the boundaries of normal womanhood means stepping outside the boundaries of patriarchal protection. All the punishments meted out to aberrant women are liable to be levied at this threatening non-woman, who provokes even greater wrath than the woman who is caught out doing girl because she does not attempt to conceal her rejecting or subversive stance. The most obvious example of this is in the castigation of 'the lesbian' in science and the law discussed earlier. We also see it in social discrimination or in threats of violence or abuse thrown at lesbians:

> 'We were in the park the other day, Hyde Park, and these three blokes were following us all the way round the park . . . they stood in a group watching us, pointing at us . . . they stopped . . . and one was behind us and one walked straight past us and he had a black thing . . . it looked like a riding crop.'[16]

Openly rejecting heterosexuality – the only crime of this interviewee was to be in a public place with her girlfriend – appears to be a licence to attack. Heterosexual women who reject or subvert femininity may also find themselves falling under this umbrella, being positioned *as* lesbian because of their independent stance – since the first wave of feminism, 'lesbian' has stood as a term of abuse (and a licence *to* abuse) for any strong-minded woman.

Reframing Femininity – Reframing Sex

There may be penalties for stepping out of line, but few women today completely abide by the strictures laid out in the traditional feminine script. However, trying to capture the complexity of this continuous process of negotiation and resistance is an inherently problematic process. None of these four positions are concrete or fixed. They are not how women *should* be, but one possible description of the different ways in which women deal with the fantasies of femininity which frame their lives, how they negotiate the various scripts which prescribe what it is to be 'woman'. I could have described eight, ten or even twenty different positions – why stop at four? Few women will find themselves described simply and neatly within any one of these different positions – these are scripts of femininity which are fluid and shifting, always open to modification and change. Women will move between different positions at different points in their lives or in different situations. They may adopt more than one position simultaneously – the boundaries between these different positions are flexible, not fixed. Indeed, as women rewrite and rescript what it is to be 'woman', the boundaries of gender and sexuality are remade and reframed. Trying to capture the 'truth' of femininity is impossible. If we try to tie it down we will be left with nothing but a shadow of what it actually is. So, whilst I have stopped at these four positions, as they seem to capture the essence of the main strategies of negotiation and resistance in which women currently engage, I am in no way saying that this is the end of the matter. Or that these are the only ways in which women can reframe femininity. This is a continuous and creative process, and adopting a reflexive or knowing stance can only encourage this creative construction and reconstruction to develop even more. My aim is not to close down discussion, nor to establish particular unitary 'types' of strategies adopted by women, but to draw attention to the myriad ways in which femininity is regulated, as well as the myriad ways in which women actively resist.

This is not to suggest that women's adoption of a particular strategy of negotiation or resistance is an arbitrary process or that women now have complete freedom in choosing to do, be, reject or subvert girl. No performance of femininity can be seen as separate from the cultural context in which a woman lives, and at any point in time there is always a limited range of possible scripts to follow or subvert. I hit puberty in the early seventies, at the height of the second wave of feminism. Growing up in Derby, a medium-sized English town, 'feminism' might as well have been happening on another planet. We may have worn hot-pants, unleashed our nascent sexuality by screaming at pop stars and harboured aspirations to higher education – things which were inconceivable to previous generations of women. In the decade after the birth of the 'sexual revolution' sex might have been mandatory rather than forbidden. But beneath the veneer of egalitarianism, very little had really changed. When I looked around me to find out what it was to be a 'woman', I was presented with a very traditional and narrow script. Woman as mother, housewife, or sexual object to be ogled or admired. Resistance or subversion in that context took the form of refusing to be the little woman at home, of wanting to live an independent existence or of wanting to have a career and be able to carve a life that was not centred on the attentions or approval of a man – strategies which are so taken for granted by women today that they would hardly be deemed resistance.

As I reflect now on the process of my own negotiation of femininity, I sometimes envy the adolescent girls of today, who seem to have far more possible ways of doing or rejecting girl than were available in my own teenage years. There are also many different scripts available within the different subcultures that now exist (riot grrls replaced goths, who replaced punks, who replaced . . .), and across different social-class groups. This is always situationally specific – the college co-ed living in California has a different range of possibilities open to her than the lesbian avenger living in London's Hackney. But perhaps I shouldn't feel envy, for there are still many commonalities across contexts and across time. As we have seen, the meaning of what it is to be 'woman' or 'man' is invariably constructed within a phallocentric frame; both femininity and masculinity are still constructed and regulated within the boundaries of heterosexual sex and romance. Whilst we may applaud women's active resistance, we must also acknowledge that there are always boundaries which determine how far this resistance may extend.

One might ask how and why a woman chooses a particular form of resistance. Clearly, whether any one woman achieves a 'fit' with the version of 'girl' she adopts (or subverts), whether she dates boys or 'shags' girls (or vice versa), will be influenced by her own psychological history and investments. 'Culture' or symbolic representation is not simply imposed from outside, with women merely slotted into the categories and roles available in their own particular cultural milieu. It is a continuous negotiation actively carried out by the woman herself, who will work with the available representations of femininity to find her own fit. The practice of doing girl is not just a case of surface appearance, a mask we take on or off as the mood takes us, something we can modify or vary as we change our hairstyle or our clothes. It is always rooted in the tension or resonance between psychological and cultural influences.[17] The way in which we adopt or resist the scripts which are available to us is always related to our unconscious needs, fears and desires, in the same way as the representations of masculinity and femininity which act to provide the boundaries of the scripts reflect the unconscious fantasies and fears of women and men.

The psychoanalyst Joan Rivere first argued this in 1929 when she introduced the concept of femininity as masquerade to describe the mask of femininity women adopt as a defence against the anxiety provoked by their being successful or intellectual in a world where only men were allowed or expected to take up that role. In one case study she described a woman academic who would give highly polished, impersonal public lectures and then behave in a coquettish, flirtatious manner towards the men in her audience immediately afterwards, as an unconscious attempt to ward off any reprisals or vengeance which might result from her challenging masculine authority. Rivere linked this to early unconscious fears of provoking the wrath of the father, and stated that femininity was in these cases a defensive escape from anxiety, which develops as a means of appeasing men: 'Womanliness . . . could be assumed and worn as a mask, both to hide the possession of masculinity and to avert the reprisals expected if she was found to possess it.'[18] Today, we might want to link women's taking on of a particular version of the masquerade to many other unconscious fears and desires, such as desire for power or for pleasure, anger with men or women, fear of intimacy, desires to denigrate women or men or desires to reproduce the fantasy family of origin.

As there are many contradictions and conflicts in our unconscious desires, and in the representations which reflect and reinforce them, there will always be many contradictions in the performance of feminin-ity. There will never be one perfect way of doing femininity or one meaning of 'woman' which will work for all women or girls. Indeed, as needs, desires and conflicts change with experience and across time, the 'fit' that a woman finds will inevitably shift and change. As one interviewee who is now in her fifties commented:

'I grew up at a time when nice girls *didn't*. We looked to men to provide the answers to our dreams. I believed it all. Yet I lived through the Pill, changing laws on abortion, "free love", and everyone I know getting divorced . . . Now I'm on my own, without a man, without children at home, and I can honestly say I'm happier than I've ever been in my life. If a miracle happens, I might meet someone else. But it doesn't seem very important these days. I wish I'd known this at twenty, when I could think of nothing else but getting a man. But at least I know it now.'

There is a complex interaction at play here between the changing fantasies and desires of the woman herself and the social world in which she lives. So whilst we may look to the life of the unconscious to attempt to explain or understand the adoption of a particular feminine script, we must never neglect the social world in which the meaning of femininity and, indeed, the meaning of unconscious desire itself is framed.

The reactions of others to the scripts women adopt may influence whether they continue to identify in a particular way. So the heterosexual woman who is doing girl, yet wants to enjoy sex outside a monogamous commitment to a man is in a potentially invidious position, her behaviour likely to be read as 'promiscuous' or the behaviour of a 'slag'. She can only continue to be sexual without being condemned if she conceals her desire and her sexual history. She may eventually move to a position of rejecting girl as a way of being autonomously sexual without manipulation or deceit. Or she may escape into the safety of monogamous marriage, attempting to do girl, and avoid condemnation or shame. In contrast, in a social context where rejecting girl is the norm, women will find it more easy (and rewarding) to play out this role. As one interviewee said:

'I've had a lot of lovers. I know I'm good at sex – I've had enough practice. I'm not really into just shagging girls I meet – but I wouldn't have any problem if I wanted to be. It's easy if you're confident, and obviously know what you're doing, and if people know you know the ropes.'

Would a heterosexual woman talk so openly about her sexual expertise and her past lovers? Perhaps today she would – at least if she read teenage magazines.

The interpretation of the specific performance of femininity a woman adopts will vary with both the context in which she enacts her display and the intentions which underpin her actions. A person dressed in the full garb of feminine beauty – 'big' hair, make-up, sexy clothes – may signify sexual availability to men, she may be following fashion or she may signify parody – as a 'lipstick lesbian' or drag queen do. Taken out of context, without explanation, we cannot easily determine what is signified. The 'femme' who stands beside her butch girlfriend and is in no way residing in the closet might be read very differently from the 'femme' who is attempting to 'pass' as girl, to keep any knowledge of her sexuality from those who are outside her intimate circle. She may do girl to pass at work; she may subvert girl through 'camping it up' in a gay bar at night. Even if we take one woman, one apparent sexual identity, the *meaning* and intention behind her particular performance of girl cannot be assumed from an outside glance. What we see is not always what we get.

Our own reading of a particular performance will inevitably be affected by how we position ourselves. If we are knowing players of a particular mode of performance (the subtleties of doing or subverting girl . . .), we will be able to recognize (and respect) this performance when it is displayed by others. If not, we may make the wrong reading – at least from the point of view of the woman herself. The case of woman being 'read' by men as sexually available, or as 'slags', when their expressed intentions are to celebrate and enjoy their own sexuality, without any reference to men, is the easiest example to draw on here. It is also the excuse given by many men in rape cases, 'She wanted it,' being the interpretation of any vaguely sexual image adopted by any woman.

As I reach the end of this journey through fantasies of femininity and sexuality I have to confess that my feelings about what has been uncovered can only be described as mixed. On the one hand it is heartening to be able to adopt a stance where women are not positioned as victims or dupes, to be able to argue with some confidence that women actively negotiate and resist archetypal (and archaic) representations of what it is to be 'woman'. Yet when we see the ways in which women who openly resist phallocentric power are often punished or condemned, it is hard not to end on a despondent or disheartened note.

However, when we weigh these costs up against the mass of women's resistance – in reframing representations of 'woman', political campaigns, academic critiques and in the negotiation of the scripts of femininity carried out continuously by individual women – it is clear that the balance is finally tipping in women's favour. Whilst we must not lose sight of the scale of the objectification and abuse of individual women, we can at the same time confidently say that this is at long last beginning to be outmatched by women's active reframing of the very meaning of femininity and, as a consequence, of the very boundaries of 'sex'.

Reframing femininity and 'what it is to be 'woman' outside the hegemonic boundaries of 'sex' may dethrone the phallus. It may subvert the traditional order of sexual difference in which 'woman' stands as foil and fantasy for man. This may unsettle our whole social sphere, as so much is based on this rigid hierarchy of sexually differentiated power. But for women at least this can only be a positive thing. When *women* are finally able to write their own scripts of femininity and of 'sex', to define in their own terms what it means to be 'woman', who knows what other changes will be brought about? Unsettling it may be, but it is an unstoppable process which is already well underway.

NOTES

1. The term 'subjectivity' is used by many critics (i.e. Henriques, J., Hollway, W., Urwin, C., Venn, C. & Walkerdine, V., *Changing the Subject: Psychology, Social Regulation and Subjectivity*, London: Methuen, 1984; Hollway, W., *Subjectivity and Method in Psychology: Gender, Meaning and Science*, London: Sage, 1989) in order to move away from the notion of a single identity. In a post-structuralist framework it is recognized that identity is multiple, fragmented and often contradictory. It is easier then to talk of identities, or of subjectivity.

2. This may appear to assume heterosexuality. However, the fear and dread of woman is not merely a result of current desire, but is associated with deep-rooted fears arising from early development and from the continuous circulation of woman as sign.

3. In terms of semiotic theorizing, 'man' and 'woman' as sign; men and women as that which is signified.

4. These are comments most frequently aimed at traditional radical feminist

arguments which document the systematic oppression and denigration of women are seen as being too extreme and unrepresentative.

5. See Faludi, Susan, *Backlash: The Undeclared War against American Women*, London: Vintage, 1992, for a thorough analysis of the backlash against women.

6. Griffin, Chris, 'I'm Not a Women's Libber but . . . : Feminism, Consciousness and Identity', in Skevington, S. & Baker, D., *The Social Identity of Women*, London: Sage, 1989; Belloff, H., Hepburn, A., MacDonald, M. & Siann, G., 'Convergence and Divergences: Gender Differences in the Perception of Feminism and Feminists', paper presented at the British Psychological Society Annual Conference, Blackpool, 5–7 April 1993.

7. It is also true that many women experience the law as a second rape if they attempt to bring their assailant to trial. The positioning of female sexuality in the law (as invisible, or as cause of male violence), may be a regulation which operates at the level of the symbolic, but it has clear material effects.

8. See Coward, R., *Our Treacherous Hearts*, London: Virago, 1993.

9. There is no *one* female gaze. There are many gazes which have reframed the meaning of what it is to be 'woman' and the meaning of 'sex'.

10. Butler, Judith, *Bodies that Matter: On the Discursive Limits of Sex*, New York: Routledge, 1993, p. 231.

11. *Dangerous Liaisons*, Stephen Frear, 1988.

12. Polly is described as a key figure on the London club scene and was interviewed by Polhemus, Ted, for *Style Surfing*, London: Thames & Hudson, 1996.

13. See Butler, Judith, *Gender Trouble: Feminism and the Subversion of Identity*, London: Routledge, 1990.

14. Both SM quotes from interviews conducted by Taylor, Gary Wilson, *Making Sense of SM: A Social Constructionist Account*, 1995, unpublished thesis.

15. Interviewed by Catherine Johnson.

16. Interview conducted by Julie Mooney-Somers.

17. I am following Butler, 1993, p. 234, here, who argued:

> Gender is neither a purely psychic truth, conceived as 'internal' and 'hidden', nor is it reducible to a surface appearance; on the contrary, its undecidability is to be traced as the play *between* psyche and appearance (where the latter domain includes what appears in *words*). Further, this will be a 'play' regulated by heterosexist constraints, though not, for that reason, fully reducible to them.

18. Rivere, Joan, 'Womanliness as Masquerade', *International Journal of Psychoanalysis*, vol. 10; reprinted in Burgin, V., Donals, J. & Kaplan, C., *Formations of Fantasy*, London: Methuen, 1986, pp. 35–44.

FURTHER READING

Abramson, P. R. (1990), 'Sexual Science: Emerging Discipline or Oxymoron?' *Journal of Sex Research*, 27, 147–65.

Abramson, P. R. & Pinkerton, S. D. (1995), 'Introduction: Nature, Nurture and In-Between', in *Sexual Nature, Sexual Culture*, P. R. Abramson & S. D. Pinkerton (eds.), Chicago: University of Chicago Press.

Adams, P. (1989), 'Of Female Bondage', in *Between Feminism and Psychoanalysis*, T. Brennan (ed.), London: Routledge.

Adler, Z. (1987), *Rape on Trial*, London: Routledge & Kegan Paul.

Alias, A. G. (1995), '46 XY, 50 Alpha-Reductase Deficiency: A (Contrasting) Model to Understanding the Predisposition to Male Homosexuality?' Paper presented at the twenty-first annual meeting of the International Academy of Sex Research, Provincetown, Massachusetts.

Altman, M. (1984), 'Everything They Always Wanted You to Know: The Ideology of Popular Sex Literature', in *Pleasure and Danger: Exploring Female Sexuality*, C. Vance (ed.), London: Routledge & Kegan Paul.

Alzate, H. & Londono, M. L. (1984), 'Vaginal Erotic Sensitivity', *Journal of Sex and Marital Therapy*, 10 (1), 49–56.

Ang, I. (1985), *Watching Dallas. Soap Opera and the Melodramatic Imagination*, London: Routledge.

Archer, J. (1994), 'Evolutionary Psychology', in *Male Violence*, J. Archer (ed.), London: Routledge.

'Attorney-General's Commission on Pornography. Final Report', Washington, DC, 1985: US Government Printing Office.

Bagley, C. & Ramsey, R. (1986), 'Sexual Abuse in Childhood: Psychologic Outcomes and Implications for Social Work Practice', *Journal of Social Work and Human Sexuality*, 5, 33–47.

Bailey, J. M. (1995), 'A Twin Registry Study of Sexual Orientation', paper presented at the twenty-first annual meeting of the International Academy of Sex Research, Provincetown, Massachusetts.

Bailey, J. M. & Pillard, R. C. (1991), 'A Genetic Study of Male Sexual Orientation', *Archives of General Psychiatry*, 48, 1089–96.

Bailey, J. M., Pillard, R. C., Neale, M. C. & Agyei, Y. (1993), 'Heritable Factors Influence Sexual Orientation in Women', *Archives of General Psychiatry*, 50, 217–23.

Baker, P. (1993), 'Maintaining Power: Why Heterosexual Men Use Pornography', in *Pornography: Women, Violence and Civil Liberties*, C. Itzen (ed.), Oxford: Oxford University Press.

Baker, A. W. & Duncan, S. P. (1985), 'Child Sexual Abuse: A Study of Prevalence in Great Britain', *Child Sexual Abuse and Neglect*, 9, 457–67.

Bancroft, J. (1983), *Human Sexuality and Its Problems*, London: Churchill Livingstone.

Banta, M. (1987), *Imagining American Women: Ideas and Ideals in Cultural History*, New York: Columbia University Press.

Baron, L. & Straus, M. A. (1987), 'Four Theories of Rape: A Macrosociological Analysis', *Social Problems*, 34, 467–89.

Barthes, R. (1972), *Mythologies*, New York: Hill & Wang.

Bartky, S. (1988), 'Foucault, Femininity and the Modernisation of Patriarchal Power', in *Feminism and Foucault: Reflections on Resistance*, I. Diamond & L. Quinby (eds.), Boston: Northeastern University Press.

Baudrillard, J. (1990), *Seduction*, New York: St Martin's Press.

Beggs, V. E., Calhoun, K. S. & Wolchik, S. A. (1987), 'Sexual Anxiety and Female Sexual Arousal: A Comparison of Arousal during Sexual Anxiety Stimuli and Sexual Pleasure Stimuli', *Archives of Sexual Behaviour*, 16 (4), 311–19.

Benjamin, J. (1984), 'Master and Slave: The Fantasy of Erotic Domination', in *Desire: The Politics of Sexuality*, A. Snitow, C. Stansell & S. Thompson (eds.), London: Virago.

Benjamin, J. (1988), *Bonds of Love: Psychoanalysis, Feminism and the Problem of Domination*, New York: Pantheon.

Benton, D. & Wastell, V. (1986), 'Effects of Androstenol on Human Sexual Arousal', *Biological Psychology*, 22 (2), 141–47.

Berger, J. (1972), *Ways of Seeing*, London: Penguin.

Berline, F. (1988), 'Issues in Exploration of Biological Factors Contributing to the Etiology of the "Sex Offender" Plus Some Ethical Considerations', in

Human Sexual Aggression: Current Perspectives, R. A. Prentky & V. L. Quinsey (eds.), New York: New York Academy of Sciences.

Blair, L. M. (Spring 1977), 'The Problem of Rape', *Police Surgeon*.

Bordo, S. (1990), 'Reading the Slender Body', in *Body Politics: Women and the Discourses of Science*, M. Jacobus, E. Fox Keller & S. Shuttleworth (eds.), London: Routledge.

Bottigheimer, R. (1987), *Grimms' Bad Girls and Bold Boys. The Moral and Social Vision of the Tales*, New Haven: Yale University Press.

Boyle, M. (1994), 'Gender, Science and Sexual Dysfunction', in *Constructing the Social*, T. R. Sarbin & J. I. Kitzinger (eds.), London: Sage.

Bradford, J. (1988), 'Organic Treatment for the Male Sexual Offender', in *Human Sexual Aggression: Current Perspectives*, R. A. Prentky & V. L. Quinsey (eds.), New York: New York Academy of Sciences.

Briere, J. & Malamuth, N. (1983), 'Self-Reported Likelihood of Sexually Aggressive Behaviour: Attitudinal versus Sexual Explanations', *Journal of Research in Personality*, 17, 315–23.

S. Bright & J. Posner (eds.) (1996), *Nothing but the Girl: The Blatant Lesbian Image. A Portfolio and Exploration of Lesbian Erotic Photography*, London: Cassell.

Brown, G. & Harris, T. (1978), *Social Origins of Depression*, London: Tavistock.

Brown, J. (1986), *Immodest Acts*, Oxford: Oxford University Press.

Browne, A. & Finkelhor, D. (1986), 'Impact of Child Sexual Abuse: A Review of the Research', *Psychological Bulletin*, 99 (1), 66–77.

Browne, E. (1980), *When Battered Women Kill*, London: The Free Press.

Bryant, J. (1985), *Testimony to the Attorney-General's Commission on Pornography Hearings*, Houston, Texas. Unpublished manuscript.

Burgess, A. & Holstrom, L. L. (1974), 'Rape Trauma Syndrome', *American Journal of Psychiatry*, 131, 981–86.

Burns, J. 'The Psychology of Lesbian Health Care', in Nicolson, P. & Ussher, J. M., *The Psychology of Women's Health and Health Care*, London: Macmillan, 1992.

Butcher, H., Coward, R., Evaristi, M., Garber, J., Harrison, R. & Winship, J. (1980), *Images of Women in the Media*, Birmingham: CCCS.

Butler, J. (1990), *Gender Trouble: Feminism and the Subversion of Identity*, London: Routledge.

Byers, J. (1988), 'Gazes/Voices/Power: Expanding Psychoanalysis for Feminist Film and Television Theory', in *Female Spectators: Looking at Film and Television*, D. Pribram (ed.), London: Verso.

Byrne, D. (1986), 'Introduction: The Study of Sexual Behaviour as a Multidisciplinary Venture', in *Alternative Approaches to the Study of Sexual Behaviour*, D. Byrne & K. Kelley (eds.), Hillsdale, New Jersey: Erlbaum Associates.

Cahill, C., Llewelyn, S. P. & Pearson, C. (1991), 'Long-Term Effects of Sexual Abuse which Occurred in Childhood: A Review', *British Journal of Clinical Psychology*, 30, 117–30.

Caldwell, J. & Caldwell, P. (1983), 'The Demographic Evidence for the Incidence and Course of Abnormally Low Fertility in Tropical Africa', *World Health Statistics Quarterly*, 36, 2–34.

Califa, P. (1988), 'The Calyx of Isis', in Califa, P., *Macho Sluts*, Boston: Aiyson Publications.

Califa, P. (1988), 'The Surprise Party', in Califa, P., *Macho Sluts*, Boston: Aiyson Publications.

Campbell, J. (1992), 'If I Can't Have You No One Can. Power and Control in Homicide of Female Partners', in *Femicide: The Politics of Women Killing*, J. Radford & D. Russell (eds.), Buckingham: Open University Press.

Camps, F. E. (1962), 'The Medical Aspects of the Investigation of Sexual Offences', *Practitioner*, 189, 1129, 31–5.

Caputi, J. (1987), *The Age of Sex Crime*, London: The Women's Press.

Carbaugh, D. (1988), *Talking American: Cultural Discourses on DONAHUE*, Norwood, New Jersey: Ablex.

Carlson, C. (1984), *Intrafamilial Homicide*, Unpublished B.Sc. thesis, McMaster University.

Carter, E. (1988), 'Intimate Outscapes: Problem Page Letters and the Remaking of the 1950's West German Family', in *Becoming Feminine: The Politics of Popular Culture*, L. Roman & L. K. Christian Smith, Sussex: Falmer Press.

Catalan, J., Bradley, M., Gallawey, J. & Hawton, K. (1981), 'Sexual Dysfunction and Psychiatric Morbidity in Patients Attending a Clinic for Sexually Transmitted Diseases', *British Journal of Psychiatry*, 138, 292–96.

Chadwick, W. (1990), *Women, Art and Society*, London: Thames & Hudson.

Cherin, K. (1981), *The Obsession: Reflections on the Tyranny of Slenderness*, New York: Harper & Row.

Chesebro, J. W. (1982), 'Communication, Values and Popular Television Series – A Four Year Assessment, in *Television: The Critical View*, H. Newcomb (ed.), Oxford: Oxford University Press.

Chicago, J. (1993), *Through the Flower: My Struggle as a Woman Artist*, New York: Penguin.

Chodorow, N. (1994), *Femininities, Masculinities, Sexualities. Freud and Beyond*, London: Free Association Books.

Cobbe, F. P. (April 1878), 'Wife Torture in England', *Contemporary Review*, 55–87.

Cole, M. (1988b), 'Sex Therapy for Individuals', in *Sex Therapy in Britain*, M. Cole & W. Dryden (eds.), Milton Keynes: Open University Press.

M. Cole & W. Dryden (eds.), *Sex Therapy in Britain*, Milton Keynes: Open University Press.

Conran, S. (1979), *Lace*, London: Penguin.

Constantine, L. L. (1979), 'The Sexual Rights of Children: Implications of a Radical Perspective', in *Love and Attraction: An International Conference*, M. Cook & G. Wilson (eds.), Oxford: Pergamon.

Contratto, S. (1987), 'Father Presence in Women's Psychological Development', in *Advances in Psychoanalytic Sociology*, G. M. Platt, J. Rabow & M. Goldman (eds.), Malaber: Krieger.

Cooper, G. F. (1988), 'The Psychological Methods of Sex Therapy', in *Sex Therapy in Britain*, M. Cole & W. Dryden (eds.), Milton Keynes: Open University Press.

Corrine, T. (1987), *Dreams of the Woman who Loved Sex. A Collection*, Austin, Texas: Banned Books.

Coward R. (1992), *Our Treacherous Hearts. Why Women Let Men Get Their Way*, London: Faber & Faber.

Cowie, E. (1992), 'Pornography and Fantasy: Psychoanalytic Perspectives', in *Sex Exposed: Sexuality and the Pornography Debate*, L. Segal & M. McIntosh (eds.), London: Virago.

Crabbe, A. (1988), 'Feature Length Sex Films', in *Perspectives on Pornography: Sexuality in Film and Literature*, G. Day & C. Bloom (eds.), London: Macmillan.

Craik, J. (1993), *The Face of Fashion. Cultural Studies in Fashion*, London: Routledge.

Crompton, L. (1985), 'The Myth of Lesbian Impunity', in *The Gay Past: A Collection of Historical Essays*, J. Licasta & R. Peterson (eds.), New York: Howorth Press.

De Lauretis, T. (1984), *Alice Doesn't: Feminism, Semiotics, Cinema*, London: Macmillan.

Dell, S. (1984), *Murder into Manslaughter*, Oxford: Oxford University Press.

Dietz, P. E. & Sears, A. E. (1987–8), 'Pornography and Films Sold in American Cities', *University of Michigan Journal of Law Reform*, 21 (1&2).

Dobash, R. E. & Dobash, R. (1979), *Violence Against Wives. A Case against the Patriarchy*, London: Open Books.

Donnerstein, E. (1980a), 'Aggressive Erotica and Violence Against Women', *Journal of Personality and Social Psychology*, 39, 269–77.

Douglas, S. (1995),*Where the Girls Are: Growing up Female with the Mass Media*, London: Penguin.

Dworkin, A. (1972), *Woman Hating*, New York: Dutton.

Dworkin, A. (1993), 'Against the Flood: Censorship, Pornography and Equality', in *Pornography: Women, Violence and Civil Liberties*, C. Itzen (ed.), Oxford: Oxford University Press.

Dworkin, A. & MacKinnon, C. (1988), *Pornography and Civil Rights: A New Day for Women's Equality*, Minneapolis: Organizing Against Pornography.

Earls, C. (1988), 'Aberrant Sexual Arousal in Sex Offenders', in *Human Sexual Aggression: Current Perspectives*, R. A. Prentky & V. L. Quinsey (eds.), New York: New York Academy of Sciences.

Eddings, B. M. (1980), 'Women in Broadcasting (US) de jure, de facto', in *Women and Media*, H. Baehr (ed.), Oxford: Pergamon Press.

Edwards, S. (1981), *Female Sexuality and the Law*, Oxford: Martin Robertson.

Ehrenreich, B. & English, D. (1978), *For Her Own Good: 150 Years of Experts' Advice to Women*, New York: Anchor Doubleday.

Eisenstein, Z. H. (1988), *The Female Body and the Law*, California: University of California Press.

Ellis, H. (1893), *Men and Women*, London: Contemporary Science Series.

Ellis, H. (1946; 1st edn 1933), 'Sexual Deviation', in Ellis, H., *Psychology of Sex*, London: Heinemann.

Estrich, S. (1987), *Real Rape*, Cambridge, Mass.: Harvard University Press.

Evans, A. (1978), *Witchcraft and the Gay Counterculture*, Boston: Fag Rag Books.

Faderman, L. (1985), *Surpassing the Love of Men*, London: The Women's Press.

Faderman, L. (1993), *Odd Girls and Twilight Lovers*, London: Penguin.

Fedoroff, J. P. et al. (1995), 'A GnRH Test of Androphiles, Gynphiles, Heterosexual Pedophiles and Homosexual Pedophiles', paper presented at the twenty-first annual meeting of the International Academy of Sex Research, Provincetown, Massachusetts.

Fidelis, M. (1989), *A Misogynist's Source Book*, London: Jonathan Cape.

Firth, S. & McRobbie, A. (1978), 'Rock and Sexuality', *Screen Education*, 29.

Firth, S. & Goodwin, A. (1990), *On Record. Rock, Pop and the Written Word*, London: Routledge.

Fogel, A. (1986), 'Talk Shows: On Reading Television', in *Emerson and His Legacy: Essays in Honour of Quentin Anderson*, S. Donadio, S. Railton & O. Seavey (eds.), Carbondale: Southern Illinois University Press.

Foucault, M. (1976), *The History of Sexuality Vol. 1*, London: Penguin.

Fox Keller, E. (1985), *Reflections on Gender and Science*, New Haven, Conn.: Yale University Press.

Fraser, A. (1992), *The Six Wives of Henry the Eighth*, London: Mandarin.

Frederick, C. (1907), 'Nymphomania as a Cause of Excessive Venery', *American Journal of Obstetrics and Diseases on Women and Children*, 56 (6), 742–44.

Frieze, I. H. (1983), 'Investigating the Causes and Consequences of Marital Rape', *Signs*, 8 (3), 532–53.

Fromuth, M. E. (1983), *The Long-Term Psychological Impact of Childhood Sexual Abuse*, Unpublished doctoral dissertation, Auburn University.

Frosh, S. (1994), *Sexual Difference: Masculinity and Psychoanalysis*, London: Routledge.

Gallichan, W. M. (1927), *Sexual Apathy and Coldness in Women*, London: T. Werner Laurie.

Garber, M. (1996), *Vice Versa: Bisexuality in Everyday Life*, London: Hamish Hamilton.

Garde, K. & Lunde, I. (1980), 'Female Sexual Behaviour: A Study in a Random Sample of 40-Year-old Women', *Maturitas*, 2, 225–40.

Garratt, S. (1984), 'Teenage Dreams', in Firth, S. & Goodwin, A. (1990), *On Record. Rock, Pop and The Written Word*, London: Routledge.

Garrett-Gooding, J. & Senter, R. (1987), 'Attitudes and Acts of Sexual Aggression on a University Campus', *Sociological Enquiry*, 59, 348–71.

Gerber, P. N. (1990), 'Victims Become Offenders: A Study of the Ambiguities', in *The Sexually Abused Male, vol. 1. Prevalence, Impact, Treatment*, M. Hunter (ed.), Lexington: Lexington MA.

Gerin, W. (1967), *Charlotte Brontë: The Evolution of Genius*, Oxford: Oxford University Press.

Gilbert, H. (1993), 'So Long as It's Not Sex and Violence. Andrea Dworkin's *Mercy*', in *Sex Exposed: Sexuality and the Pornography Debate*, L. Segal & M. McIntosh (eds.), London: Virago.

Gilbert, S. & Gubar, S. (1979), *The Madwoman in the Attic: The Woman Writer and the Nineteenth-Century Imagination*, New Haven: Yale University Press.

Goldstein, M. J., Judd, L., Rice, C. & Green, R. (1970), 'Exposure to Pornography and Sexual Behaviour in Deviant and Normal Groups', *Technical Report of the Commission on Obscenity and Pornography, vii, Washington DC*.

Golombok, S., Spencer, A. & Rutter, M. (1983), 'Children in Lesbian and Single-Parent Households: Psychosexual and Psychiatric Appraisal', *Journal of Child Psychology and Psychiatry*, 24, 551–72.

Gordon, M. T. & Riger, S. (1991), *The Female Fear*, Urbanna: University of Illinois Press.

Graham, H. & Oakley, A. (1981), 'Competing Ideologies of Reproduction: Medical and Maternal Perspectives on Pregnancy', in *Women, Health and Reproduction*, H. Roberts (ed.), London: Routledge & Kegan Paul.

Griffin, S. (September 1971), *Rape: The All-American Way*, Ramparts.

Griffin, S. (1981), *Pornography and Silence*, London: The Women's Press.

Groneman, C. (1994), 'Nymphomania: The Historical Construction of Female Sexuality', *Signs*, 19 (2), 337–67.

Groth, A. N. & Burgess, A. W. (1982), 'Rape: A Sexual Deviation', in *Male Rape: A Casebook of Sexual Aggression*, Sacco Jr (ed.), New York: AMS Press.

Hall, S. (1980), 'Encoding/Coding', in *Culture, Media and Language*, S. Hall, D. Hobson, A. Lowe & P. Willis (eds.), London: Hutchinson.

Halleck, S. L. (1971), *Psychiatry and Dilemmas of Crime*, LA: University of California Press.

Hamer, D. (1995), 'Sexual Orientation, Personality Traits and Genes', paper presented at the twenty-first annual meeting of the International Academy of Sex Research, Provincetown, Massachusetts.

Hanmer, J. & Saunders, S. (1983), 'Blowing the Cover of the Protective Male: A Community Study of Violence to Women', in Garmanikow, E., Morgan, D., Purvis, J. & Taylorson, D. (1983), *The Public and the Private*. London: Heinemann.

Harding, S. (1991), *Whose Science? Whose Knowledge? Thinking from Women's Lives*, Milton Keynes: Open University Press.

Harvey S. (1980), 'Women's Place in the Absent Family of Film Noir', in *Women in Film Noir*, A. Kaplan (ed.), London: BFI.

Haskell, M. (1974), *From Reverence to Rape: The Treatment of Women in the Movies*, New York: Penguin Books.

Hawton, K. (1985), *Sex Therapy: A Practical Guide*, Oxford: Oxford University Press.

Henry, G. W. (1948), *Sex Variants: A Study of Homosexual Patterns*, New York: Paul B. Hoeber Inc.

Herdt, G. (1984), *Ritualised Homosexuality in Melanesia*, Berkeley: University of California Press.

Herdt, G. (1987), *The Sambia: Ritual and Gender in New Guinea*, New York: Holt, Rinehart & Winston.

Holbrooke, D. (1989), *Images of Women in Literature*, New York: New York University Press.

Holland, P. (1987), 'When a Woman Reads the News', in *Boxed in: Women and Television*, H. Baehr & G. Dyer (eds.), London: Pandora.

Holloway, W. (1993), 'Differences and Similarities in a Feminist Theorisation of Heterosexuality', paper presented at the British Psychological Society, Blackpool.

Holmstrom, L. L. & Burgess, A. W. (1979), 'Rapists Talk: Linguistic Strategies to Control the Victim', *Deviant Behaviour*, 1, 105–6.

Honore, T. (1978), *Sex Law*, London: Duckworth.

Hoon, P., Murphy, D. W. & Laughter, J. S. (1984), 'Infrared Vaginal Photoplethysmography: Construction, Calibration and Sources of Artifact', *Behavioural Assessment*, 6, 141–52.

Horney, K. (1967), *Feminine Psychology*, London: Norton.

Hoskins, E. (1979), 'The Hoskins Report: Genital and Sexual Mutilation of Females', *Women's International Network*, USA: Lexicon.

Howitt, D. (1989), 'Pornography: The Recent Debate', in *Measure of Uncertainty: The Effects of Mass Media*, G. Cumberbatch & D. Howitt (eds.), London: Libbey.

Howitt, D. (1992), *Child Abuse Errors*, Hemel Hempstead: Harvester Wheatsheaf.

Howitt, D. & Cumberbatch, G. (1990), *Pornography: Impacts and Influences*, London: Home Office Research and Planning Unit.

Humm, M. (1989), *Feminisms: A Reader*, Hemel Hempstead: Harvester Wheatsheaf.

Hyde, M. H. (1972), *The Other Love: An Historical and Contemporary Survey of Homosexuality in Britain*, London: Mayflower Books.

Itzen, C. (1993), 'Entertainment for Men: What it is and What it Means', in *Pornography: Women, Violence and Civil Liberties*, C. Itzen (ed.), Oxford: Oxford University Press.

Itzen, C. (1993), *Pornography: Women, Violence and Civil Liberties*, Oxford: Oxford University Press.

Itzen, C. (1993), 'Pornography and the Social Construction of Sexual Inequality', in *Pornography: Women, Violence and Civil Liberties*, C. Itzen (ed.), Oxford: Oxford University Press.

Itzen, C. & Sweet, C. (1993), 'Women's Experience of Pornography', in *Pornography: Women, Violence and Civil Liberties*, Oxford: Oxford University Press.

Janney, K. (1988), *The Pirate's Lady*, London: Mills & Boon.

Jeffreys, S. (1985), *The Spinster and Her Enemies. Feminism and Sexuality 1880–1930*, London: Pandora.

Jeffreys, S. (1987), *The Sexuality Debates*, London: Routledge & Kegan Paul.

Jeffreys, S. (1990), *Anticlimax: A Feminist Perspective on the Sexual Revolution*, London: The Women's Press.

Jehu, D. (1984), 'Impairment of Sexual Behaviour in Non-Human Primates', in *The Psychology of Sexual Diversity*, Howells (ed.), Oxford: Blackwell.

Kallman, F. J. (1952), 'Comparative Twin Study on the Genetic Aspects of Male Homosexuality', *Journal of Nervous Disorder*, 115, 282–98.

Kaplan, A. (1980), 'Introduction', in *Women in Film Noir*, A. Kaplan (ed.), London: BFI, 1–5.

Kaplan, A. (1983), *Women in Film. Both Sides of the Camera*, London: Methuen.

Kaplan, A. (1992), *Motherhood and Representation. The Mother in Popular Culture and Melodrama*, London: Routledge.

Kaplan, C. (1989), 'The Thorn Birds: Fiction, Fantasy, Femininity', in *Formations of Fantasy*, V. Burgin, J. Donald & C. Kaplan (eds.), London: Routledge.

Kaplan, H. S. (1974), *The New Sex Therapy*, New York: Brunner/Mazel.

Kaplan, L. J. (1991), *Female Perversions*, London: Penguin.

Kelkar, G. (1985), 'Women and Structural Violence in India', *Women's Studies Quarterly*, 13, 3–4, 16–18.

Kendrick, W. (1987), *The Secret Museum*, London: Viking.

Kent, S. (1985), 'Scratching and Biting Savagery', in *Women's Images of Men*, S. Kent & J. Morreau (eds.), London: Writers and Readers Publishing.

Kent, S. & Morreau, J. (1985), 'Preface', in *Women's Images of Men*, S. Kent & J. Morreau (eds.), London: Writers and Readers Publishing.

Kinder, M. (1974–5), 'Review of *Scenes from a Marriage* by Ingmar Bergman', *Film Quarterly*, 28 (2), 48–53.

Kinsey, A., Pomeroy, W. & Martin, C. (1948), *Sexual Behaviour in the Human Male*, Philadelphia: Saunders.

Kinsey, A. C., Pomeroy, W. B., Martain, C. E. & Gebhard, P. H. (1953), *Sexual Behaviour in the Human Female*, Philadelphia & London: Saunders.

Kiss and Tell (Blackbridge, P., Jones, L. & Stewart, S.) (1994), *Her Tongue on My Theory. Images, Essays and Fantasies*, Vancouver: Press Gang Publishers.

Kitzinger, C. (1987), *The Social Construction of Lesbianism*, London: Sage.

Knight, B. (1972), *Legal Aspects of Medical Practice*, London: Churchill Livingstone.

Kokken, S. (1967), *The Way to Married Love: A Happier Sex Life*, London: Souvenir Press.

Koss, M. P., Gidycz, C. A. & Wisniewski, N. (1987), 'The Scope of Rape: Incidence and Prevalence of Sexual Aggression and Victimisation in a

National Sample of Higher Education Students', *Journal of Consulting and Clinical Psychology*, 55, 162–70.

Koss, M. P. & Leonard, K. E. (1984), 'Sexually Aggressive Men: Empirical Findings and Theoretical Implications', in *Pornography and Sexual Aggression*, N. Malamuth & E. Donnerstein (eds.), New York: Academic Press.

Koss, M. P. & Oros, C. J. (1982), 'Sexual Experiences Survey: A Research Instrument Investigating Sexual Aggression and Victimisation', *Journal of Consulting and Clinical Psychology*, 50, 455–7.

Kronemyer, R. (1980), *Overcoming Homosexuality*, New York: Macmillan.

Kuhn, A. (1985), *The Power of the Image: Essays on Representation and Sexuality*, London: Routledge.

Kuhn, A. (1995), *Family Secrets: Acts of Memory and Imagination*, London: Verso.

Lakoff, R. T. & Scherr, R. L. (1984), *Face Value: The Politics of Beauty*, London: Routledge & Kegan Paul.

Lamb, C. (1987), *Whirlwind,* London: Mills & Boon.

Langevin, R., Bain, J., Wortzmann, G., Hucker, S., Dickey, R. & Wright, P. (1988), 'Sexual Sadism: Brain Blood and Behaviour', in *Human Sexual Aggression: Current Perspectives*, R. A. Prentky & V. L. Quinsey (eds.), New York: New York Academy of Sciences.

Lees, S. (1992), 'Naggers, Whores and Libbers: Provoking Men to Kill', in *Femicide: The Politics of Women Killing*, J. Radford & D. Russell (eds.), Buckingham: Open University Press.

Lees, S. (1993), *Sugar and Spice*, London: Penguin.

Lees, S. (1996), *Carnal Knowledge: Rape on Trial*, London: Penguin.

Leiberman, M. K. (1986), ' "Some Day My Prince Will Come": Female Acculturation through the Fairy Tale', in Zipes, J. (1986), *Don't Bet on the Prince. Contemporary Fairy Tales in North America and England,* Hants: Gower.

Leman, J. (1987), 'Programmes for Women in 1950's British Television', in *Boxed in: Women and Television*, H. Baehr & G. Dyer (eds.), London: Pandora.

Lesage, J. (1986), 'Political Aesthetics of the Feminist Documentary Film, in *Films for Women*, C. Brunson (ed.), London: BFI.

Le Vay, S. (1993), *The Sexual Brain*, Massachusetts: MIT Press.

Linden, R. R., Pagano, D. R., Russell, D. E. H. & Leigh Star, S. (1982), *Against Sado-Masochism. A Radical Feminist Analysis*, California: Frog in the Well.

Livingstone, S. & Lunt, P. (1994), *Talk on Television: Audience Participation and Public Debate*, London: Routledge.

Lloyd, A. (1995), *Doubly Deviant, Doubly Damned. Society's Treatment of Violent Women*, London: Penguin.

Lovelace, L. (1976), *Inside Linda Lovelace*, New York: Four Square Books.

Mailer, N. (1971), *A Prisoner of Sex*, London: Sphere Books.

Malamuth, N. & Check, J. V. P. (1980), 'Penile Tumescence and Perceptual Responses to Rape as a Function of Victim's Perceived Reactions', *Journal of Applied Social Psychology*, 10, 528–47.

Malamuth, N., Heim, M. & Feshback, S. (1980), 'Sexual Responsiveness of College Students to Rape Depictions: Inhibitory and Disinhibitory Effects', *Journal of Personality and Social Psychology*, 38, 399–408.

Malamuth, N. (1981), 'The Effects of Mass Media Exposure on Acceptance of Violence Against Women: A Field Experiment', *Journal of Research in Personality*, 15, 436–46.

Malson, H. (1996), *The Thin Body*, London: Routledge.

Marcus, S. (1974), *The Other Victorians: A Study of Pornography in Mid-Nineteenth Century England*, New York: American Library.

Martin, E. (1989), *The Woman in the Body: A Cultural Analysis of Reproduction*, Milton Keynes: Open University Press.

Masciarotte, G. J. (1991), 'C'mon Girl: Oprah Winfrey and the Discourse of Feminine Talk', *Genders*, 11, 81–110.

Master, R. E. L. & Lea, E. (1963), *Sex Crimes in History: Evolving Concepts of Sadism, Lust, Murder and Necrophilia from Ancient to Modern Times*, New York: Julian Press.

Masters, W. H. & Johnson, V. J. (1970), *Human Sexual Inadequacy*, Boston: Little Brown.

McClintock, A. (1992), 'Gonad the Barbarian and the Venus Flytrap: Portraying the Male and Female Orgasm', in *Sex Exposed: Sexuality and the Pornography Debate*, L. Segal & M. McIntosh (eds.), London: Virago.

MacKinnon, C. (1982), 'Feminism, Marxism, Method and State: An Agenda for Theory', *Signs*, 7 (3), 515–44.

MacKinnon, C. (1983), 'Feminism, Marxism, Method and State: Towards Feminist Jurisprudence', *Signs*, 8 (4), 635–58.

McMahon, K. (1990), 'The Cosmopolitan Ideology and the Management of Desire', *The Journal of Sex Research*, 27 (3), 381–96.

McRobbie A. (1978), 'Working-Class Girls and the Culture of Femininity', in *Women Take Issue*, Women's Studies Group, Centre for Contemporary Cultural Studies (ed.), London: Hutchinson.

McRobbie, A. (1989), *Feminism and Youth Culture*, Basingstoke: Macmillan Education.

Mellencamp, P. (1995), *A Fine Romance: Five Ages of Film Feminism*, Philadelphia: Temple University.

Melman, A. (1978), 'Development of Contemporary Surgical Management for Erectile Impotence', *Sexuality and Disability*, 1, 272–81.

Mendal, M. P. (1995), *The Male Survivor. The Impact of Sexual Abuse*, London: Sage.

Merck, M. (1993), 'From Minneapolis to Westminster', in *Sex Exposed: Sexuality and the Pornography Debate*, L. Segal & M. McIntosh (eds.), London: Virago.

Mill, J. S. (1955; first published in 1869), *The Subjugation of Women*, London: Dent.

Millar, J. (1861), *Hints on Insanity*, London: Henry Renshaw.

Miller, H. (1965), *Nexus*, New York: Gove Press.

Modleski, T. (1984), *Loving with a Vengeance. Mass-Produced Fantasies for Women*, New York: Routledge.

Moffat, M. (1989), *Coming of Age in New Jersey*, New Brunswick: Rutgers University Press.

Mohr, J. W., Turner, R. E. & Jerry, N. B. (1964), *Paedophilia and Exhibitionism*, Toronto: Toronto University Press.

Money, J. (1988), 'Commentary: Current Status of Sex Research', *Journal of Psychology and Human Sexuality*, 1, 5–15.

Monter, W. (1981), 'Sodomy and Heresy in Modern Switzerland', *Journal of Homosexuality*, 6.

Moore, R. (1975), 'From Rags to Riches: Stereotypes, Distortion and Anti-Humanism in Fairy Tales', *Interracial Books for Children*, 6, 1–3.

Morgan, R. (1980), 'Theory and Practice: Pornography and Rape', in *Take Back the Night: Women on Pornography*, L. Lederer (ed.), New York: Morrow.

Morgan-Taylor, M. & Rumney, P. (1994), 'A Male Perspective on Rape', *New Law Journal*, 144 (669), 1490–93.

Morris, P. (1993), *Literature and Feminism*, Oxford: Blackwell.

Mulvey, L. (1975), 'Visual Pleasure and Narrative Cinema', *Screen*, 16 (3), 1–16.

Murphy, T. F. (1992), 'Redirecting Sexual Orientation: Techniques and Justification', *The Journal of Sex Research*, 29 (4), 501–23.

Nadler, R. N. (1988), 'Sexual Aggression in the Great Apes, in *Human Sexual Aggression: Current Perspectives*, R. A. Prentky & V. L. Quinsey (eds.), New York: New York Academy of Sciences.

Nead, L. (1987), 'The Magdalen in Modern Times: The Mythology of the Fallen Woman in Pre-Raphaelite Painting,' in *Looking on: Images of Femininity in the Visual Arts and Media*, R. Betterton (ed.), London: Pandora.

Neil, J. (1993), *Flames of Love*, London: Mills and Boon.

Nestle, J. (1995), 'Woman of Muscle, Woman of Bone', in *Tangled Sheets. Stories and Poems of Lesbian Lust*, R. Elwin & K. X. Tulchinsky (eds.), Toronto: The Women's Press.

Nochlin, L. (1988), *Women, Art and Power: And Other Essays*, London: Thames & Hudson.

J. O'Faolain & L. Martain (eds.), (1974), *Not in God's Image: Women in History*, London: Virago.

O'Sullivan, C. (1991), 'Acquaintance Rape on Campus', in Parrot, Andrea & Bechhofer, L. (1991), *Acquaintance Rape: The Hidden Crime*, New York: Wiley.

Pacteau, F. (1994), *The Symptom of Beauty*, London: Reaktion Books.

Parker, R. & Pollock, G. (1981), *Old Mistresses: Women, Art and Ideology*, London: Pandora.

Parrot, A. & Bechhofer, L. (1991), *Acquaintance Rape: The Hidden Crime*, New York: Wiley.

Parrot, A. & Link, R. (1983), 'Acquaintance Rape in a College Population', paper presented at the Eastern Regional meeting of the Society for the Scientific Study of Sex, Philadelphia, P A.

Pasini, W. (1977), 'Unconsummated and Partially Consummated Marriage as Sources of Procreative Failure', in *Handbook of Sexology*, J. Money & H. Musaph (eds.), Amsterdam: Elsevier/North Holland.

Pattatucci, A. M. L. & Hamer, D. H. (1995), 'The Genetics of Sexual Orientation: From Fruitflies to Humans', in *Sexual Nature, Sexual Culture*, P. R. Abramson & S. D. Pinkerton (eds.), Chicago: University of Chicago Press.

Pavlka, M. S. & McDonald, S. (1995), 'Sexual Nature: What Can we Learn from a Cross-Species Perspective?', in *Sexual Nature, Sexual Culture*, P. R. Abramson & S. D. Pinkerton (eds.), Chicago: University of Chicago Press.

Persons, E. S. (1988), *Dreams of Love and Fateful Encounters: The Power of Romantic Passion*, New York: Norton.

Place, J. (1980), 'Women in Film Noir', in *Women in Film Noir*, A. Kaplan (ed.), London: BFI.

Pollock, G. (1988), *Vision and Difference: Femininity, Feminism and Histories of Art*, London: Routledge.

Porter, R. (1990), 'Men's Hysteria in Corpore Hysterico?' paper presented at the Wellcome Institute Symposium on the History of Medicine: History of Hysteria, London.

Poulter, J. S. (1991), *Peers, Queers and Commons: The Struggle for Gay Law Reform from 1950 to the Present*, London: Routledge.

Pumphrey, M. (1987), 'The Flapper, the Housewife and the Making of Modernity', *Cultural Studies*, 1 (2), 179–94.

Radford, J. (1992), 'Retrospect on a Trial', in *Femicide: The Politics of Women Killing*, J. Radford & D. Russell (eds.), Buckingham: Open University Press.

Radway, J. (1987), *Reading the Romance: Women, Patriarchy and Popular Literature*, London: Verso.

Réage, P. (1980), *The Story of O*, London: Corgi.

Rivera, R. R. (1991), 'Sexual Orientation and the Law', in *Homosexuality: Research Implications for Public Policy*, J. C. Gonsiorek & J. D. Weinrich (eds.), London: Sage.

Robson, R. (1992), 'Legal Lesbicide', in *Femicide: The Politics of Women Killing*, J. Radford & D. Russell (eds.), Buckingham: Open University Press.

Rosenfeld, Q., Nadelson, C., Krieger, M. & Backman, J. (1979), 'Incest and Sexual Abuse of Children', *Journal of the American Academy of Child Psychiatry*, 16, 327–39.

Rowe, K. (1986), 'Feminism and Fairy Tales', in Zipes, J. (1986), *Don't Bet on the Prince. Contemporary Fairy Tales in North America and England*, Hants: Gower.

Rubin, G. (1984), 'Thinking Sex', in *Pleasure and Danger: Exploring Female Sexuality*, C. Vance (ed.), London: Pandora, 1996.

Rumney, P. N. S. & Morgan-Taylor, M. P., *The Legal Problems Associated with Males as Victims of de facto Rape* (forthcoming).

Russell, D. (1984), *Sexual Exploitation: Rape, Child Sexual Abuse and Workplace Harassment*, London: Sage.

Russell, D. (1993), 'Pornography and Rape: A Causal Model', in *Pornography: Women, Violence and Civil Liberties*, C. Itzen (ed.), Oxford: Oxford University Press.

Russell, D. E. H. (1982), *Rape In Marriage*, New York: Macmillan.

Russell, D. E. H. (1982), 'The Prevalence and Incidence of Rape and Attempted Rape of Female', *Victimology*, 7, 81–93.

Russell, D. E. H. (1986), *The Secret Trauma: Incest in the Lives of Girls and Women*, New York: Basic Books.

Russell, D. E. H. (1991), 'Wife Rape', in Parrot, Andrea & Bechhofer, L. (1991), *Acquaintance Rape: The Hidden Crime*, New York: Wiley.

Russo, V. (1981), *The Celluloid Closet: Homosexuality in the Movies*, New York: Harper & Row.

Ryder, R. (1989), 'Child Abuse', *The Bulletin of the British Psychological Society*, 2 (8), 333.

Sarrell, P. M. & Masters, W. H. (1982), 'Sexual Molestation of Men by Women', *Archives of Sexual Behaviour*, 117, 117–31.

Saunders, D. (1985), *The Woman's Book of Love and Sex*, London: Sage.

Schow, M. (1994), 'Backlash and Appropriation', in *The Power of Feminist Art: Emergence, Impact and Triumph of the American Feminist Movement*, N. Broude & M. D. Garrard (eds.), New York: Harry N. Abrams.

Scully, D. (1990), *Understanding Sexual Violence. A Study of Convicted Rapists*, London: Unwin Hyman.

Segal, L. (1983), 'Sensual Uncertainty, or Why the Clitoris is Not Enough', in *Sex and Love: New Thoughts on Old Contradictions*, S. Cartledge & S. Ryan (eds.), London: The Women's Press.

Segal, L. (1992), 'Sweet Sorrows, Painful Pleasures. Pornography and the Perils of Heterosexual Desire', in *Sex Exposed: Sexuality and the Pornography Debate*, L. Segal & M. McIntosh (eds.), London: Virago.

Segal, L. (1993), 'Introduction', in *Sex Exposed: Sexuality and the Pornography Debate*, L. Segal & M. McIntosh (eds.), London: Virago.

Segal, L. (1994), *Straight Sex*, London: Virago.

Seiter, E., Borchers, H., Kreutzner, G. & Warth, E. M. (1991), *Remote Control: Television, Audiences and Cultural Power*, London & New York: Routledge.

Senn, C. Y. (1993), 'The Research on Women and Pornography. The Many Faces of Harm', in *Making Violence Sexy. Feminist Views on Pornography*, D. Russell (ed.), Buckingham: Open University Press.

Senn, C. Y. (1993), 'Women's Multiple Perspectives and Experiences with Pornography', *Psychology of Women Quarterly*, 17, 319–41.

Seward, J. & Green, W. (1990), *Rape: My Story*, London: Bloomsbury.

Showalter, E. (1987), *The Female Malady*, London: Virago.

Shrimpton, J. (1990), *Jean Shrimpton: An Autobiography*, London: Ebury Press.

Silverman, D. & McCombie, S. (1980), 'Counselling the Mates and Families of Rape Victims', in *The Rape Crisis Intervention Handbook*, S. McCombie (ed.), New York: Plenum Press.

Simpson, K. (1962), *A Doctor's Guide to Court*, London: Butterworths.

Smart, C. (1976), *Women, Crime and Criminology: A Feminist Critique*, London: Routledge.

Smith, D. (1988), 'Feminist as Discourse', in *Becoming Feminine: The Politics of Popular Culture*, L. Roman & L. K. Christian Smith (eds.), Sussex: Falmer Press.

Smith, L. (1991), *Sexuality in Western Art*, London: Thames & Hudson.

Smyth, C. (1992), *Lesbians Talk. Queer Notions*, London: Scarlet Press.

Soloman-Godeau, A., 'Living with Contradictions, Critical Practices in the Age of Supply-Side Aesthetics', in Squire, 1989.

Spence, J. (1978), 'Father–Daughter Incest: A Clinical View for the Correction Field', *Child Welfare*, 57, 581–90.

Spence, J. (1995), *Cultural Sniping. The Art of Transgression*, London: Routledge.

Squiers, S. (ed.) (1990), *The Critical Image*, New York: Bay Press.

Squire, C. (1989), *Significant Differences: Feminism in Psychology*, London: Routledge.

Squire, C. (1991), 'Is the Oprah Winfrey Show Feminist Television?', paper presented at the International Women's Studies Congress, New York.

Squire, C. (1994), 'Empowering Women? The Oprah Winfrey Show', *Feminism and Psychology*, 4 (1), 63–79.

Stanko, E. A. (1985), *Intimate Intrusions. Women's Experience of Sexual Violence*, London: Routledge & Kegan Paul.

Steele, V. (1985), *Fashion and Eroticism: Ideals of Feminine Beauty from the Victorian Era to the Jazz Age*, Oxford: Oxford University Press.

Steinem, G. (1983), *Outrageous Acts and Everyday Rebellions*, East Toledo Publications, Inc.

Steinmetz, S. (1977), *The Cycle of Violence*, New York: Praeger Publishers.

Steward, S. & Garrett, S. (1984), *Signed, Sealed and Delivered. True Life Stories of Women in Pop*, London: Pluto Press.

Stiglmayer, A. (1994), *Mass Rape: The War Against Women in Bosnia Herzegovina*, Lincoln & London: University of Nebraska Press.

A. Stiglmayer (ed.) (1994), 'The Rapes in Bosnia Herzegovina', in *Mass Rape: The War Against Women in Bosnia Herzegovina*, A. Stiglmayer (ed.), Lincoln & London: University of Nebraska Press.

Stoller, R. & Levine, I. S. (1993), *Coming Attractions: The Making of an X-Rated Movie*, New Haven: Yale University Press.

Storer, H. (1856), 'Cases of Nymphomania', *American Journal of Medical Science*, 32 (10), 378–87.

Straus, M. A., Gelles, R. J. & Steinmetz, S. (1980), *Behind Closed Doors: Violence in the American Family*, New York: Doubleday.

Surrey, J., Sweet, C., Michaels, A. & Levin, S. (1990), 'Reported History of Physical and Sexual Abuse and Severity of Symptomatology in Women Psychiatric Outpatients', *American Journal of Orthopsychiatry*, 60, 412–17.

Sussman, L., *The Ultimate Sex Guide: A Bedside Book for Lovers*, BPPC Paperbacks, 1993.

Sweet, C. (1993), 'Pornography and Addiction: A Political Issue', in *Pornography: Women, Violence and Civil Liberties*, C. Itzen (ed.), Oxford: Oxford University Press.

Symons, D. (1995), 'Beauty is in the Adaptions of the Beholder: The Evolutionary Psychology of Human Female Sexual Attractiveness', in *Sexual Nature, Sexual Culture*, P. R. Abramson & S. D. Pinkerton (eds.), Chicago: University of Chicago Press.

Tait, R. L. (1889), *Diseases of Women and Abdominal Surgery*, Leicester: Richardson.

Tate, T. (1993), 'The Child Pornography Industry', in *Pornography: Women, Violence and Civil Liberties*, C. Itzen (ed.), Oxford: Oxford University Press.

Taylor, A. S., 'The Principles and Practice of Medical Jurisprudence', London: John Churchill, 1865.

Taylor, H. (1989), *Scarlett's Women: Gone with the Wind and its Female Fans*, London: Virago.

Teifer, L. (1986), 'In Pursuit of the Perfect Penis', *American Behavioural Scientist*, 29 (5), 579–99.

Teifer, L. (1991), 'Commentary on the Status of Sex Research: Feminism, Sexuality and Sexology', *Journal of Psychology and Human Sexuality*, 43 (3), 5–42.

Terry, J. (1990), 'Lesbians under the Medical Gaze: Scientists Search for Remarkable Differences', *The Journal of Sex Research*, 27 (3) 317–99.

Thompson, S. (1990), 'Putting a Big Thing in a Small Hole: Teenage Girls' Accounts of Sexual Initiation', *The Journal of Sex Research*, 27 (3), 341–61.

Threadgold, T. & Cranny Smith, A. (1990), *Feminine and Masculine Representations*, Sydney: Allen & Unwin.

Tickner, L. (1987), *The Spectacle of Woman: Imagery of the Suffrage Campaign 1907–1914*, London: Chatto & Windus.

Tieger, T. (1981), 'Self-Rated Likelihood of Raping and Social Perception of Rape', *Journal of Research in Personality*, 15, 147–58.

Tong, R. (1987), *Women, Sex and the Law*, New Jersey: Rowman & Alanheld.

Treadwell, N. (1984), *Sex Female: Occupation Artist. The Contemporary Women*, Womenswold, Kent: Nicolas Treadwell Publishing.

Trivelpiece, J. (1990), 'Adjusting the Frame: Cinematic Treatment of Sexual Abuse and Rape of Men and Boys', in *The Sexually Abused Male, vol. 1. Prevalence, Impact, Treatment*, M. Hunter (ed.), Lexington: Lexington MA.

Ussher, J. M. (1989), *The Psychology of the Female Body*, London: Routledge.

Ussher, J. M. (1991), *Women's Madness: Misogyny or Mental Illness*, Hemel Hempstead: Harvester Wheatsheaf.

Ussher, J. M. (1993), 'The Construction of Female Sexual Problems: Regulating Sex, Regulating Women', in Ussher, J. M. & Baker, C., *Psychological Perspectives on Sexual Problems: New Directions in Theory and Practice*, London: Routledge.

Ussher, J. M. (ed.) (1997), *Bodytalk: The Material and Discursive Regulation of Sexuality, Madness and Reproduction*, London: Routledge.

Ussher, J. M. & Baker, C. (1993), *Psychological Perspectives on Sexual Problems: New Directions in Theory and Practice*, London: Routledge.

Ussher, J. M. & Dewberry, C. (1994), 'The Nature and Long-Term Effects of Childhood Sexual Abuse: A Survey of Adult Women Survivors in Britain', *British Journal of Clinical Psychology*, 34, 177–92.

Vance, C., (1993), 'Negotiating Sex and Gender in the Attorney-General's Commission on Pornography', in *Sex Exposed: Sexuality and the Pornography Debate*, L. Segal & M. McIntosh (eds.), London: Virago.

Veith, I. (1965), *Hysteria: The History of a Disease*, Chicago: University of Chicago Press.

Walkerdine, V. (1990), *Schoolgirl Fictions*, London: Verso.

Wallen, K. (1995), 'The Evolution of Female Desire', in *Sexual Nature, Sexual Culture*, P. R. Abramson & S. D. Pinkerton (eds.), Chicago: University of Chicago Press.

Walters, D. R. (1975), *Physical and Sexual Abuse of Children*, Bloomington: Indiana University Press.

Weeks, J. (1981), *Sex, Politics and Society. The Regulation of Sexuality since 1800*, London: Longmans.

Weibel, K. (1977), *Mirror, Mirror: Image of Women Reflected in Popular Culture*, New York: Anchor Books.

Weidegar, P. (1985), *Histories Mistress: A New Interpretation of a Nineteenth-Century Ethnographic Classic*, London: Penguin.

Weir, J. (Jr) (1895), 'The Effects of Female Suffrage on Posterity', *American Naturalist*, 24 (345), 815–25.

Wigmore, J. H. (1940), *A Treatise on the Anglo-American System of Evidence in Trials at Common Law*, (3rd edn.), vol iii, Boston: Little Brown.

Wilbanks, W. (1986), 'Criminal Homicide Offenders in the US: Black vs White', in *Homicide among Black Americans*, D. F. Hawkins (ed.), New York: University Press of America.

Wilkinson, S. & Kitzinger, C. (eds.) (1993), *Heterosexuality: A Feminism and Psychology Reader,* London: Sage.

Williams, L. (1990), *Hard Core,* London: Pandora.

Williams, L. M. (1994), 'Recall of Childhood Trauma: A Prospective Study of Women's Memories of Child Sexual Abuse', *Journal of Consulting and Clinical Psychology,* 62 (6), 1167–76.

Williamson, J. (1987), *Decoding Advertisements: Ideology and Meaning in Advertising,* London: Marion Boyars.

Wilson, G. D. (1988), 'The Socio-Biological Basis of Sexual Dysfunction', in *Sex Therapy in Britain,* M. Cole & W. Dryden (eds.), Milton Keynes: Open University Press.

Wilson, M. & Daly, M. (1992), 'Till Death Us Do Part', in *Femicide: The Politics of Women Killing,* J. Radford & D. Russell (eds.), Buckingham: Open University Press.

Wilson, P. R. (1981), *The Man They Called a Monster,* North Ryde, Australia: Cassell.

Winship, J. (1987), *Inside Women's Magazines,* London: Pandora.

Wittig, M. (1980), 'The Straight Mind', *Feminist Issues,* 1 (1).

Wittig, M. (1992), *The Straight Mind and Other Essays,* Hemel Hempstead: Harvester Wheatsheaf.

Wright, R. & West, D. J. (1981), 'Rape: A Comparison of Group Offences and Lone Offences', *Medicine, Science and the Law,* 21, 25–30.

Wyre, R. (1993), 'Pornography and Sexual Violence', in *Pornography: Women, Violence and Civil Liberties,* C. Itzen (ed.), Oxford: Oxford University Press.

Young, J. (1976), 'Wife Beating in Britain: A Socio-Historical Analysis 1850–1914', paper presented to the American Sociological Association, August, New York City.

Zillman, D. & Bryant, J. (1984), 'Effects of Massive Exposure to Pornography', in *Pornography and Sexual Aggression,* N. Malamuth & E. Donnerstein (eds.), Orlando, Florida: Academic, 1984.

Zipes, J. (1986), *Don't Bet on the Prince. Contemporary Fairy Tales in North America and England,* Hants: Gower.

INDEX